DO-IT-YOURSELF
MEDICALTESTING

DO-IT-YOURSELF MEDICAL TESTING

240 TESTS YOU CAN PERFORM AT HOME

THIRD EDITION

Cathey Pinckney
and
Edward R. Pinckney, M.D.

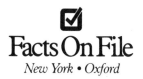

Facts On File

New York • Oxford

FOR CATHEY LEE PINCKNEY

Great Librarian, Great Shooter, but *still* a Bum*

[On second thought, after your experience, better a bum?]

*(From Neil Simon's *Come Blow Your Horn*)

Do-It-Yourself Medical Testing

Copyright © 1989 by Cathey Pinckney and Edward R. Pinckney, M.D.

Facts On File, Inc.
460 Park Avenue South
New York, New York 10016

Library of Congress Cataloging-in-Publication Data

Pinckney, Cathey.
  Do-it-yourself medical testing: 240 tests you can perform at home
/ Cathey Pinckney and Edward R. Pinckney.—3rd ed.
    p. cm.
  Includes index.
  ISBN 0-8160-1928-2. —ISBN 0-8160-2085-X (pbk.)
  1. Diagnosis. 2. Self-examination, Medical. I. Pinckney, Edward
R. (Edward Robert). II. Title.
RC71.3.P56   1989
616.07′5—dc19

British CIP data available on request

Printed in the United States of America

10 9 8 7 6 5 4 3 2 1

NOTICE

The tests described in this book are not intended to be diagnostic; no medical test by itself can be used to make a diagnosis. The nature of medical testing is that it is constantly evolving and subject to interpretation. Therefore, while the authors of this book have done their best to ensure the accuracy and completeness of the material presented, the reader is advised that no claim can be made that all relevant information concerning the medical tests described in this book is included here. Additionally, the reader is advised that this book is not a manual for self-diagnosis or self-treatment and is further advised to consult with his or her physician in search of answers or treatment for any medical problems. The authors and publisher also disclaim liability for any loss or risk, personal or otherwise, resulting, directly or indirectly, from the use, application or interpretation of any of the contents of this book. *Do-It-Yourself Medical Testing* is not to be considered a substitute for the professional judgment of a physician.

The names of various products such as test devices, equipment and supplies are given in this book for informational purposes only. Inclusion of a particular product does not imply approval or endorsement by the authors; exclusion of a product does not imply disapproval, disparagement or criticism. It is also quite possible that a test described here will no longer be available by the time this book is published. The marketer of a home test kit may go out of business within months after introducing the kit; this could be from a lack of public enthusiasm or, more likely, from a Food and Drug Administration (FDA) order barring the product's sale. At the same time, new home test kits are being introduced monthly; information about such tests may not have been available just prior to publication.

Should you have any untoward symptoms (pain, breathing difficulty, weakness, vision problems, to cite a few examples) or signs (skin rashes or growths and bleeding anywhere are among the many possibilities) or any discomfort or disability that is bothering you, do not rely on any home test before seeking medical attention.

Should you have any problem with a medical test device or supplies, after assuring yourself that the test was performed properly, you can help yourself and others by reporting that problem to the Medical Device & Laboratory Product Problem Reporting Program. Call toll-free anytime: (800) 638-6725.

The following are some problems that have already been reported and in most instances corrected:

- The test's directions were unclear or inadequate or seemed to be wrong.
- The test was difficult to perform.
- The device or test material did not seem to perform properly.
- The device or test material did not seem safe to handle or operate.
- The device, or parts of it, broke easily.
- The test results did not seem appropriate or consistent, especially after the user checked with his or her doctor's office or a commercial laboratory.
- The container or bottle provided as part of the test kit could easily be mistaken for some other medicinal product.
- The product was mislabeled.

At the time this book's manuscript was sent to the printer, there was a great deal of confusion concerning the availability of many home tests. The federal Food and Drug Administration, without whose express permission virtually no medical test apparatus may be marketed—albeit the accuracy of the test is not considered—has, during the past two years, been formulating new rules and changing old ones, leaving do-it-yourself test makers and sellers in a constant dilemma. The home AIDS test is a prime example. After allowing many companies to research and make ready for sale a simple blood-collecting kit that would easily permit do-it-yourself AIDS testing, the FDA suddenly, and without due warning or explanation, declared the sale of any form of AIDS self-testing to be illegal. Several manufacturers of other home tests were in essence also "discouraged" by the FDA from making their tests easily available to the public. Thus, although all the tests in this book were once openly available for home use, it is possible that a few may no longer be readily obtainable; in some cases, it may be necessary to go through a doctor to obtain a particular test.

CONTENTS

x CONTENTS

Water Response
Elimination Diet

PREFACE TO THE THIRD EDITION

When the first edition of this book was published in 1983, sales of home testing kits in the United States were recorded at $300 million. The following year, when the revised edition was published, the public spent almost $400 million on home tests. During the present year, 1989, health-conscious consumers are expected to spend more than $1 billion purchasing do-it-yourself medical monitoring devices, and marketing consultants predict that such purchases will reach $2 billion annually within the next few years.

The primary reason for such an aggressive growth in this particular aspect of "self-care" is the increasing responsibility that patients, and even potential patients, are taking for preventing illness and, should illness occur, sharing with their doctors all aspects of therapy—especially its effectiveness. And while there are a few within the medical establishment who openly admit their fear of a reduction in income or loss of a God-manque image when patients perform medical tests at home, the vast majority of practicing physicians welcome the participatory patient; not only will the patient's active involvement lower the total cost of health care, it will also allow the medical profession to focus its time and attention on more serious medical problems.

But more than anything else, performing medical tests at home will enhance one's knowledge of disease—its cause, its course and the way it is usually treated. Such basic information is still the best approach to the prevention of illness and ultimately the maintenance of good health. And then there is the matter of privacy—keeping suspicion of a problem to oneself and avoiding the embarrassment of letting even the doctor know of a possible indiscretion. Pregnancy and certain sexually transmitted diseases are good examples; if they do in fact exist, medical treatment is justified. If they are not present, no one need know your fears.

To a greater extent than ever before, the same tests performed by doctors are now available to the public; in most instances the test material is identical to that used by professionals. Thus, accuracy is assured—assuming, of course, that the directions are precisely followed by whoever performs the test. And do-it-yourself medical testing can save lives. Cancer specialists have estimated that if everyone performed home tests to detect occult (invisible) blood in the stool regularly, at least 60,000 deaths from colon cancer could be prevented each year. If every woman who could possibly be pregnant tested herself for pregnancy before having an X-ray or taking any drug, it has been estimated that birth defects could be reduced by at least 50 percent. If everyone with a blood pressure problem measured his or her own blood pressure at home regularly, at least one out of three could give up dangerous antihypertensive drugs.

With each passing month, at least one new home medical test will probably be introduced; 75 new tests have become available in the six years since this book was first published. What such tests can offer is a better, less mysterious understanding of both health and disease, a means to alleviate much illness, an avenue of cooperation with one's doctor never before possible and, not just incidentally, a sharp reduction in expenditures for medical care.

GENERAL INFORMATION

There is nothing new about home medical testing. If you have ever taken your own or your child's temperature or simply felt the warmth of a forehead, you have performed no less of a medical test than your doctor does when he or she takes your blood pressure or taps your knee with a rubber reflex hammer—both of which you can also do. You can just as easily measure how much glucose (sugar) is in your blood and urine, examine your feces for hidden blood and worms, evaluate your vision and hearing, and even appraise how well your heart and lungs are functioning. In fact, there are more than 200 medical tests that can be performed at home.

In most instances the cost of testing at home is far less than the cost of testing carried out in a doctor's office, hospital or commercial laboratory. But of even greater importance, the test results can be far more accurate. According to the Public Health Service, about one in every seven professionally performed medical tests is either in error or unreliable for practical application—which means that that little bit of extra care and attention you provide when you test yourself can make quite a difference as far as accuracy is concerned. For example, blood glucose values are much more precise and useful when they reflect your typical daily activities rather than the apprehension you feel in your doctor's office or the effects you experience after lying in a hospital bed for several days.

Have you been told you have a blood pressure problem? Before starting on a course of dangerous drugs to treat your alleged hypertension, take your own blood pressure at home. You might discover that your ostensible illness is really a "white-coat" disease—that is, high blood pressure as a consequence of your anxiety whenever you face your doctor. Have some doubts about this? Can you remember ever lying in bed late at night and thinking you heard strange sounds as if someone were trying to break in? How soon did you feel your heart pounding? The few seconds it took for you to react apprehensively to what you imagined were more than enough time for a surge of adrenalin to pass through your body, making your pulse speed up and your blood pressure rise. The same thing can happen to anyone who harbors the remotest fear of a doctor's examination. And it has been reliably estimated that one out of every three people now being treated for high blood pressure really needs no drugs at all.

The lowest reading of one's blood pressure is known to be the most accurate. If you feel unsure about blood pressure measurements taken in a doctor's office, why not perform that test yourself at home? You can easily do it; all you need is a sphygmomanometer (the medical term for the cuff that goes around your upper arm and its attached measuring device), available at almost every pharmacy or through many mail-order catalogs for as little as $9.95. This could be a small price to avoid the large cost, and potential dangers, of a lifetime of taking one or more medicines.

Have you had unexplained bouts of dizziness lately—perhaps along with occasional faintness, headaches, lapses of memory and moments of impaired judgment that your doctor has been unable to diagnose? You could test your environment for carbon monoxide (CO). This colorless, odorless deadly gas can enter a home from a faulty furnace, an improperly vented hot water heater, an attached garage or even a barbecue that is used indoors. It can enter a car from a faulty exhaust pipe or a poor ventilation system. It can also come from smoking. For less than the cost of a few packs of cigarettes, you can test for this common cause of a variety of bizarre symptoms by placing a carbon monoxide monitor in your home and car. Do-it-yourself testing of your surroundings can contribute toward a diagnosis by capturing "scene-of-the-crime" evidence that would ordinarily escape detection by the usual office or laboratory tests.

WHAT MEDICAL TESTS DO

Most people think medical tests make diagnoses. The tests alone do not. They are rarely specific about any disease. Tests may help confirm the cause of an illness, usually by pointing more toward one condition than others that can cause similar symptoms. They may aid in locating the source of pain or discomfort. They can, at times, assist in relieving the anguish that accompanies so many medical conditions. (It is a known fact that some people feel completely cured of their complaints without any therapy whatsoever, simply after undergoing one or more tests.) But in all but a very few instances, medical tests do not supply a precise diagnosis.

The detection of hidden blood (also called occult blood, meaning that it is not visible to the naked eye) in your bowel movement, for instance, does not necessarily mean disease—least of all colon cancer. The occult blood test can be positive for several days after you eat rare meat; after you brush your teeth, especially if you brush your gums properly; even after you take aspirin or iron tablets. Or occult blood could come from parasites acquired simply by going barefoot; dogs can deposit worms in backyards or on lawns, and these worms can bore through the skin of your feet and settle in the intestines.

The fact that most medical tests are ambiguous is only one drawback. Their accuracy and usefulness are further compromised by a variety of bodily aberrations, routine activities and environmental conditions. Whether you sit, stand or lie down when you take a test can alter the resulting value, as can what you have eaten or drunk. A loud noise or a pretty nurse can so distort a blood cholesterol test's outcome as to result in unnecessary diet changes, dangerous drugs and altered lifestyles. In other words, do not rely on medical tests alone. If the test results corroborate your medical history (your description of your illness, including your past health record and that of your family, is the most important of all clues that ultimately lead to a diagnosis), and if they parallel the direction of your signs and symptoms (signs are objective indicators, such as a rash; symptoms are subjective, such as pain), then the test results become just another link in the chain that should support a correct clinical conclusion followed by successful specific therapy.

HEALTH MAINTENANCE

Where home medical testing can be of real value is in screening for little-thought-of hidden sources of illness and for early warning signs of some inconspicuous or latent diseases—especially when timely detection can prevent disability. Home testing can be of equal value when used to monitor and help control some existing illnesses. When people with diabetes were taught to test their own blood glucose levels at home, the dangerous consequences of diabetic coma were reduced by almost 70 percent, and the number of emergency visits to doctors and hospitals was halved. In another self-care program for patients with an inherited blood disease, the cost of medical treatment was reduced by over half, and the life span of those patients was more than doubled.

Many medical tests consist of nothing more than observation: The secret simply lies in knowing what to watch for and what the perceived information could mean. If all parents would kiss the cheeks and foreheads of their infants regularly and learn to discern any unusual saltiness on the skin surface, many of the tragic lung and intestinal problems that can result from cystic fibrosis could probably be prevented. If family members would learn to observe each other's ears, eyes, throats and skin, they could at times become aware of medical versus nonmedical conditions and relieve themselves of much anxiety—not to mention expense. Simple, systematic scrutiny of one's breasts, hair, feces, teeth, temperature, testicles, urine and weight are home medical tests that can repay the effort a thousandfold in physical and financial peace of mind. Knowing what questions to ask an elderly family member who is behaving in a seemingly abnormal manner could help differentiate between a physical and a psychological basis for the problem. Using the right questionnaire has been known to prevent tragic social and financial consequences in many a family where stress, malnutrition, alcoholism and incipient brain and liver abnormalities had been overlooked.

If home medical testing does nothing more than prompt you to seek medical care early enough to allow a simple, relatively comfortable cure, it is more than justified. And lest you think that the medical profession discourages this seeming intrusion into its hallowed halls, direct participation in one's own health care, as well as in the care of family members, is now accepted within most of the medical profession; there are exceptions, to be sure. Many doctors, however, encourage their patients to play a part in arriving at a diagnosis and welcome shared responsibility in making treatment choices. They have found that this not only increases patient compliance, allowing a more rapid, more successful outcome, but it also is an effective means of preventing related health problems.

SOME PRECAUTIONS

While most of the medical tests described in this book are fairly easy to perform, and the equipment or supplies needed are relatively inexpensive, they should not be thought of as playthings. Directions that accompany test material should be followed exactly. It is recommended that the first time any test is performed, it be done in consultation with your doctor. Let him or her watch you take your blood pressure initially; let your physician show you how to take your own blood sample; let him or her demonstrate visual field testing, the use of the reflex hammer, tuning fork, otoscope and any other instrument you contemplate using. In this way, you can avoid many misunderstandings and errors.

Practice using your instruments at home on family and friends whom you know are in good health. Look at normal eardrums or throats; observe the effect of reflex testing; observe urine consistency, body blemishes and contours as often as possible. The more familiar you become with such things, the more accurate your test results will be.

Because so many of the tests depend on color comparisons, be sure you have normal color vision as well as good visual acuity. Do not attempt to evaluate color changes if you have any doubt about your ability to discriminate between colors.

Always keep in mind, too, the possibility of false-positive and false-negative results. A false-positive test is one that indicates the possible presence of a disease or condition that does not in fact exist. The more sensitive a test, the greater the likelihood that it will produce a false-positive result. Diet, physical activity, emotional upset, the medicines you take and a failure to follow test directions exactly are also apt to alter or falsify a test's results. A false-negative test is one that fails to show a positive result even though some disease or condition exists that should cause a positive value. More often than not, a false-negative result comes from carelessness in performing a test.

Good doctors insist that any abnormal medical test result be confirmed by a second test before incorporating that result into their record of related evidence. Unless you are performing a home test while under a doctor's care (such as with asthma, diabetes or stomach ulcers or during pregnancy), it is considered good practice to repeat home medical tests—even those yielding negative results—at least twice until you feel sufficiently self-assured about your technique.

MEDICAL CONSULTATION VERSUS MEDICAL ATTENTION

Considering that most home testing will be of the screening or health-monitoring variety, the chances of true-positive test results are slim. But should a medical test and its repeat show a positive result suggesting some disease or condition, professional confirmation should be sought. Most positive tests do not indicate an emergency (there are exceptions if you are diabetic, pregnant, etc.) and only warrant a medical consultation. That could mean nothing more than a phone conversation with your doctor to describe your findings and have the doctor weigh your test results in light of his or her knowledge of your past medical history and his or her last examination of you. It could also mean an office visit to allow additional procedures to confirm or disprove your test findings.

A medical test result that warrants medical attention is not diagnostic, but it could indicate the possibility of some serious or even life-threatening condition as well as a disease that could be dangerous to others around you. If the discussion of a test in this book advises that medical attention is warranted based on certain test results, this means you should seek immediate medical care, either from your own doctor or—should your personal physician not be available—from a hospital or community emergency facility.

SELF-CARE

Self-care does not necessarily mean assuming total and absolute responsibility for your health; it really means taking a greater interest in, and sharing responsibility for, maintaining good health and participating in diagnosis and therapy. The more you know and understand about disease, the greater your opportunity to apply appropriate measures to avoid illness. Home medical test monitoring can be thought of as a type of preventive maintenance for your body. Remember, no single medical test—whether performed at home, in your doctor's office, in a hospital, or at a commercial laboratory or other test location (X-ray facility, health fair, research center)—should be considered diagnostic. This book is not about self-care, as such, but rather provides information on only one small aspect of health maintenance. It is not a handbook for self-diagnosis but only a guide to help you and your doctor help yourself. A medical test in itself is relatively meaningless until it is interpreted in light of your medical history, your signs and symptoms, and your doctor's training and experience applied to his or her observations after examining you.

WARNINGS

If you have any gross abnormality (pains or persistent aches, growths on your skin, obvious blood in a bowel movement or unexplained bleeding anywhere, difficulty in breathing, inability to coordinate your movements, problems in seeing or hearing, or any discomfort or disability that is more than you have had or are used to), do not rely on any home test before seeking medical attention; call or visit your doctor or emergency center immediately.

Never assume that the result of your medical test is definitive; if you have any doubt about either a positive or a negative test result, consult your physician and share your doubts as well as your test result with him or her.

Every medical test includes some degree of risk; in most instances it is virtually negligible, but every test should be considered from the standpoint of the possible harm it might cause as well as the information it might provide.

- One risk is the possibility that additional, more dangerous tests could be performed in order to substantiate your original test findings. Before undergoing sophisticated testing, have your doctor assure you that it is really necessary; that there are no alternative, safer tests; and that the results of the tests will affect or alter your doctor's decisions.
- The other, equally serious risk is that persistent false-negative test results can provide misleading assurance that you are disease-free; never make such an absolute assumption without your doctor's confirmation.

And this is not a book on home treatment. No suggestions, recommendations or directions are meant to be offered as therapy or any other means to a cure. True, a good scrubbing in a hot tub might help eliminate fleas, lice or mites, but the real remedy for any condition comes from working with your doctor to assure that treatment is successful and possible complications are avoided. Let home medical testing be your means of maintaining your health and preventing disease; but let it be no more than your adjunct to professional diagnosis and treatment.

OPPOSITION TO DO-IT-YOURSELF MEDICAL TESTING

Not all doctors accept the idea that people should be able to participate actively in their own medical care, especially when it comes to preventing illness. The opposition seems to be based primarily on three undocumented premises. First, and evidently foremost, is the potential loss of income to the doctor and laboratory when medical tests are performed at home rather than in the doctor's office or in a commercial laboratory. Commercial laboratories are worried about the economic effects of do-it-yourself testing; one trade newsletter has come out requesting technicians to be more aggressive in trying to create apprehensiveness in those who test themselves at home. In contrast, the American Medical Association's most recent pronouncement on the subject concluded: "With physician guidance, self-testing is not only less costly for the country, but probably for the patient as well."

The second objection to home testing comes from doctors who feel that patients are too stupid to follow directions properly; surprisingly, there are still a few doctors around who like to play God. The third demurrer to do-it-yourself medical testing comes from the Food and Drug Administration— whose permission to market a test must be obtained before it can be sold to the public. The FDA has stated that all home tests must come with directions written in language that someone with no more than a sixth-grade education can easily understand. It also fears that certain home tests require the presence of a physician to explain the results—that without professional guidance right at the tester's elbow, the social consequences could be worse than the disease.

Fortunately, the majority of doctors support and even encourage do-it-yourself medical testing. Incidentally, the *Journal of the American Medical Association* has suggested that physicians as well as patients could profit from this book's contents. A California Medical Association investigator of the matter concluded: "On balance, I don't think doctors should have any serious objections to these test kits. My experience has been that the more testing that is done, the more people tend to go to the doctor because there are so many borderline results." Obviously, those borderline results may be just the ones that detect the very early onset, or latency, of an illness, thereby allowing quicker, less expensive and more effective treatment.

HOW TO USE THIS BOOK

The tests presented in this book are grouped under various categories not necessarily related to the conditions that their results can reflect. Urine tests, for example, can indicate a wide variety of bodily actions or reactions not limited to the kidneys and genitourinary system. Blood tests can suggest problems outside the circulatory system. A breath test for alcohol really has no bearing on how well the lungs function. The simplest way to decide on a test is to first ascertain its purpose. If a medical test is intended to screen for the possibility of latent disease, the "Health Maintenance Index" (see the Appendix) should be consulted. When your doctor recommends a particular test, the book's Index should suffice.

In the test descriptions, whenever you see the name of another test printed in **boldface** type, it means that that test is described in detail under its own heading.

The introduction to each test describes its general purpose, what substance or function it is supposed to indicate or measure, how the test works and any common conditions (activities, diet, drugs, etc.) that could interfere with the test results. This preliminary discussion is not intended to be all-inclusive; it is nothing more than a basic, simply worded explanation of what the test is about.

Each test description also includes the sections discussed below.

What Is Usual

Because it is almost impossible to define "normal" values without due regard for a particular individual's age, sex, height, weight, family characteristics and a host of other variables, this section describes what one would most likely find in the "average" person. Should routine activities tend to alter test values in a supposedly healthy human being, the effect of such activities is mentioned. For example, physical exercise or prolonged walking or standing may cause a positive urine protein test, but that could be a normal, rather than abnormal, test result for many people. And many test results are not simply positive or negative; some show quantitative changes, such as when measuring how much air the lungs can hold. In almost all medical tests, *usual* values can fluctuate widely and still be usual.

What You Need

Personal abilities as well as required equipment and/or supplies are listed, along with approximate costs. For some tests the price of the material will seem high, either because the manufacturer packages the material only in large quantities at this time or because the necessary apparatus is costly. To offset the cost of expensive items, many people form groups or use clubs or other organizations to share the cost and use of such paraphernalia. Others weigh the cost against the time and expenditures for repeated visits to the doctor's office when the same test can be performed at home; for example, a device to monitor asthma and other chest ailments can pay for itself just by eliminating one office visit.

The cost of equipment or supplies can vary tremendously from one pharmacy or medical supply store to the next. There are no fixed prices for the test material, so it can pay to shop around. The prices cited in this book were typical at the time of publication.

In a great many instances health insurance plans or government-sponsored medical care programs will reimburse you, in part or fully, for the purchase of a medical device or test material when recommended by a physician. "At-home" blood glucose monitors and blood pressure measuring devices are only two examples of medical equipment whose rental or purchase is usually covered by insurance reimbursement.

The easiest place to find most of the items needed for testing is your local pharmacy. While not every item will always be carried in stock, pharmacists have access to wholesale medical supply houses. Check the yellow pages of your telephone directory under the heading "Hospital Equipment & Supplies" for sources of items unavailable at or through your pharmacy. Many home health care businesses also rent expensive test apparatus. Some direct-mail catalogs include a variety of medical test devices, and there are new companies that deal exclusively in home testing. If you have a good relationship with your doctor, he or she can easily order anything and everything you could need from a pharmaceutical supply house at the lowest possible cost.

At times you may be confronted by a pharmacist or medical supply sales representative who will refuse to sell you a test item unless you present a doctor's prescription. With very few exceptions, the test material described in this book does not, by law, require a doctor's permission for purchase. Where such devices are so restricted, however, most doctors usually supply the device directly. You can always contact your local Food and Drug Administration (FDA) office to determine the status of any specific device.

What to Watch Out For

The majority of the caveats mentioned in this section reflect the mistakes and problems people have experienced when performing a particular test.

They are primarily observations regarding mechanical difficulties to be avoided, but they also include commonly overlooked possible interferences with proper test procedures as well as other obstacles that may arise.

Although the products and supplies mentioned in this book were available at the time of publication, it is possible that technological developments might well cause a particular device or test material to be withdrawn from the market or replaced by something different—usually something easier to use and more effective. The home diagnostics field is growing so rapidly that it is difficult to keep track of every new device.

You should always watch out for expiration dates on supplies that require them. Be sure that the material you buy will have a reasonable shelf life. And be sure that the product is properly sealed; many chemicals become useless or deteriorate fairly rapidly when exposed to air or moisture.

What the Test Results Can Mean

The conditions described in this section are suggestive of the most common causes of abnormal or unusual test results. You should never attempt to interpret a "positive," or abnormal, test result yourself. As but one example, a lower-than-normal blood hemoglobin test, while most likely signifying an anemia, does not even hint at what is causing the anemia. Medical textbooks list anemia as part of, or the consequence of, several hundred unrelated diseases. Then again, the test result could have come from your having squeezed your fingertip too tightly and diluted the drop of blood with other tissue fluids.

Although any one of the implications noted here may seem quite plausible, it would be a foolish waste of time and testing to accept such test results as conclusive. Should a test result warrant a medical consultation, it would be a disservice to yourself and your family not to contact your doctor and discuss the matter. Should a test result warrant medical attention, it would be irresponsible not to proceed immediately to your doctor or nearest emergency facility.

If, however, your test results do not indicate ill health, and you take pleasure in monitoring and maintaining your health as well as preventing illness, enjoy!

Reliability

In essence, the reliability of a test is more than simply how often the test or observation will reveal the presence of the substance or situation being tested for, or how precise the measurement is; it also involves how often the test is right (or "positive") when the disease or condition suspected is really there and just as right (or "negative") when the disease or condition does not exist. The true accuracy of any medical test—whether performed at home or in the most sophisticated laboratory—takes into account its *sensitivity* (how often it correctly indicates the presence of an actual disease and does not give a false-negative result), its *specificity* (how often it properly fails to show the presence of a nonexistent disease and does not give a false-positive result) and the *prevalence* of a suspected condition in the "community" of the patient being tested. A test is more apt to show a positive result if it is used to help diagnose a disease that is quite common—in or near where the patient lives or within the patient's particular parameters (age, sex, race, etc.). The reliability figures cited for the tests in this book take all these factors into account, primarily as reported in the medical literature, as well as based on actual test application.

Again, no matter how reliable a medical test is, it never allows for a specific diagnosis—either by you or by a physician. And you might keep in mind that more than half of all professionally performed medical tests are less than 80 percent accurate. Moreover, when medical tests are performed by professionals, be it at a commercial clinical laboratory or in a doctor's office, the chances of an accurate result range from less than 50 percent at worst to about 85 percent at best. The very best laboratories are known to make mistakes in one out of every seven tests. It is actually possible, if an individual is careful, to be more accurate at home than so-called experts in the medical testing field.

To be sure, never accept the results of a single test, even if it has been performed by a physician or clinical laboratory—especially if those results could affect your way of life. And in the long run, it is not expensive to confirm an abnormal test result with another physician or laboratory; always keep in mind that the primary purpose of home testing is to screen for nothing more than clues to latent illness, with the goal of uncovering disease before it becomes a disability.

ENVIRONMENTAL TESTS

There is no place like home to practice preventive medicine through do-it-yourself testing. It may come as quite a surprise to learn that a great many illnesses—and the discomfort, pain and suffering that accompany them—come from your environment: the home you live in, the atmosphere around you, the things you take for granted such as your drinking water, foods, building materials, cleaning and pesticide products, and even pets. Because smog has become commonplace, you can now monitor the outside air yourself—especially if you suffer from a breathing problem. The monitoring of indoor air, however, is relatively new; testing for pollutants coming from within the place where you live and where, if you are a homemaker or a small child, you may well spend almost 24 hours a day can help you avoid a host of dangers and diseases. More than half of all fatal poisonings in the United States are attributed to carbon monoxide (CO); deaths among children under 5 years of age due to this indoor pollutant have more than doubled in the past 10 years. Especially if you have any sort of gas appliance, monitoring for this substance alone, at a cost of less than $10.00 a year, can not only save your life but also prevent a great many illnesses that are all too often attributed to the "flu."

Testing for harmful loud noises, lead in your dishes, poisons in your water and whether you are being affected by someone else's smoking are simple but very effective health maintenance measures. It has been estimated that almost half of all common illnesses come from such environmental causes—even the workplace, of course, is essentially a home during employment hours. Learn to monitor your environment and you may well prevent most of those illnesses; of equal importance, you can help avoid the exacerbation or worsening of existing diseases.

AIR POLLUTION
(Detecting the active ingredients of smog)

People with respiratory problems are well aware of the breathing difficulties they suffer when air quality is diminished. Even those without unusual lung sensitivity can have adverse symptoms when any or all of the main ingredients of air pollution (smog) reach excessive levels. Smog chemicals can also cause a fibrotic lung condition called bronchiolitis obliterans (at one time a very rare condition), which requires prolonged steroid treatment. The four most common air contaminants are ozone, nitrogen dioxide, sulfur dioxide and carbon monoxide (see Environmental Tests, **Carbon Monoxide** for details regarding this dangerous air pollutant).

Ozone. The most active ingredient of smog is ozone (O_3), a colorless, highly reactive gas that forms when by-products of combustion (such as nitrogen dioxide) and certain organic compounds (such as paint vapors and as-yet-unburned gasoline fumes) are struck by sunlight (which is why it is worse in summer months); some say it comprises 95 percent of smog. Ozone can also be produced by lightning and other electrical discharges. It is really a more active form of normal oxygen (O_2) comprised of three oxygen atoms instead of two, and that third atom is what makes the gas extremely irritable to the eyes and lungs. It can cause difficulty in seeing clearly, especially at night, and can even cause double vision.

While asthmatics will have greatly increased attacks when ozone is present, even those without lung disease can have difficulty breathing; marathon runners show a marked reduction in their ability as ozone levels in the air increase. Some compare ozone damage to radiation damage (see Environmental Tests, **Radiation Monitoring**), since it can destroy body cells and cause chromosome (genetic) defects. In general, ozone levels should never exceed 0.12 parts per million (ppm), and even this "acceptable" amount can harm the body over one hour's time; yet most large cities regularly have twice this level of ozone in the air. Los Angeles exceeded acceptable ozone standards during 148 days in 1987. When ozone reaches 0.3 ppm, it can cause coughing and other breathing difficulties; it can cause lung damage at 0.6 ppm. The cabin of a passenger airplane can reach 1.0 ppm; if you are flying and notice the characteristic odor of ozone (like the smell of freshly sun-dried clothes), you should tell the airline personnel and the pilot can change altitude to reduce the ozone concentration. And it has been reported in medical journals that people who eat large amounts of polyunsaturated fat show even greater lung, skin and red blood cell damage when ozone concentrations increase.

Nitrogen dioxide. The second harmful component of smog is nitrogen dioxide (NO_2). This gas helps contribute to the brownish haze when air pollution is severe. Nitrogen dioxide comes primarily from combustion, especially gasoline, diesel and jet engines; from the decomposition of plant material and agricultural wastes; and even from burning cigarettes. It also comes from using the gas stove, furnace and water heater inside your home. This gas, too, causes lung irritation and damage by combining with water in the lungs and turning into nitrous acid. Some feel it injures tissues to a far greater degree than ozone, causing asthmatics to have more severe attacks.

One of the first nonrespiratory symptoms of nitrogen dioxide intoxication is weakness that seems to have no explanation; this is usually associated with cyanosis (decreased oxygen in the blood, causing the skin to have a bluish color). After a single exposure to a large amount of the gas, or after a few weeks of small, repeated exposures, **Pulmonary Function Measurements** (see Breath and Lung Tests) will show lower-than-normal test results. More recently, medical research has revealed that regular exposure to nitrogen dioxide results in a greater amount of colds and bronchitis, and there are other reports linking it to cancer and heart disease. Although not too much attention has been paid to nitrogen dioxide, at present it is believed that any amount greater than 0.053 ppm is dangerous; so far only the city of Los Angeles regularly exceeds that concentration. It is said that some people can "taste" the sweetness of the gas when it reaches 1 ppm, and it is known to cause chest pains at 15 ppm. Concentrations greater than 100 ppm can be fatal.

Sulfur dioxide. The third basic component of smog is sulfur dioxide; it too, comes from engine combustion, but it also comes from gasoline and sugar refining, chemical plants and cleaning agents. And it, too, causes respiratory difficulties, including more frequent and more severe asthmatic attacks; it can mimic asthma in people without that disease, and it seems to be more irritating in cool rather than warm weather and whenever there is fog. As little as 1 ppm can bring on an asthmatic attack in someone who has the disease, but it seems to take 5 ppm to have the same effect on someone without asthma. It is also believed that sulfur dioxide in the air can turn to sulfuric acid, the basic component of acid rain.

It is possible to test one's environment for the main ingredients of smog and to detect excessive amounts of these gases long before they are reported in newspapers (many cities offer daily air-quality reports showing when ozone, nitrogen dioxide and carbon monoxide exceed clean-air standards, but these reports are normally a day late).

What Is Usual

Unfortunately, what should be usual—clean air—is a rarity. A recent report from Concerning Cars/Information in the Public Interest (P.O. Box 450, Pound Ridge, N.Y. 10576) showed that just about every city with a population of over a half-million was in violation of the Clean Air Act of 1963 (last amended in 1977) for ozone and carbon monoxide. The report also points out that 1 ppm is the same as one drop of vermouth in 80 "fifths" of gin, to give an idea of how small a quantity of a pollutant can be harmful.

Smog reporting. In most areas of the country, newspapers carry reports of smog ingredient levels—and predictions of how much of each pollutant will be present in the air the following day. The reports generally appear under the headline "Air Quality" and cite the "usual" levels of one or all of smog's basic constituents. Most often, the amounts in the air are expressed as the PSI, or pollutant standard index; this number translates parts per million of each substance into a "standard" measurement. From 0 to 50 is considered good air quality; 50 to 100 reflects a moderate air quality rating; anything over 100 is unhealthful, with more than 200 *very* unhealthful and 275 or more hazardous. Unfortunately, the amount of each toxic gas—ppm—in the air is not the same for each PSI; for example, only 1 ppm of carbon monoxide equals 11 on the PSI scale, and it takes only 9 ppm of CO to reach unhealthful levels. An ozone PSI of 50 reflects only 0.06 ppm, and 0.12 ppm (about one-tenth as much CO) is considered unhealthful. A PSI of 10 for nitrogen dioxide equals only 0.01 ppm, and more than 0.1 ppm is unhealthful. Thus, anytime any air-quality ingredient is predicted to exceed 100 PSI, it should be considered a warning—in particular for those with existing heart and/or lung problems.

What You Need
Carbon monoxide detectors and monitors are described under Environmental Tests, in the detailed discussion of **Carbon Monoxide.** Detecting monitors for ozone and nitrogen dioxide are available from many sources. One is the American Gas & Chemical Company (220 Pegasus Ave., Northvale, N.J. 07647); a badge holder with 10 test papers costs $16.00. These test papers will detect ozone at a concentration of 0.1 ppm per hour (1 ppm immediately) and nitrogen dioxide at a minimum of 5 ppm within a 15-minute period. The company also sells a hydrogen sulfide badge and indicators that will detect that gas at 10 ppm within a 10-minute period; although hydrogen sulfide is not the same thing as sulfur dioxide, it can be dangerous to the lungs at 10 ppm and is an indirect indication of sulfur in the air. Unopened, the test papers have a shelf life of six months.

What to Watch Out For
Most monitors can accumulate very small doses of the gases over a period of time, and the length of time that the monitor was exposed must always be taken into account; if there is any doubt about the reading, change the disposable monitor and keep track of the time it is exposed. Although some monitors can be reused after small exposures, it is best not to try to reuse them once they show a distinct color change.

What the Test Results Can Mean
When the test monitors show a toxic amount of a smog element, it is best to try to close off your home from the outside air and stay inside. If appro-

priate, you might consult your physician and make advance arrangements for specific medications when smog ingredients reach irritant levels. If, when no smog is evident, the monitors show the presence of toxic gases, it warrants a more technical search for in-house sources of those gases (call your gas company to look for leaks). If you have persistent breathing problems, it warrants a medical consultation regardless of what the monitors show.

Reliability
All the monitors claim to meet Occupational Safety and Health Administration (OSHA) standards and are considered about 90 percent accurate.

INDOOR AIR POLLUTION
(Testing for the possible cause of frequent "colds")

The air inside your home can be as great a cause, if not a greater cause, of lung irritation (constant coughing, sneezing, sinusitus and other allergic manifestations) and skin rashes as outdoor **air pollution** (see Environmental Tests), or smog. In addition to **carbon monoxide, asbestos, formaldehyde, nitrogen dioxide, radon** (all discussed under Environmental Tests) and the irritating ingredients of smog, other pollutants may be part of the air you breathe. A common but rarely considered contributor to breathing problems is the mold (fungi) that forms in air-conditioning and heater filters, in humidifiers and behind wallpaper that is constantly moistened by the damp air coming from humidifiers or from the frequent boiling of water in the kitchen. The more humid a house is kept, the greater the possibility of mold spores' forming. And humidity can also help the house dust mite to flourish in furnace filters, upholstered furniture, mattresses and box springs. This almost invisible insect, which is part of house dust and looks somewhat like a pubic louse (see Body Observations, **Skin Infestations: Pediculosis (Lice)**, Figure 11), albeit even smaller, while not in itself harmful, can make many people hypersensitive to its feces and cause severe allergic-type breathing problems when carried about the air in the house, whether alive or dead. Other indoor pollutants include cockroaches, whose presence is now known to cause asthma; the dried saliva from pets (see Allergy Tests, **Patch Testing**); and even chemicals used around the house (chemical air fresheners; bleaches; glues; hair sprays; aerosol products, such as deodorants and insecticides; paints; polishes); and of course, smoking. In essence, many so-called chest conditions and allergies, including dermatitis, can be caused by a polluted home environment rather than simply being "a virus" or a strictly medical malady. In turn, uncovering such a source of sickness can easily lead to its cure.

Regular inspections of humidifiers, heater/air-conditioning filters and areas that are moister than normal can reveal mold formations. If you are experiencing an unusual problem, you can take your air-conditioner or furnace filter to any local analytical or testing laboratory (see the yellow pages) to determine whether your environment is overrun with the house dust mite, a particular kind of mold or even the bacteria that cause Legionnaires' disease.

What Is Usual

It is hardly unusual to have spray chemicals, cleaning compounds and dust around the house. Generally, they do not bother the occupants. If you try to keep your home moist (humidified), especially in cold weather, it is usual to have mold formations (excessively moist air has not been proved to prevent colds or allow asthmatics to breathe easier).

What You Need

Most of all, you need a willingness to diligently search your home for mold and dust, a willingness to acknowledge the use of potentially irritating—even toxic—chemicals within your home and a willingness to take dust samples and samples from your air filters for analysis.

There are companies that specialize in evaluating indoor air quality, and their costs, while relatively expensive, must be compared with virtually endless professional/medical testing of an individual that may well end up being totally useless. One such company, Occupational Medical Center (OMC) (490 L'Enfant Plaza East, SW, Washington, D.C. 20024; [202] 488–7990), will discuss a possible indoor air problem by mail or phone to help determine an evaluation cost. It will perform analysis of mold/fungi samples for $50.00.

Of particular interest, especially to homebuyers, in 1989 the National Draeger company (P.O. Box 120, Pittsburgh, PA 15230) introduced a Home Inspection Kit that offers a simple way of testing for toxic gases and vapors in a home. In this way a prospective home purchaser (or renter) can know if indoor pollution could be a problem. The kit tests for **carbon monoxide,** natural gases (leaks from stoves or heaters), nitrous fumes (see **nitrogen dioxide**) and **formaldehyde** (tests for many other potentially dangerous substances—depending on the geographical area and ambient air are also available). The initial test kit costs $341.75 but that includes a basic bellows pump for precise air measurements and sufficient spare parts to last for years along with sufficient test material for 10 carbon monoxide tests and five natural gas tests. In general, each subsequent test for any substance averages $3.00.

Some real estate agents offer such testing, including **radon** measurements, without charge; it is good preventive medicine not to complete a home purchase without an indoor air pollution evaluation. Existing homeowners could avoid much discomfort, not to mention illness, by surveying their home on an annual basis; the initial cost of the test equipment can be shared by several families.

What to Watch Out For
Most of all, you should be alert for rooms that are too moist or damp, especially where moisture comes from commercial humidifiers, since the water is always added but rarely changed and the device is rarely cleaned. Check with a testing laboratory beforehand to be sure it understands how to search for house dust mites. Such a search should cost from $25.00 to $50.00.

What the Test Results Can Mean
If you find mold and/or house dust mites and eliminate them, you stand a good chance of relieving many allergy-like symptoms. If there is an allergy to dried pet saliva, a medical consultation is warranted; there have been reports of immunotherapy's successfully reducing that allergic response. Your doctor can also give you a protocol for eradicating the house dust mite. If, after not using household chemicals for a week or two, your symptoms lessen or disappear, you might well be able to uncover the specific chemical that caused your problem by adding each potential offender, one by one, and seeing whether it provokes any respiratory or skin irritation.

Reliability
Indoor air pollutants are a major cause of asthma, sinusitus and dermatitis. In general, the search for house dust mites in filters is 90 percent accurate; that is, they are easy for a trained observer to detect. If mold and house dust mites were found and eliminated, many allergists say that at least half of all allergies could be "cured."

Note: You can help eliminate a great deal of indoor air pollution by installing highly efficient air filters either in a central air conditioning/heating system or as a portable room unit. The filter that comes with most heating systems is relatively useless in eliminating dust particles, mold and plant spores and pollens. In contrast, electronic precipitators (Honeywell, Sears and Trion make them), high-efficiency particulate air (HEPA) filters (Enviracaire, (800) 332-1110; Space-Gard, (800) 356-9652) or electrostatic air cleaners that act like electronic precipitators but do not require electricity (Newtron, (800) 543-9149) can filter out some or most of the tiniest allergens and irritants. A few of these filters include charcoal prefilters that can help clear odors, tobacco smoke and some smog ingredients. Each type of filter may also have some potentially adverse effect. Electronic precipitators are said to give off about 0.01 ppm **ozone** and they do require regular, time-consuming, maintenance; they are the most expensive. Room air filters can be disturbingly noisy to some people; they, of course, are the least expensive. Some allergists feel that such filters are quite worthwhile and you might consult your own doctor, or an allergist, for his recommendation; however, professional allergy associations now report that these devices do not show a statistically significant improvement in many allergic patients. Keep in mind that, for allergy and/or dust relief, these filters must operate 24 hours a day. And, you must check with your air conditioner/heater installer for its air flow (cubic feet per minute or cfm); some filters lose their efficiency if too much, or too little, air is circulated by the blower motor.

ASBESTOS
(A cause of breathing problems and cancer)

Although asbestos is not commonly found in the home, it can be part of the insulation material around furnaces, pipes and electrical coverings. In many instances it is sprayed into buildings, usually between the walls, as fireproofing. It is also used in brake linings, paint, paper and cement manufacture, and even some types of cloths; obviously, workers in these fields are much more apt to be exposed. In Japan, where rice is preferred when coated with talc, the talc has been found to contain asbestos. It is even found in the air in many cities; New York City, for example, has shown up to 60 nanograms (ng) of asbestos in a cubic meter (a space about the size of a large refrigerator); and each nanogram represents about 1 million asbestos fibers the size of one's hairs. Asbestos exposure is usually measured in fibers per cubic centimeter (cc), with the present safety level being less than 3 fibers per square inch of space.

Asbestos (the word means "incombustible") is a combination of metals, most commonly magnesium and silicones, and can cause lung and stomach cancers as well as difficulty in breathing, especially after prolonged exposure. The first signs of asbestos damage are usually bronchitis and wheezing; the condition can progress to total respiratory failure.

It is now possible to self-test one's home for the presence of asbestos; even solid pieces of hidden asbestos can break down into invisible air-borne fibers if they are jarred or in the path of air gusts.

What Is Usual
Although asbestos fibers are not really normal, they may be found almost everywhere, but more so in industrial manufacturing areas. Recently, some rural areas have shown levels of up to 30 ng per cubic meter. Still, the presence of any asbestos in a home is not considered usual.

What You Need
The simplest test for asbestos in the home is the Asbestest Kit, available from E–C Apparatus Corp. (3831 Tyrone Blvd. N., St. Petersburg, Fla.

33709). Because of the way these tests are packaged, it is necessary to purchase a kit of 55 tests for $135.00 (about $2.45 a test), so it is best to share this test with others in order to reduce the price. The test takes about five minutes, and although it involves the use of several chemicals, no experience is required.

What to Watch Out For
Most of all, if you suspect an object of containing asbestos, be careful how you handle the specimen so that the fibers cannot be inhaled. While tiny solid pieces are best for testing, it is possible to test carpets and clothing by gathering a sufficient-size sample. Be careful of the chemicals used to perform the test; they can be poisonous and can burn the skin.

What the Test Results Can Mean
Any indication of asbestos in your home environment calls for more technical testing to verify your findings. Should asbestos actually be present, it requires very specialized removal. If you are suffering from dyspnea (difficulty in breathing), it warrants a medical consultation regardless of whether asbestos is present; should it be present, however, it may explain your symptoms.

Reliability
The Asbestest is known to detect as little as 1 percent asbestos (the upper limit permitted by the Environmental Protection Agency). It is possible to have a false-positive test result, but any positive test justifies the use of additional, more sophisticated techniques.

CARBON MONOXIDE (CO)
(A rarely thought of, but quite common, cause of a host of sickness symptoms and signs; it is replacing syphilis as the "great imitator" of dozens of different diseases.)

If someone in your family has suddenly started having angina symptoms (vicelike pains and/or a sensation of burning or pressure in the chest and/or arms); if the man of the family has developed impotency problems; if anyone, or especially if everyone, seems to be suffering from the "flu" (headaches, dizziness, nausea, mental confusion); and if your doctor has been unable to find the cause, you might want to check the concentration of carbon monoxide (CO) in your home—especially if you have a gas-burning appliance (stove, heater, dryer, etc.) inside, or even in a garage or room adjacent to, your home.

In a recent random survey of 1,000 homes, 1 out of 10 showed sufficient CO indoors to be the previously unsuspected cause of a variety of illnesses.

Other studies have revealed that 1 out of every 20 people who seek emergency medical care, especially during the winter months, turns out to have CO poisoning—something rarely even considered by most doctors. The Public Health Service says that at least 10,000 people a year are known to experience CO intoxication, with more than 10 percent dying from a single accidental exposure. In fact, CO is the leading cause of death due to poisoning in the United States.

That a diagnosis of CO poisoning is easily missed is understandable; not only can it be the cause of heart pains, sexual problems and "flu" symptoms, but even a minute amount of inhaled CO can be misdiagnosed as a perfect imitation of pneumonia, a gall bladder attack, epilepsy and, all too often, food poisoning, unless an alert doctor happens to think of CO. CO exposure also causes dyspnea (shortness of breath), giddiness, impaired vision and judgment (especially dangerous when driving), memory loss, muscle paralysis and ringing in the ears. A recent study has shown that CO inhalation causes significant hormone changes; hormones from the adrenal gland in particular are markedly altered in a way that is similar to a severe reaction to stress. The increased amount of the hormone aldosterone, following CO inhalation, is associated with hirsutism (excessive hair growth) in women. Carbon monoxide alone, as well as cigarette smoke, whose primary toxic ingredient is CO, are now definitely linked to decreased estrogens (female hormones) along with an earlier-than-normal menopause and an increased risk of osteoporosis (weakened bone structure); there have been reports of ovarian failure (sterility). In men it is known that CO causes an increase in atherosclerosis (which can block the arteries to the penis as well as the heart), along with a severe loss of oxygen to those organs; testosterone production is also reduced in male smokers—all of which could be the basis for impotence. And after someone has been exposed to, and has seemingly recovered from, an excess of CO, there can—even years later—be personality changes, such as irritability, violence and psychoses, as well as direct damage to nerves, causing weakness, blindness, deafness and even parkinsonism symptoms. For someone with a known heart condition, inhalation of almost any CO can be fatal.

Carbon monoxide is a colorless, odorless, tasteless gas that comes primarily from combustion. Some specific sources include:

• A gas stove (range) in your home. CO can even come from the pilot light alone, but much more is produced when the stove is in use.
• Any gas-burning or kerosene-burning appliance inside the home—a gas dryer, water heater or general heating system, such as a wall or floor heater. Gas appliances adjacent to the home (in an attached garage, utility room, etc.) if not properly vented can allow CO to seep through walls and ceilings.

- Any internal combustion (gasoline, diesel) engine, such as an automobile, generator or lawn mower.
- Home fireplaces where burning is not complete and the flues are not properly installed or become clogged.
- Charcoal fires, such as barbeques.
- Industrial plants where organic chemicals are manufactured and refineries where coke is burned.
- Some paint removers and solvents containing methylene chloride (the evaporating fumes can change to CO).
- Smoking—tobacco or any other substances.

Obviously, in garages and automobile tunnels and on heavily trafficked streets, the concentration of CO is greatly increased.

Carbon *mon*oxide (CO) must be distinguished from carbon *di*oxide (CO_2); an example of carbon dioxide is the harmless bubbles in soft drinks. The two gases are frequently confused; even *The New York Times* insisted in a health article that it was carbon *di*oxide that came from combustion, and it was months before the paper, quite reluctantly, admitted its error.

Carbon monoxide does its damage by replacing normal oxygen-carrying hemoglobin in the blood with carboxyhemoglobin (COHb), a compound that prevents life-supporting oxygen from reaching the heart, brain and the other body organs. One part of carboxyhemoglobin can replace 200 or more parts of normal hemoglobin. It then requires 200 times as much oxygen for each part of carboxyhemoglobin just to bring things back to normal; that oxygen, however, may not always correct any damage that was done.

One particular problem arises when gas appliances are used in newer homes that are insulated so completely that air leakage to the outside is kept to a minimum. Recent central air-conditioning/heating systems may not allow for the introduction of any fresh air into the ducts; in the past most systems brought in up to 25 percent fresh air. Thus, if CO is present in only one room, it is recirculated undiluted throughout the home. If you live in such a home, you should consider opening windows and doors on a regular basis.

Although being inside a house containing CO is most often to blame for the signs and symptoms of CO poisoning, there is one report of a man who suffered severe exacerbation of his heart disease whenever he cut his grass by walking behind his gasoline-powered mower. Tests revealed that he was breathing in extensive amounts of CO given off by his mower's engine exhaust.

Carbon monoxide monitoring. It is easy, and relatively inexpensive, to check your home, garage, work environment and even your automobile for carbon monoxide. It could be lifesaving to have CO monitors at critical locations in your home and attached garage. If you have an unvented gas space heater, of which the Consumer Product Safety Commission says there are at least 8 million still in use, your chances of dying from CO are increased 1,000 times. You can also carry CO monitors with you to places such as ice-skating rinks, where gasoline-powered ice-resurfacing machines are known to exceed safe CO exposure, or while camping if you use gas or gasoline stoves, lamps or lanterns. Some parents have their children carry CO monitoring badges when traveling in school buses; excessive CO in the buses is known to cause many different symptoms, nonspecific illnesses and learning problems.

Carbon monoxide breath monitoring. While most blood tests for carbon monoxide are complicated and expensive laboratory procedures, it is fairly simple to detect and measure the amount of carboxyhemoglobin in the blood by testing for the amount of carbon monoxide in the breath. It usually requires at least a 50 percent concentration of carboxyhemoglobin to cause fainting or unconsciousness, but over 2 percent can cause heart pains and mental impairment. It takes no more than 10 percent to cause a headache and shortness of breath; over 30 percent can make you dizzy, impair your judgment and vision, and make you extremely agitated; over 60 percent can be fatal.

Smoking when pregnant can cause a marked decrease in oxygen and an increase in CO to the brain and body of the fetus—proportionately much more than to the expectant mother. And the loss of oxygen to the unborn baby can persist for hours after the mother stops smoking. Severe CO poisoning can also cause miscarriage and stillbirth.

What Is Usual

Carbon monoxide in the air is measured primarily by parts per million (ppm). While there should never be any evidence of CO in your environment, with today's motor vehicle and industrial exhausts, it is not unusual to find anywhere up to 15 ppm in residential areas, from 5 ppm to 50 ppm in a car while driving and, of course, even greater amounts in an urban setting. The ambient air around Los Angeles frequently exceeds 27 ppm for more than eight hours a day, while Denver averages 21 ppm and New York City averages 16 ppm; New York also leads the nation in the number of days of CO pollution with greater-than-allowable CO concentrations—more than 80 days a year. At the customs and immigration check points between Mexico and California, CO levels of 50 ppm to 60 ppm over an eight hour period are usual where travellers can wait in line, car engines idling, for up to four hours before crossing the border; many federal officials there vomit, pass out and regularly suffer from CO poisoning. At the present time health authorities say the air inside a home should never exceed 9 ppm over an eight-hour period; in contrast, the Occupational Safety and Health Administration (OSHA) allows 50 ppm per hour, with a maximum of 400 ppm for eight hours, but only in the workplace.

More recently, based on the many and severe cardiovascular effects of CO that have been reported in the medical literature, the National Institute for Occupational Safety and Health (NIOSH)—a group that advises OSHA— has recommended that present OSHA limits on CO exposure at work be reduced from 50 ppm per hour, averaged over an eight-hour period, to 35 ppm per hour, with a maximum allowable exposure of 200 ppm over an eight-hour period, or half the present standard of 400 ppm.

A recent government survey of blood carboxyhemoglobin levels showed that as a possible result of air pollution, just about everyone—even children under 3 years of age—shows the consequences of exposure to CO; the average blood COHb levels were from 1 percent to 2 percent. Because cigarette, cigar and pipe smoke regularly contain about 400 ppm of CO, those who smoke had blood carboxyhemoglobin levels more than four times higher than nonsmokers; 10 percent COHb was not unusual, and this amount can come from no more than one pack of cigarettes a day.

What You Need

The simplest, and least expensive, way of detecting CO in the home is by using a color-indicator monitor.

- The Quantum Eye is a business-card-size device that will last for up to a year (much depends on how many times it indicates CO). It is insensitive to other common gases such as natural cooking gas and can be reused by exposing it to fresh air. It costs $9.95, plus postage, from the Quantum Group (11211 Sorrento Valley Rd., San Diego, Calif. 92121). This company also makes small, battery-operated models for $50.00 and up that sound an alarm when a dangerous amount of CO is present; color-change monitors must be constantly observed for an indication of the gas. Both monitors—those that show a color change and those that sound an alarm—will indicate the presence of 50 ppm of CO within seven hours (well within government safety standards); they will, of course, show the presence of greater amounts in a much shorter time (300 ppm in 25 minutes).
- The DeadStop monitor is available for $1.95 each from several mail-order sources; one is Sporty's Tool Shop (Clermont Airport, Batavia, Ohio 45103). This indicator is supposed to show a color change in the presence of 40 ppm of CO after 15 minutes. Once opened, the indicators are good for about a month; if unopened, they are claimed to have a shelf life of three years.
- The Leak-Tec badge is a holder that uses replaceable CO detector but-

tons that should show a color change after a five-minute exposure to 50 ppm; they cost $30.00 for one badge and 10 buttons from American Gas & Chemical Co. (220 Pegasus Ave., Northvale, N.J. 07647). Once a button is taken from its sealed package, it is good for about a month. Unopened, it has a shelf life of six months.

• Extremely precise spontaneous or continuous-reading digital display monitors are available from many sources at a cost of from $300.00 to $1,500.00. They give immediate results and can help locate the exact source of the carbon monoxide. Contact National Draeger Inc. (P.O. Box 120, Pittsburg, Pa. 15275).

Carbon monoxide breath testing can be performed with a National Draeger CO breath test kit that includes a special glass tube into which you exhale; the cost is $36.00 for 10 tubes. Although the price of each test then comes to $3.60, there is an initial cost of $190.00 for a special Bellows Pump (necessary for standardization of the amount of breath to be measured). Most laboratories charge at least $30.00 for a single blood COHb test. Obviously, the cost must be taken into account, but it can be considered relatively inexpensive if it justifies the stopping of smoking and subsequently relieves previously unexplained symptoms. It can be of even greater value if a positive breath test leads to home or work areas that contain dangerous CO levels, thus preventing future damage or revealing the cause of one or more physical or emotional problems. No technical training is needed to perform the test.

National Draeger also sells a combination digital-reading area monitor with a breath-measurement kit accessory for about $1,100.00; this equipment can of course, be shared with others to help reduce the cost.

What to Watch Out For

Be alert for potentially misleading information: Some gas stove manufacturers will tell you that their stoves are "permitted" to have up to 800 ppm of CO coming from them when in use; you should know that this is their own "certification" and that such CO levels can be dangerous. In the case of one particular gas stove, the pilot light alone constantly gave off 59 ppm of CO; this, in turn, caused CO levels of from 30 ppm to 40 ppm throughout the home during the day and up to 60 ppm during the night, when there was no usual activity such as opening doors. That stove turned out to be the specific cause of angina attacks, and when it was replaced with an all-electric stove, the angina completely disappeared.

If you do have gas appliances, and you see any flame—even a pilot light—with an orange or yellow color, it could be giving off excessive CO, and you should call your gas company for adjustments as well as CO measurements; there usually is no charge. If you have to relight a pilot light on a cold appliance, leave the pilot light burning for half an hour before turning the appliance on; a sudden flame on cold metal markedly increases the level of CO in the air. More than anything else, if you have gas heaters, especially of the wall type, do not plug up the vents to the outside (many people do this to avoid drafts when the heater is not in use); this act has caused thousands of fatalities. And of course, *never use a gas oven to warm your home.*

Some CO detectors will react in the presence of strong gasoline fumes and alcohol vapors; one electronic detector will give off an alarm if you cook with wine. Some detectors react if hydrogen sulfide or nitrous oxide fumes (components of smog) are present in large quantities. Most will react if you smoke near them. Always check to see to just what substances, other than CO, a monitor will react.

Do not perform the breath test in an environment where carbon monoxide might exist, such as one's place of work, a room at home that is suspect or even a room where someone is, or has recently been, smoking. It could cause false-elevated breath values.

What the Test Results Can Mean

Any indication of CO in your environment from any monitor means that your home could be dangerous. Open all windows to permit the entry of fresh air and leave the premises. You must then locate the source (heater, water heater, stove, garage exhaust, etc.); to do so, you may need an expert with more technical equipment. Contact your gas company and public health department immediately. If you feel at all unusual or sick, medical attention is warranted.

Although the presence of more than 5 percent of carboxyhemoglobin in one's breath is not absolute proof that carbon monoxide gas is the basis for certain symptoms, it does warrant a medical consultation. Any test value greater than 10 percent warrants medical attention, even if no symptoms are evident. Carboxyhemoglobin levels ranging around 10 percent can be the cause of leg cramps—especially at night—and shortness of breath, even while resting. It should also be assumed that if one family member has a high concentration of carboxyhemoglobin, everyone in the same environment (possibly with a faulty heater) could be so affected. Children and pets show symptoms with much lower area/breath CO concentrations than do adults. If the test is positive as an apparent result of exposure at one's place of work, especially if there is reason to suspect CO poisoning, it is even more probable that all those in the same environment will be affected.

Smokers who show an elevated carboxyhemoglobin level and know that they are not exposed to carbon monoxide gas from any other source will find that their carboxyhemoglobin level will decrease almost immediately after they stop smoking; within a short time of their becoming nonsmokers (and not being exposed to smokers in the immediate vicinity), their carboxyhemoglobin level will return to nearly 1 percent. Incidentally, it takes no more than 70 ppm of CO in the air to cause a 10 percent carboxyhemoglobin level in the blood; each 7 ppm CO in the air is thought to raise the blood carboxyhemoglobin level by 1 percent.

One particular application of CO home monitoring can best be illustrated by the home-sickness syndrome. There are many reports of people who particularly seemed to feel sick over weekends and during vacation time spent at home. Once they returned to work, usually on a Monday, they always felt better. What it came down to was that they were exposed to high levels of CO while at home—it may surprise you to learn that studies have revealed that most people spend about 90 percent of their time indoors when they are at home—and obtained relief from CO concentrations while at work. A somewhat similar situation occurs when you call your doctor to discuss your illness symptoms and are told to "Take it easy and stay in bed for a few days." If your home has excessive CO levels, being at home—and even worse, staying in bed—may be the very reason for your symptoms; getting out of the house and into fresh air could be the cure.

Reliability

Of the relatively inexpensive CO monitors, only the Quantum Eye was consistently accurate when measured against extremely precise digital-reading devices. Some of the others did not always respond as claimed; humidity in the air can affect them and it may be necessary to breathe on the indicator to supply humidity before use. Breath CO measurements were always better than 90 percent accurate.

Note: Sudden deliberate or severe accidental carbon monoxide intoxication—to the point of unconsciousness—often turns the skin bright red; the pupils are usually dilated; the breathing is more like snoring; the pulse is fast and hard, with each beat seeming sharper and more hammerlike than usual. Obviously, immediate emergency medical attention is mandatory.

Observation: Dr. Prescott H. Haralson, a specialist in family practice from Amarillo, Texas, wrote in a medical journal warning his colleagues because of a personal experience: If you find flies in a room dying for no apparent reason, get out fast—the cause could be carbon monoxide.

One of the most effective forms of preventive medicine you can practice is to install smoke and carbon monoxide detectors in your home.

FORMALDEHYDE
(Even your furniture can be hazardous)

Formaldehyde-containing products can include the cement used to hold plywood layers together in home construction, the adhesive that makes up particle board (this material could be part of your walls, paneling or insulation) and even the glue that is used for furniture and cabinets. Synthetic-fiber carpets, drapes and even permanent-press clothing may contain the chemical. It is also the same substance used as a disinfectant and embalming fluid that you may remember smelling in hospital corridors. Formaldehyde in products (called formalin when diluted) can decompose over the years, return to a gaseous state and become part of the air you breathe. If and when it does, it can destroy body cells; it changes into formic acid once it gets into the body.

Usually, the first indication of formaldehyde in the home environment is eye irritation that seems to have no logical explanation. This is most often followed by throat and lung irritation, such as difficulty in talking along with coughing. These symptoms, together with skin rashes, can even come from tiny, unnoticeable amounts of formaldehyde in the air. Ultimately, there may be stomach pains, vomiting and diarrhea, vision difficulties (spots before the eyes), headaches and memory defects, numbness and ultimately death. Formaldehyde can trigger asthmatic attacks and is now believed to be a cause of cancer.

There are home tests that will tell you whether formaldehyde is part of your home air; they can even reveal the particular room where only one piece of furniture may be at fault.

What Is Usual

Although there should be no formaldehyde in the air in one's home, it is not unusual to detect such fumes in homes that have been built since 1980, when energy conservation was at its peak, in recently remodeled homes and especially in older mobile homes, where formaldehyde was the main ingredient in the insulation. Exposure to more than 0.5 parts per million (ppm) over an eight-hour period is considered dangerous. More than 0.1 ppm at any time can cause eye and throat irritation. The Occupational Safety and Health Administration (OSHA) has set a permissable formaldehyde exposure level in the workplace of 1 ppm over an eight-hour period as a time weighted average and where there is a limited, short-term exposure, no more than 2 ppm during any 15-minute period; however, OSHA admits that exposure to 0.5 ppm within eight hours is dangerous to one's health.

What You Need

One way of testing your home, or a particular room, is by placing a formaldehyde monitor in the area for a specific period of time and then having that monitor analyzed. The 3M (Minnesota Mining and Manufacturing) Company, through its affiliate AFS (P.O. Box 10752, White Bear Lake, Minn. 55110), will send you a monitor, directions for use, a prepaid return envelope and, ultimately, a detailed report indicating whether formaldehyde exists and how much you are exposed to; you must send the company a cashier's check or money order for $45.95. It has local safety equipment distributors (see the yellow pages telephone directory) that will sell you the monitor for about $60.00. Envirotech Services Inc. (547 Park Ave., Prairie du Sac, Wis. 53578) will send you a two-test kit that allows you to test your home and see the results immediately (while the results are not expressed in quantities as precise as those provided by the 3M test, they are nonetheless adequate for screening purposes); the price is $40.00.

What to Watch Out For
Be sure to test your home area the way it is normally used; do not overventilate or seal off a room.

What the Test Results Can Mean
It may well be that discovering formaldehyde in your home will explain various symptoms you are having. It does seem that it takes prolonged, continuous exposure to the gas before symptoms develop; however, the greater the concentration, the sooner symptoms occur. There are ways to seal off, or remove, formaldehyde-containing products from your home and to treat clothing and fabrics to eliminate the chemical; your local health department can give you detailed instructions. If your symptoms persist and no formaldehyde is detected, or if they persist after formaldehyde is removed, a medical consultation is warranted. At present, formaldehyde insulation is no longer legal.

You might also want to test your lung function (see Breath and Lung Tests, **Pulmonary Function Measurements**) as a means of detecting one possible consequence of formaldehyde exposure.

Reliability
While only the 3M monitor now meets Occupational Safety and Health Administration standards for accuracy, both the 3M and Envirotech Services monitors are accurate enough for home use. The Envirotech monitor will reveal formaldehyde levels as low as 0.1 ppm in one hour's time; the 3M monitor will show 0.1 ppm in eight hours' time.

RADON
(A possible cause of lung cancer)

Since 1984 radon has become one more environmental hazard to hit the headlines. Yet right after the turn of this century—nearly 90 years ago—this colorless, odorless, radioactive gas was already associated with lung cancer in miners. In 1978 warnings about this gas, then called the "deadly wind," were made public, but few people listened. It was not until 1984, however, when a nuclear power plant engineer set off a radiation-detection device during a decontamination survey and then discovered that his contamination came from his home rather than his job, that public health authorities stood up and took notice.

Radon comes from the natural decay of radium and uranium; these minerals are found virtually everywhere on earth but not always in the same concentrations. Some areas of the country are virtually radon-free, while others contain more radon than in radium mines. The gas is usually harmless when diluted in the open air; it is when it becomes concentrated in the less ventilated basement or rooms of a home that its radioactive effects can be dangerous. Radon can enter a home through cracks in concrete floors or foundations, alongside loose-fitting pipes and drains that run from the inside to the outside of the house and even through bricks and blocks that are porous. If the water source is a well surrounded by radium/uranium-containing soil, radon can even come in with the water. Because it ends up as a gas, its primary path for damage is through the lungs, simply by being breathed in.

The dangers from radon are the dangers of alpha ray radioactivity (see Environmental Tests, **Radiation Monitoring**); at this time the emphasis is on its association with lung cancer. Depending on whose statistics you accept, exposure to excessive radon (the precise amount is still under study) could result in from 3,000 to 30,000 lung cancer deaths a year. It has been recommended that every house in the country be tested for radon; and subsequent to all the scary headlines, an endless number of companies have sprouted up offering an almost infinite variety of ways to test your house for you. But before you decide which test is the most practical for your purposes, contact your regional Environmental Protection Agency (EPA) office and obtain three booklets: (1) *A Citizen's Guide to Radon*, (2) *Radon Reduction Methods: A Homeowner's Guide* and (3) *Radon Measurement Proficiency Report* (which lists companies that have demonstrated they can properly test for radon).

If, however, you cannot wait to learn more than you probably ever wanted to know about radon, you can easily find a radon-detection service that offers you a device to place in your home for several days; it is then sent back to the company and analyzed, and the findings are made known to you. This is probably the simplest, and at present the most effective, way to begin a home radon survey.

It must be kept in mind that radon is not always present in the same concentration from day to day; weeks can go by without any being detected. And two adjacent, identically built homes may not show similar radon levels.

What Is Usual

Obviously, no detectable radioactivity would be the ideal. Unfortunately, as with cosmic radiation, there will always be some radon gas present; the ideal then becomes a home where radon radioactivity is prevented from entering. At present the EPA has decided that 4 picocuries of radiation per liter of air from radon should be the limit (this quantity is expressed as 4 pCi/L); roughly translated, it means that in every quart of air in your home, there should only be about 10 radioactive particles every minute. This is two to five times less than most other countries allow. A *curie,* named for Marie Curie, the discoverer of radium, is the radioactivity of 1 gram of radium; a picocurie is one-trillionth of a gram. While it is admitted that this small amount could still be dangerous, it is felt that considering costs, 4 pCi/L is about as low a level as can be achieved in the presence of typical radium/ uranium soils.

What You Need

A radon-gas trap of one kind or another is all that is required. Such a device can cost from $10.00 to $100.00. The least expensive can be as effective as the most costly. It is best to contact your local or state health department; most have lists of the more than 200 companies whose devices are known to work. Then again, some health departments will supply you with a radon-detection device without charge as a means of uncovering problem areas. There are companies that will do everything for you—for a price; they will come to your home, place and remove the containers, and evaluate the results. A continuously operating monitor that sounds an alarm when radon levels become dangerous can cost $250.00. The ultimate detection apparatus is the hand-held Radon Sniffer, which you can purchase for $2,250.00; it will give you regular, repeated, on-the-spot measurements.

What to Watch Out For

Make sure the radon detector stays in place for enough days to permit you to average out your radon exposure—with the preferable duration being one week. Be sure the room(s) being tested are in their usual condition; if the windows are always closed, leave them that way. If your home is usually well ventilated during the summer, it is best to test for radon during the winter months. Do not hesitate to place several detectors throughout your home, especially in rooms most frequently occupied. Most radiation monitors (Geiger counters) that restrict themselves to beta and gamma radiation cannot detect radon gases, so be certain the device you use will register the presence of radon.

What the Test Results Can Mean

Should the tests reveal levels of radon gases greater than 4 pCi/L, your home is probably among the one out of every five believed to be so contaminated. If the first test lasted for only a few days and was positive, you should arrange for a second test to last for at least a month. The latest assumption concerning the dangers of living in a home containing just 4 pCi/L is that it will cause lung cancer in 1 out of every 100 people; obviously, the greater the amount of radon, the greater the odds of lung cancer. Just as obviously, if you smoke and live with radon gases, you may well quadruple your odds of acquiring cancer. Knowing you have been exposed to radon gases for many years warrants a medical consultation to ascertain your lung status and to keep a close watch on your pulmonary function (see Breath and Lung Tests, **Pulmonary Function Measurements**)—but do not automatically submit to chest X-rays as a means of routinely checking for a lung problem. Excessive amounts of radon in the home mostly warrant corrective measures to seal out the gases and adequately ventilate the home.

Reliability
Properly processed radon-detection tests are 90 percent accurate, if and when radon is present.

SMOKING
(Are you being injured by secondary smoke?)

If you smoke, be it tobacco or marijuana, you are probably well aware of the potential damage caused by the smoke and, most likely, tend to overlook the risks. If you do not smoke, you can still suffer the same ill effects from "passive," or involuntary secondary, smoking. Perhaps the best example of secondary smoke dangers comes from a recent Japanese study showing that nonsmoking wives of smokers had a death rate from lung cancer twice that of nonsmoking wives of nonsmokers. While the hazards to a fetus from the mother's smoking are well documented, less is heard about the fact that children in homes where smoking is routine suffer a far greater incidence of wheezing, coughing, ear infections, headaches and hospital admissions for lung disease; newer findings now also relate such smoking to heart disease in infants and young children. Of particular interest to nonsmokers is the fact that since the smoke from the burning end of a cigarette has not passed through unburned tobacco and/or filters, it is not only as disease-causing as smoke drawn through the unlit end of the cigarette but in some cases it contains chemicals that are even *more* dangerous than those in smoke that is inhaled. Smoke from marijuana may contain even greater amounts of toxic substances than tobacco; **carbon monoxide** (see Environmental Tests) is but one such ingredient. And someone who has been in a room where marijuana has been smoked can show a false-positive test for the drug for weeks, even if he or she stayed several feet away from the smoker.

It is estimated that nearly 50 million Americans over the age of 17 are regular smokers. It is also estimated that each year well over 300,000 people die as a direct consequence of smoking, while up to 5,000 people who never smoke also die annually from lung cancer alone as a consequence of secondary smoke.

There is a simple way to find out whether you are affected by secondary smoke (sometimes referred to as "sidestream" smoke). The **Thio-Screen** test measures the amount of thiocyanate in your saliva (thiocyanate is the end product of the cyanide in tobacco); smokers usually have three times as much thiocyanate as nonsmokers, who, if not around smokers, rarely show any measurable amount. This is the same test used by some life insurance companies as a means of determining the degree of an applicant's risk. It has also been used to help evaluate a possible cause of illness in infants and teenagers.

Another test can reveal whether smoke is indirectly in your environment—even in alleged no-smoking areas. By wearing a color-change Smoke-Check badge, you can measure any accumulated exposure to certain tobacco-smoke products. You can also monitor home and work areas for clandestine smoking.

What Is Usual

In general, people who do not smoke will show less than 0.5 micromoles per liter (μmol/L) of thiocyanate in their saliva. It is extremely difficult to avoid smoke entirely, and certain vegetables—such as cabbage, garlic, horseradish, mustard and turnips—as well as almonds can increase thiocyanate in saliva. Those who smoke, even an average of only one pack of cigarettes a week, usually show a saliva thiocyanate content greater than 0.5 μmol/L.

What You Need

A **Thio-Screen** test kit can be obtained from David Diagnostics Inc. (4601 Broadway, Astoria, N.Y. 11103); material for 25 tests costs $12.00. The test takes less than one minute.

Three Smoke-Check badges are available from Assay Technology (935 Industrial Ave., Palo Alto, CA 94303) for $9.95; larger quantities are much less expensive.

What To Watch Out For

Do not perform the test until the person to be tested has gone at least 30 minutes without eating or drinking. Keep in mind the foods that can imitate a positive smoking reaction. In addition, foods containing certain color additives may color the test solution and give a false-positive result as can blood in the mouth at the time of testing. The use of aspirin products as well as some antihistamines and tranquilizers may also mask the appropriate color reaction and wrongly indicate a positive test.

What The Test Results Can Mean

With the understanding that this is only a screening test to ascertain whether tobacco is in fact being used by and/or affecting individuals, a positive result could well be sufficient warning of the dangers of smoking; it is not a specific diagnostic test to reveal the presence of a disease. As more and more studies are conducted, it is becoming obvious that smoking also contributes to cancer of organs other than the lung, larynx and trachea; cancers of the esophagus, stomach, pancreas, cervix, bladder and kidney are increased in smokers when compared to the rates for non-smokers. Ulcers and many forms of heart disease (it is now known that smoking increases the clotting of blood) are more definitely associated with smoking. And there is new evidence that smoking, especially while a woman is pregnant, can damage DNA and cause defective embryonic growth and development. If someone is suffering unexplained symptoms and signs, especially related to the lungs, the test results could be of help to a doctor in directing his or her investigation. A positive test result in an infant or teenager warrants a medical consultation to help determine whether smoke is in fact adversely affecting the young person's health.

Reliability

With smokers the test is considered 95 percent accurate; the amount of smoking does influence the test result, with some very light smokers showing a negative response. When it comes to testing the effect of passive or secondary smoke on non-smokers, much depends on the condition under which the smoking takes place (room size, ventilation, frequency of smoking, etc.); in general, the test has been shown to be at least 75 percent accurate in detecting the effects of secondary smoke.

The Smoke-Check badge will indicate exposure equivalent to the smoke from one cigarette.

Tobacco and smoking dependence (addiction). In May 1988 the surgeon general of the United States (the nation's chief public health officer) declared smoking to be an addiction similar to the abuse of illegal drugs such as cocaine. There is a test you can take that indicates your degree of smoking tolerance (physical dependence). It was developed by Dr. Karl-Olav Fagerstrom of Uppsala, Sweden, and while it has been reported on in many medical journals, the most definitive description is found in the *International Review of Applied Psychology* 32 (1983): 29–52. To complete this test, called the Fagerstrom Nicotine Tolerance Scale (see Figure 1), you need only answer eight questions.

To find out your score, or how dependent you are on nicotine:

Figure 1. Fagerstrom Nicotine Tolerance Scale.

	A	B	C
1. How soon after you wake up do you smoke your first cigarette?	After 30 min	Within 30 min	—
2. Do you find it difficult to refrain from smoking in places where it is forbidden, such as the library, theater, doctor's office?	No	Yes	—
3. Which of all the cigarettes you smoke in a day is the most satisfying one?	Any *other* than the first one in the morning	The first one in the morning	—
4. How many cigarettes a day do you smoke?	1–15	16–25	More than 26
5. Do you smoke more during the morning than during the rest of the day?	No	Yes	—
6. Do you smoke when you are so ill that you are in bed most of the day?	No	Yes	—
7. Does the brand you smoke have a low, medium, or high nicotine content?	Low	Medium	High
8. How often do you inhale the smoke from your cigarette?	Never	Sometimes	Always

• Assign no points for each answer in column A.
• Give yourself 1 point for each answer in column B.
• Give yourself 2 points for each answer in column C. (*Note:* There are only three questions in column C.)

A score of 7 or more indicates you are highly dependent on nicotine. A score of from 1 to 6 indicates a relatively low, but existing, dependence.

Various validations of this questionnaire have shown it to be as reliable as physical measurements in indicating drug dependence. And it has been shown that those with the highest scores seem to be more successful with therapy to eliminate the addiction. The higher your score, the greater your need for a medical consultation.

RADIATION MONITORING
(Detecting X-ray hazards before they cause permanent damage)

Exposure to radiation or radioactivity can be extremely dangerous to your health. The sources of possible exposure include:

- Nuclear power plants.
- Testing of nuclear weapons.
- X-rays and radioactive chemicals for medical diagnosis and treatment.
- Disposal of radioactive or nuclear wastes.
- Microwave ovens.
- Radio and television transmission waves.
- Old television receiving sets (especially color sets manufactured prior to 1970).
- Jewelry made with radioactive metals (old gold and some irradiated blue sapphires from Africa; ceramic and cloisonne objects from Taiwan).
- Irradiation of feeds (for purposes of sterilization and preservation).
- Some smoke detectors.
- Some static eliminators used to treat film and phonograph records.
- Pottery glazed with uranium oxides (it is usually colored orange or red); some kitchen and bathroom tiles made immediately after World War II.
- Old clocks and watches painted with luminous radium.
- Some camping lanterns.
- Cigarette smoke.
- The atmosphere (from cosmic radiation and radioactive material in the ground; see Environmental Tests, **Radon**).
- Old buildings constructed with radioactive materials.

The damage that can occur to and in your body from exposure to radioactivity, even if only very tiny amounts are involved, is such that there is sufficient reason to measure your environment constantly to detect how much radiation you are being exposed to and how much of that radiation your body absorbs.

There are two basic kinds of radiation: ionizing and nonionizing. Ionizing radiation comes from X-ray machines, radioactive chemicals, nuclear generators and weapons, and "background" sources such as cosmic radiation, from the sun and atmosphere, and earthly radiation, from radioactive material in the ground, in water and even in some foods, all acquired from naturally occurring radioactive substances such as uranium.

Nonionizing radiation comes from radio and television emissions, microwave generators such as radar, ultrasound devices, power lines, household appliances and computers—to mention but a few sources. Once believed to be innocuous, this form of radiation is now considered potentially quite harmful (see Environmental Tests, **Electromagnetic Pollution**).

Ionizing radiation refers to that form of radioactivity which in very minute amounts can ionize, or break down and destroy, the cells that make up body tissues. Ionizing rays are usually described as alpha, beta and gamma. Alpha rays can be stopped by a piece of paper and are usually not harmful unless they get inside the body, primarily via the lungs or stomach, where they are extremely dangerous. Beta rays can cause skin burns and internal damage but can usually be stopped by a thin sheet of metal. Gamma rays are high-energy penetrating rays such as X-rays and nuclear radiation (as from a bomb), which can only be partially stopped by very dense shielding, such as thick layers of concrete and lead. All three types of rays are normally emitted at the same time and from the same source, but cosmic radiation consists mostly of alpha and beta rays.

Ionizing radiation may be recorded in different ways. The basic measurement unit is the *roentgen*, abbreviated *R*, which indicates the amount of radioactivity being emitted by the source (an X-ray machine, a nuclear weapon, etc.). Usually, unless a cumulative dose is being measured, R is measured in relation to time and is expressed as R per hour to indicate exposure. But because radioactive emissions are generally much smaller than 1 R, they are most commonly reported as milliroentgens, or mR, per hour (R = 1,000 mR).

When calculating the amount of radioactivity the body absorbs, the unit of measurement is the *rad* (radiation *a*bsorbed *d*ose); the international term for rad is *Gray* (Gy), and 1 Gray equals 100 rads. In general, direct exposure to 1 R of gamma rays, such as X-rays, results in the body's receiving and absorbing 1 rad. A third term, used mostly in medicine, is the *rem* (radiation dose *e*quivalent in *m*an); the international term for rem is *Sievert* (Sv), and 1 Sievert equals 100 rems, which reflects the estimated biological effect or damage from the radiation absorbed dose, or rad. A rem takes into account the damaging effect of the different kinds of rays (alpha rays, once ingested or inhaled, can cause 10 times as much tissue damage as gamma or X-rays).

Whether or not radiation causes damage depends on several other factors: the distance from the source of the rays; physical obstacles in the way of the rays, such as clothing or protective shielding; whether the source of the radioactivity is performing properly (a correctly calibrated X-ray machine); and whether radioactive material is ingested, inhaled or injected.

A few examples: A single chest X-ray, taken with the machine 6 feet away, depending upon the technician's skill, can cause the body to absorb from 0.05 to 25 rads (sometimes expressed as 50 millirads to 25,000 millirads; 1 rad = 1,000 millirads). A GI (gastrointestinal) series—in which the esophagus, stomach and small intestine are fluoroscoped and X-rayed continually—can cause the body to absorb from 4 rads to 6 rads each minute that the test is being conducted (usually such a test lasts from 10 minutes to 20 minutes). And it is not unusual for some medical diagnostic procedures such as cardiac catheterizations to cause body absorption of from 50 rads to 100 rads each time. The use of radioactive iodine to treat hyperthyroidism can deliver 5,000 rads to 10,000 rads; it is also known to cause retinal damage. And it is now known that X-rays of the chest cause damage to, and obstruction of, the coronary arteries that supply the heart and could be the cause of heart attacks; X-rays of the neck can cause atherosclerosis of the carotid arteries, which nourish the brain.

A recent congressional report on X-ray exposure concluded that the greatest source of excessive, dangerous radiation is unnecessary X-ray examinations, most often performed by unskilled and untrained technicians using poorly maintained equipment. As but one example, over 4 million gastrointestinal series are performed in the United States every year—more as a routine procedure than as a specific diagnostic test. And 75 percent of all nonhospital X-rays in the United States are taken by doctors and technicians who have not had specialized training in the science of radiant energy and its effects. These nonradiologists who own their own X-ray machines perform twice as many X-ray examinations as radiology specialists. Medical radiology contributes 10 times as much radiation exposure to the public as all other man-made sources combined.

Governmental and scientific studies indicate that individuals over 18 years of age should not be exposed to more than 300 mR (0.3 R) a week nor to more than a total of 5 R a year. There is a formula to indicate excessive radiation exposure after the age of 18: Using 5 R as the maximum, simply subtract 18 from your age and multiply by 5. Thus, by the time you reach the age of 19, your total cumulative exposure since birth should not have exceeded 5 R. By age 30 it should be no more than 60 R and by age 50 no more than 160 R. These figures could also be measured as rads. Children under the age of 18 should not be exposed to more than 100 mR per year. Of interest, some color television sets manufactured before 1970 can emit an average of 2.7 mR per hour at the screen's surface. A child who regularly uses that television set as part of a video game or computer screen can, while close to the screen, receive an eye and thyroid gland radiation biological effect of from 800 millirems (mrem) to 900 millirems per year (1 rem = 1,000 mrem).

Some other consequences of radiation: Exposure of a fetus to only 1 R during pregnancy increases by 50 percent the child's chance of having cancer before reaching the age of 12; from 2 R to 5 R can cause malformation of a fetus and chromosome damage; 50 accumulated R can double one's chances of having leukemia; 200 R can stop sperm production in a man and menstruation in a woman; 400 R can be fatal, although death may not occur until months later. All ionizing radiation is accumulative; small doses over a period of time can add up to a damaging amount.

Other sources of ionizing radiation include gold rings and jewelry made, resized or repaired during the 1930s and 1940s that may be contaminated with radioactive material. Irradiated gold that had once been used to treat cancers was subsequently recycled and used by 30 to 40 manufacturers in the making of jewelry. People who purchased objects made from this recycled gold have since been treated for dermatitis and skin cancers, necessitating skin grafts and amputation of ring fingers. Cigarette smoke contains radiation, and this radioactive smoke can also be inhaled by nonsmokers in the same room; it has been linked to lung cancer (see Environmental Tests, **Smoking**). Smoking 1½ packs of cigarettes a day for a year produces a level of radioactivity exposure equivalent to 300 chest X-rays. Uranium mining is believed to be the cause of an excessive amount of stomach cancer in Navajo Indians; this disease was once very rare in that group.

Radiation sickness, sometimes called acute radiation syndrome, comes most often from exposure to excessive diagnostic or therapeutic X-rays and can cause extreme weakness, loss of appetite, nausea, vomiting, hair loss, pigmentation and atrophy of the skin, and dilated blood vessels on the skin, similar to spider angioma (see Body Observations, **Skin Observations**). These consequences are not always permanently damaging, and most disappear after treatment.

Unlike radiation sickness, radiation damage from ionizing radiation permanently injures the body by interfering with its ability to manufacture blood cells and by destroying the walls of blood vessels and the lining of the intestinal tract, causing severe anemia; an inability to fight off infections and cancers; an inadequate blood supply to the brain and spinal cord; and swelling, ulceration and hemorrhage of the stomach and intestines. It has been postulated that up to 3 percent of all cancers come from cosmic radiation.

Damage from ionizing radiation affects various body organs and tissues quite differently (the breast and thyroid gland are far more sensitive and more easily damaged than the kidney or brain), and any organ damage may not become evident for several hours to several years after exposure.

With all this in mind, you should know that although cosmic radiation in Denver is more than twice what it is in New York City (because of its high altitude, Denver averages from 75 millirads to 140 millirads annually; at sea level in New York City, averages from 15 cosmic radiation millirads to 35 millirads), New Yorkers still have twice as much cancer as do inhabitants of Denver. This only serves to show how limited our knowledge of actual radiation effects still is. When exposure to **radon** (see Environmental Tests) is added on, the amount of radiation exposure can be doubled.

What Is Usual

Although it may not seem normal, it is usual to be exposed to some cosmic and earthly radiation at all times; the amount can depend on where you live and how much structural and other shielding there is. For every 5,000-foot rise in altitude above sea level, the rate of cosmic radiation is about doubled.

If you were to measure radiation on a meter, it would not be unusual to detect about 50 mR (0.05 R) when you are standing outdoors at sea level. Occasional traveling in an airplane could expose you to some additional radiation, but because of the brief periods at high altitude and some shielding from the metal fuselage, it averages only 1 mR (0.001 R) per trip; airline personnel, however, can more than quadruple the amount of their natural background radiation. Some televisions are still said to expose the viewer to 0.15 rem per hour of viewing.

Depending upon your work, you could be exposed to three or four times more radiation than in your nonwork environment, especially if you work with X-rays, nuclear chemicals and other electronic equipment, or near nuclear test sites. Radiation from medical, dental and industrial sources is not considered a usual exposure, albeit it may be helpful or necessary.

What You Need

To test for exposure, you will have to obtain a radiation-detection device; such devices are sold under many different names: dosimeter, home or personal Geiger counter, radiation alert monitor, radiation contamination detector, radiation meter, radiation survey meter. They can come with the ability to test for radiation exposure in various ranges—anywhere from 0 R to 600 R (some show how many mR strike you per hour). Most personal dosimeters are calibrated in mR (one-thousandth of an R) and go to 1,000 mR. They usually measure and total the cumulative radiation exposure while being used. Area radiation detectors commonly have both low and high ranges, from 0 mR to 50 mR per hour; they indicate momentary exposure but do not total the dose. Most meters test for all three types of ionizing radiation, but there are meters that are limited to only one form, should you want to test only your food or the water in your fishbowl.

Dosimeters are usually worn on the body (similar to a fountain pen) and have optical gauges that can be read in a way that resembles how one looks through a telescope; they are considered the most accurate radiation-monitoring devices and are used primarily for medical-legal purposes; doctors, nurses and technicians who use X-rays wear them. They also usually require separate chargers to reset them back to zero for reuse. Geiger counters or radiation alert monitors are hand-held, less-than-pocketbook-size instruments that have direct-reading number gauges, digital displays and colored lights to indicate various ranges of immediate radioactivity translated into what the rate of hourly exposure would be; some also have light and sound alarms that can be preset to go off when a specified amount of radiation is detected.

There are so many different monitors available that it would be impossible to list them all; suffice it to say that they range in price from $60.00 to $90.00 for a dosimeter (plus $90.00 for a charger to reset it back to zero) and from $69.00 to $300.00 for personal Geiger counters and general radiation exposure monitors, which can test air, water, buildings, food, and so on and do not require recharging. A reliable Geiger counter radiation-detection meter called the DX-1 is available from RDX Nuclear (203 E. Southern Ave., Tempe, Ariz. 85282) for less than $100.00. It reads from 0.1 mR per hour to 10 mR per hour and will "beep" when exposed to greater amounts. A tissue-equivalent dosimeter, which directly indicates how much radiation has been absorbed by the body, costs $200.00. A detector to monitor only microwaves costs from $9.00 to $20.00. A somewhat different form of radiation exposure monitoring is offered by Personal Monitoring Technologies (88 Elm St., Rochester, N.Y. 14604). For $39.00 a year it will supply you with a CompuRad Radiation Health Monitor, which you carry with you and which measures your actual exposure from environmental sources as well as from medical and dental X-rays.

To protect yourself against damaging ultraviolet radiation from sunlight, there are several devices, which cost from $3.00 to $40.00; they take into account the type of skin (for people who burn easily or only minimally) and then signal when the maximum tanning dose of radiation has been reached.

What to Watch Out For

Try to ascertain just how much radiation you will be measuring; if you are monitoring low-range amounts (cosmic, earthly or other environmental sources, X-rays or industrial emissons), you do not need high-range or multirange detectors; low-range detectors will do the job and will usually cost less. If you want to monitor all the radioactivity you are exposed to over a selected period of time, you might prefer a dosimeter that ranges from 0 R to 600 R. Be aware that while some detectors come with an on-off switch, others do not and will continuously detect any and all radioactivity—whether from an old luminous watch, television set, certain building materials or background radiation—which could distort a particular measurement. Some detectors have to be recalibrated regularly; usually, the manufacturer performs this service.

Before you undergo any X-ray procedure, be sure to find out whether there might be some other way for your doctor to make a diagnosis, and do not request X-rays purely for your own satisfaction. It has been reported in medical journals that chest fluoroscopy examinations on American women have caused breast cancers equal to the proportion suffered by Japanese women exposed to the atom bombs at Hiroshima and Nagasaki. X-ray treatments of the spine, used in some cases of ankylosing spondylitis (an inflammation of the vertebrae) are believed to cause leukemia at the same rate as those who survived the atomic bombs.

Always demand proper shielding of breasts, eyes, reproductive organs and the thyroid gland during any X-ray. When adolescent girls are X-rayed for possible scoliosis (abnormal curvature of the spine), now a common practice in schools, their breasts must be shielded against the radiation exposure.

The most important thing to watch out for is the unnecessary X-ray, with the so-called routine chest X-ray being the worst offender. A great many studies show that the risks from unnecessary X-rays are far greater than the possible benefits—not just from radiation but as much from the possibility of a false-positive interpretation. Dental X-raying of children is another example of a situation where "routine" X-rays should be avoided; there should be a definite necessity for the X-ray, and it should be limited to the tooth in question and not include the entire mouth.

Unless in a life-threatening situation, women should observe the "10-day rule": Do not allow any X-rays except during the 10 days after menstruation starts. This is to prevent harm to a possible fetus. It is also a wise preventive measure to perform a *pregnancy* test (see Urine Tests, **Clinical Analysis: Pregnancy**) before any X-ray.

Finally, watch out for the unshielded X-ray, the untrained X-ray operator and/or the uninspected X-ray machine. As but one example, in California any doctor who uses an X-ray machine as well as the technician who takes the pictures must, by law, be certified by the state. In 1987 alone, 400 California doctors and their employees were found to be taking X-rays although they were not certified (certification entails undergoing two years of formal study and training). No legal action was taken against these doctors, who were simply given letters urging them to stop; however, they are ignoring the law and continuing to use their X-ray machines. That state's radiologic certification office also admitted there were nearly 8,500 X-ray machines and operators still not inspected.

Reliability

In general, environmental radiation monitors are 90 percent accurate. Personal monitors that are carried or worn on the body are close to 100 percent accurate. Low-priced microwave-detection devices are not very accurate but could provide an early warning of oven leakage. Ultraviolet-detection devices to protect one from sunburn are considered to be 80 percent accurate.

ELECTROMAGNETIC POLLUTION

In addition to, but quite different from, ionizing radiation (see Environmental Tests, **Radiation Monitoring**), there are nonionizing electric and magnetic radiations that are also believed to be able to penetrate and affect the body—by causing hormone changes, damaging cells (making certain cells more susceptible to diseases such as cancer) and even causing a variety of neurological and mental illnesses, whose effects have included suicide. This form of electrical energy can come from radio and television broadcasting antennae, radar, microwaves (whether used for cooking or for detection), the power lines that carry electricity to industry and to your home, a host of medical diagnostic equipment and home electric appliances such as computers, vacuums and even electric blankets (also see the discussion of video display terminal radiation at the end of this entry).

Actual scientific cause-and-effect proof of injury as a result of being exposed to such electronic waves and magnetic fields is still not absolute, but there have been court awards for illness indirectly associated with living near power lines. Military personnel in the path of radar waves have been reported to have died from such exposure, and amateur radio operators have been reported to have an increased incidence of several diseases, including leukemia. As for electric blankets, and even heated water beds, an article in a 1986 issue of *Bioelectromagnetics* reported changes in fetal growth and evidently spontaneous abortions in families using these devices; whether such harmful effects are due to the heat or to the electromagnetic fields has not been determined.

While electric and magnetic waves can be produced together, they are usually measured differently. The electric waves may be expressed in hertz, or Hz, standing for cycles per second (typical house current is 50 Hz to 60 Hz; radio and television signals run from 500,000 Hz to multimillion Hz; and a cellular phone can transmit at 1 billion Hz). With radio waves, the greater the frequency (Hz), the greater the ability to penetrate buildings— but the shorter the effective range. Microwaves are reported in terms of volts per minute or power density (milliwatts per square centimeter). Magnetic field strength is measured in gauss, or G (the effect of the earth's magnetic field on a compass needle is 1 G; a toy magnet registers about 10 G; and a diagnostic magnetic resonance imaging machine can run to 20,000 G). There have been reports that 0.001 G from an electrical field can cause a biologic effect.

Diathermy is a medical procedure in which electromagnetic waves are converted to heat when they get inside the body and are used as an approach to healing injured tissue. In contrast, an electrocardiograph machine detects the natural electromagnetic fields given off by the heart's beating and records that action graphically as an aid to diagnosis.

Outside the medical field, microwaves identical to radar rapidly cook food in a microwave oven. Unfortunately, these same electromagnetic fields can also affect sensitive electronic equipment such as pacemakers, computers, navigation systems, electric garage doors and telephones, making them inoperable.

Whether electromagnetic fields are in fact a health hazard is still not absolutely resolved. Research has lately been emphasizing the search for a relationship between overhead power lines and various forms of cancer. One way of "testing" for the presence of such specific energy radiations is to note the thickness of the power lines near your residence; the thicker they are, the more current they carry and the greater the likelihood of electromagnetic fields that could have a biologic effect. Some utility companies will make specific measurements for you, without charge, or there are consultants who will provide this service (usually at a cost of several hundred dollars a day). There are instruments available, starting at about $300.00, that allow self-measurement, but these require training and constant calibration.

A new, simple-to-use electromagnetic detector that costs $75.00 and is used with a multimeter (a readily available electrical measuring device costing from $10.00 to $100.00) is available from Electrical Fields Measurement Co. (P.O. Box 326, Stockbridge, Mass. 01260). This device indicates gauss in microvolts; the better the multimeter, the smaller the amount of field that can be detected.

The distance from the source of any electromagnetic radiation is important. For example, a vacuum cleaner motor may show 0.1 m gauss within an inch of the motor but no evident gauss more than an inch away. Again, although the exact bodily effects from electromagnetic radiation are not really understood, failure of the detector to show any gauss does indicate little, if any, radiation is present.

Should you find you are living in an environment that is "bombarded" by electromagnetic radiation, there are ways of insulating your home from these nonionizing rays. Such protection must be kept in perspective; you could also screen out radio and television reception and you might have to forego the convenience of electrical appliances and lights. At present there are no "standards" for exposure, nor are specific levels of electromagnetic radiation known to be illness-causing; the field is relatively new. Still, it is yet another source of environmental pollution that must be considered a potential health hazard until proved otherwise.

Video display terminal (VDT) radiation. Video display terminals, or VDTs (televisionlike tubes such as are used to show computer data), have been found to give off low-level radiation, consisting primarily of electromagnetic emissions. There have been reports that this radiation might be the cause of miscarriages and birth defects. Although no concrete evidence has been presented to substantiate this charge, the Canadian government has requested that pregnant women not be allowed to work at or near a VDT, and in 1988 a New York county passed a law regulating exposure to VDTs in the workplace. A Food and Drug Administration (FDA) study of VDTs showed no ionizing radiation being given off but did detect nonionizing radio frequency radiation; at present there are no limitations on this type of radiation, and manufacturers can provide built-in shields against it.

There are devices that can test for VDT radiation, but they are relatively expensive for an individual ($600.00 to $800.00); their cost would not be out of line for a business, however, and if you work with a VDT, you might suggest their use to your company. For further information contact Holiday Industries (14825 Martin Dr., Eden Prairie, Minn. 55344) or EKM Associates (342 Consumers Rd., Willowdale, Ontario M2J-1P8, Canada).

COOKING OILS
(Protect your body and your senses from bad oil.)

Certain vegetable oils that are used in cooking (canola, corn, and safflower are but a few) are being promoted as more healthful because they contain polyunsaturated fatty acids as opposed to having more saturated fatty acid, as do butter or lard. *Polyunsaturate* is actually an adjective that describes the chemical makeup of certain kinds of fatty acids. When polyunsaturated fatty acids are heated for 15 minutes or more, changes can take place in the chemical structure as well as the character of such oils, which, in turn, cause a change in the flavor of foods cooked in those oils. Moreover, polyunsaturated fatty acids can be made nutritionally undesirable after heating. When a polyunsaturate is heated, it acquires a new, lower iodine number. The iodine number is one way fats are determined to be saturated or unsaturated—the lower the number, the more saturated the fat is supposed to be. Thus, when the iodine number of polyunsaturates is lowered by heating, they can be considered more saturated.

Polyunsaturated fats not only become nutritionally undesirable after long heating (and reuse), they can also become dangerous. Animal experiments reported in a number of chemical and nutritional journals have shown that long-heated oil actually enhanced atherosclerosis, caused tumors and cancers, and shortened life. There have also been a number of studies showing that people who increase polyunsaturates in their diet have a higher incidence of cancers (especially skin cancers) than those on a more balanced diet.

In the past the American Heart Association vigorously promoted virtually unlimited use of polyunsaturated fats and oils as a purported means of lowering blood cholesterol levels. The association has since retracted its strong endorsement of these particular fatty acids and now suggests that equal proportions of saturated as well as polyunsaturated fats be consumed along with an equal one-third proportion of monounsaturated fat, such as olive oil, while still keeping total fat consumption low.

Because of the increased use of polyunsaturated oils and because of their inherent dangers, ways have been developed to detect their breakdown in cooking oils. To be sure, the company that developed the technique for testing cooking oils and measuring for the content of free fatty acids has not done so primarily for health/medical reasons, but rather for the benefit of the restaurant and prepared-food industries, to improve the quality of the foods they produce while allowing them to cut costs by using cooking oils for the longest amount of time.

The test can easily be performed by anyone cooking with polyunsaturated oils, and since heated polyunsaturates can be harmful to one's health, the test can be a valuable preventive measure, by revealing at what point the oils have become dangerous and should be discarded.

What Is Usual

In many kitchens where cooking is done with oils, it is usual to use, cool and then reuse those oils. Some food establishments keep the oil heated all day; they may filter the oil or add chemicals or add an extra bit of fresh oil to the original batch from time to time to avert the off-flavor and characteristic odor of overcooked oil, with complete disregard for the detrimental effects that this practice could have on the consumer. One vending machine that offers french-fried potatoes reuses (reheats) the same soybean oil up to 200 times.

What You Need

An Oil Test Kit can be used to determine the quality of cooking oil. The test, which is based on standard American Oil Chemists' Society methods, offers a means of evaluating at what point cooking oil is becoming dangerous and should be completely replaced. The test kits are available from Fresh Oil International (5182 Old Dixie Highway, Forest Park, Ga. 30050), at $17.95 for 30 tests, including shipping. Each test takes three minutes.

What to Watch Out For

If the oil to be tested is hot, draw the oil sample from the cooking utensil and cool for approximately two minutes (to below 200° F) before testing. The oil is then put into a test bottle containing all the test materials. If, after the test bottle is shaken for 10 seconds to 15 seconds, the solution of oil and test materials is pink to red, the oil is still usable. If the solution turns colorless or has a brown-yellow color, the oil should be discarded. Since the chemical test solution is poisonous, the test bottle should be kept well away from all foods.

What the Test Results Can Mean

If the test results induce you to discard any cooking oil before it breaks down, you will never have food that tastes and smells of rancid oil, but more important, you will not be subjecting your body to the dangers inherent in overcooked oil.

Reliability

The test is considered to be 95 percent accurate in revealing potentially dangerous cooking oil.

LEAD
(A common cause of mental as well as physical illness)

Although there are a number of environmental sources of lead against which precautions are normally taken, this metal can also be found in an equal number of unexpected places. Most people are familiar with air-borne lead coming from gasoline additives and from paints; few think of dangerous amounts of lead coming from pottery and jewelry glazes, toys, the metal used for typesetting, storage batteries, cable coverings, pipe solderings and even brass fixtures. In 1988 an oil company gave away free decorative glasses with gasoline purchases; each glass contained more than 450 times as much lead as allowable. Burning old newspapers puts a tremendous amount of lead into the air (paper imprinted with colored ink is 12 times worse as a source of lead than paper imprinted with black ink). And when the hair of someone coming off a rifle or pistol range is tested, it can show a dose that would be almost fatal if that level of exposure were allowed to continue.

While most lead poisoning comes from sources in or near a workplace where lead is an integral part of a particular process (battery making, smelting, paint removing, radiator repairing), the most recently discovered source of dangerous lead exposure was electric water fountains used in schools and office buildings, where up to 40 times the allowable levels were found. While, in general, soil contains about 15 mg of lead per kg (a mg, or milligram, is about two particles of table salt; a kg, or kilogram, is almost 2¼ pounds), house dust can have 500 times as much.

Lead poisoning, sometimes called plumbism (the chemical symbol for lead is *Pb,* abbreviated from the Latin word for lead; the word *plumbing* is also derived from this source, because all early plumbing pipes were of lead), can be acute (rapid in onset) or chronic (slow-developing) from the accumulated intake of lead through eating contaminated foods or putting lead-painted objects in the mouth, from breathing in lead fumes and even from absorbing it through the skin. Children are much more susceptible to lead poisoning than adults, and this frequently reflects itself as an undiagnosed learning problem in school.

Acute lead poisoning most often comes from the sudden ingestion of a toxic amount of lead and generally manifests itself by stomach pains, vomiting and a constant metallic taste in the mouth; within a few hours or a day, diarrhea and black bowel movements usually occur. The kidneys may shut down (no urine), and then the victim can slip into a coma.

Chronic lead poisoning most commonly starts with a loss of appetite, irritability, dullness and an inability to perform mentally as well as physically. Other signs and symptoms include weakness and the possible appearance of a thin black line (lead line) on the gums. There are innumerable other manifestations of chronic lead poisoning; a few include an inability to hold up one's hand or foot, lack of coordination, convulsions and delirium.

It is believed that hundreds of children die each year, and thousands more suffer mental problems, from unsuspected exposure to lead. Pediatricians estimate that between 1976 and 1980 nearly 800,000 preschool children had toxic levels of lead in their blood.

Although there are laws prohibiting the manufacture and sale of paint containing more than 0.06 percent lead (years ago most wall paint contained up to 50 percent lead), a great many buildings still have high-lead, usually peeling, paint—something young children seem to have an affinity for putting in their mouths and chewing (it has a sweet taste). The law also forbids the manufacture and sale of dishes and pottery that give off more than from 2 parts per million (ppm) to 7 ppm of lead in a 24-hour period (depending on the size of the dish); yet in 1987 there were at least 20 recalls of dinnerware, flatware and hollowware containing dangerous amounts of lead—and not all were from foreign manufacturers. The random tests performed on imported dinnerware showed that nearly 7 out of every 100 pieces had excessive quantities of lead—and no more than 1 out of every 1 million pieces of imported dinnerware is actually checked for lead.

You can test your dishes and other glazed china at home to see whether it contains lead that is given off and becomes part of the food you eat. You can also have your water tested by your local health department, usually without charge, or by a commercial laboratory.

What Is Usual

Unfortunately, the presence of lead in the air and in substances you eat, drink or touch seems inevitable; it should not be usual. Present laws allow a certain amount of lead to be in dinnerware, drinking water, paints and various industrial products and processes. It has also been estimated that the average daily diet contains about 0.2 ppm of lead, meaning that everyone regularly eats about 0.021 mg of this metal a day, with the highest quantity being found in leafy vegetables. Other estimates indicate that the suspected *average* inhalation of lead is 0.006 mg a day and that *average* drinking water adds about 0.002 mg daily; 500 mg of lead is considered fatal, and this substance can accumulate in the body over the years.

What You Need

A home test kit to test for lead in your dishes and crockery can be obtained from Frandon Enterprises Inc. (511 North 11th St., Seattle, Wash. 98103); the cost, including postage and handling, is $24.50, and the kit will test more than 100 items. The yellow pages lists laboratories that will test your water for lead and other substances. Direct testing of water for lead and for some other chemical hazards can be arranged through Trace Minerals International (4919 North Broadway, Boulder, Colo. 80302) for $25.00 (also see Environmental Tests, **Drinking Water Analysis**).

What to Watch Out For

A positive test for lead could also mean that other metals may be present. At times it is necessary to perform additional tests specifically for lead; more often than not, however, the toxic metal is lead. Frandon Enterprises will test specifically for lead for $10.00; many health departments will test your questionable samples without charge. Because of the obnoxious gas the test can produce, it is best to perform the test outdoors. Be careful of the test solution; it is caustic.

What the Test Results Can Mean

Any color change with the Frandon solution is sufficient to conclude that the tested object is leaching lead; do not use that object for food or drink. Although the color changes can indicate the amount of lead in ppm, it must be emphasized that *any* color change should be considered a dangerous sign until proved otherwise. If you find you have been using dishes or other pottery containing lead, it warrants a medical consultation for individual blood, hair or urine testing. If, in retrospect, you identify any of the signs or symptoms of lead poisoning, especially in children, it, too, warrants individual lead testing; again, this may well be available, without charge, from your local health department.

Reliability

The test is considered 90 percent accurate as a means of alerting one to a potential lead hazard. A negative test result is considered an almost 100 percent accurate indication that no lead is being released.

NITRATES
(A water pollutant that can cause cancer and poison infants)

Although drinking water is usually, and regularly, tested for toxic materials, recent surveys have revealed that some municipal water supplies have occasionally exceeded what is believed to be a safe amount of nitrates. Nitrates most often get into a water supply from fertilizers, but they can also come from industrial waste discharge, pesticides and the manufacture of plastics. When ingested, nit*rates* can be converted to nit*rites* through the action of saliva and intestinal bacteria. The nitrites may then become nitrosamines, a compound known to cause cancer in animals.

In recent years medical journals have reported fatalities in infants whose formula was mixed with water containing nitrates; the nitrates alter normal **hemoglobin** (see Blood Tests) to a form called methemoglobin, which cannot carry oxygen, and infants are extremely susceptible to any interference with respiratory function. One of the first signs of nitrate-nitrite poisoning is cyanosis—a bluish color to the skin, lips and other mucus membranes. Other symptoms include headache, nausea, dizziness and a drop in blood pressure; in fact, nitrites, such as nitroglycerine, are used therapeutically to lower blood pressure and to dilate the heart's arteries as a treatment for angina. Of incidental interest, nitrates are a natural component of certain vegetables, such as spinach, and are used as a preservative in smoked and variety meats. It is easy and inexpensive to test your water at the faucet, and it is especially important to do so if you use the water to prepare baby formula.

What Is Usual
While drinking water should contain no nitrates, the Public Health Service does allow up to 45 parts per million (ppm); 50 ppm has caused infant deaths.

What You Need
Nitrate dipsticks are available from David Diagnostics Inc. (46-01 Broadway, Astoria, N.Y. 11103); four test strips cost $4.00, including postage (the cost is less if they are purchased in quantity). The test, which takes one minute, indicates 0 ppm, 30 ppm or 60 ppm of nitrate.

What to Watch Out For
It is best to check your tap water twice—first, right after you turn on the faucet and, second, after the water has been running for at least 10 minutes (which is more likely to indicate a distant, more common source of contamination). Be sure your water sample is not collected in a container that once held cosmetics; many cosmetics are made with nitrogen products.

What the Test Results Can Mean
Any indication of nitrate, no matter how minuscule, in drinking water warrants not drinking that water at all—more so if it is given directly to infants or mixed with their formula or fruit drinks. It has been reported that even as small a quantity as 10 ppm of nitrate in drinking water is sufficient to cause methemoglobin in an infant. Should there be any doubt about a baby's skin color, immediate medical attention is warranted. If there is doubt about one's drinking water supply and nitrates are revealed, medical attention is warranted to determine the blood's oxygen-carrying capacity.

Reliability
The test is 90 percent accurate in revealing nitrates.

SULFITES
(A test that could prevent a fatality)

Since 1983 several sudden deaths have reportedly been linked to the ingestion of sulfites, and at least one death is attributed to drinking wine with a high sulfite content. No one can even guess at how many allergic reactions due to sulfites go unrecognized or misdiagnosed, but there are increasing reports in medical journals of people's "passing out" right after eating a catered or restaurant salad. Sulfiting agents have been used profusely in many restaurant salad bars, and even the National Restaurant Association has urged its members to stop putting sodium bisulfite on foods—or at least make customers aware of its presence. Restaurant owners claim that just by having to cut fresh lettuce more frequently (without sulfites, shredded lettuce loses its crispness in a matter of hours), their food and labor costs increase threefold for that product alone.

And many food-processing substances—such as flavored gelatin, beet sugar, corn sweeteners and food starches—sometimes include sulfites. Sulfiting agents are commonly used as antioxidants and preservatives (to prevent discoloration and spoilage) in many other foods, wines, beer and pharmaceuticals (antibiotics, anesthetics, corticosteroids, some heart drugs and bronchodilators, to name but a few). Many drug manufacturers are now removing the sulfites from their products; your doctor or pharmacist can tell you which ones still contain the substance. It is estimated that from 10 percent to 20 percent of the 10 million to 20 million asthmatics in this country are dangerously sensitive to sulfites and that many usually nonallergic individuals are also at risk.

The signs and symptoms of a sulfite reaction include nausea, diarrhea, flushing, swelling (edema) of the face and throat, hives, itching, generalized dermatitis, a dangerous drop in blood pressure, shock, loss of consciousness and a total cessation of breathing—with any or all of these signs and symptoms usually occurring within 15 minutes after ingestion. Sulfites and other sulfur compounds can also cause chalkiness and brittleness of teeth, alter a great many blood test results and interfere with the absorption and usefulness of many nutrients.

As little as 5 mg of sulfites by mouth and only 1 ppm (part per million)*

---

*One ppm is a concentration equivalent to 1 mg in 1 liter (quart); an example would be one particle of fine table salt in about 3 quarts of water. Another way of expressing such minute quantities was explained to physicians in their journal *American Family Practitioner*. The article described 1 part per billion as the concentration that would result from pouring 1 ounce of ink (or bourbon) into a tank the size of a football field and 10 stories high. Make that tank a half-mile long, a half-mile wide and a half-mile high, filled with water, and then pour in that 1 ounce of ink (or bourbon), and you will have a concentration of 50 parts per quadrillion—or the amount of toxic dioxin found recently in Midland, Michigan.

of the sulfite sulfur dioxide (see the discussion of sulfur dioxide in Environmental Tests, **Air Pollution**) in the air can cause any or all of the above-mentioned symptoms, signs and other physical reactions, yet the federal government allows 350 ppm of sulfur dioxide in wine production and has yet to adequately control the use of sulfites in food. It is estimated that the "average" daily diet contains about 3 mg of sulfites and that wine and beer drinkers ingest an extra 10 mg of sulfites a day. Studies have shown that there may be as much as 100 mg of sodium metabisulfate alone in a typical restaurant meal; reactions to sulfites and other related sulfur compounds are becoming so common that they have been recognized as a real public health hazard.

In August 1986, after many years of arguing about the need for legislation, the FDA banned the use of sulfites in some fresh and dried fruits and vegetables and required certain packaged foods to be labeled if they contain 10 parts per million or more of sulfites. The FDA also set new standards lowering the amount of sulfites allowed in processed shrimp to less than 100 ppm. At present there is a proposal to ban the use of any sulfites on fresh potatoes, where this substance is commonly used, but there is no ban on the use of sulfites on canned, frozen or dehydrated potatoes.

Because several medical studies have reported adverse reactions to prescription drugs containing sulfites (which are found in about 1,100 oral, inhaled and intravenous products), warning labels are to be required where sulfites are used in the manufacture of those medications.

The Treasury Department's Bureau of Alcohol, Tobacco and Firearms (BATF) issued a statement in January 1987 that "A label declaration of sulfites in foods and beverages will enable persons who are aware of an intolerance to sulfites to minimize their exposure to these ingredients." However, the BATF allowed, first, a one-year transition period (to January 1988) before all foods will be required to carry a label showing their sulfite content and, second, an indefinite period before all alcoholic beverages will be required to carry a sulfite declaration label.

Because one death from acute asthma was caused by drinking a wine that contained only 92 parts per million of sulfites, and because that figure is well below the 350 ppm level that the federal guidelines allow, even the new regulations are not much of a protection for susceptible people. Some states (California, for one) are less strict in requiring sulfite labeling, so that even if the federal government does mandate warning labels, it would seem sensible and possibly lifesaving for individuals who know or suspect they might be at risk to test their own foods, beverages and prescription drugs.

What Is Usual
Although it may be usual to find sulfur compounds, especially sulfites, in wine and certain foods, especially lettuce and seafoods, it is not normal. The ideal is to have no measurable amounts of sulfites in any food or beverage.

What You Need

You can identify the presence of sulfites with a CHEMetrics test kit, which costs $18.00 for 30 tests; each test takes one to two minutes. The kits come with all necessary supplies, including self-filling ampoules that perform the proper dilution automatically. They can be obtained from CHEMetrics Inc. (Rt. 28, Calverton, Va. 22016).

A dipstick Sulfitest has also been developed. If sulfites are present, the dipstick will change color from white to pink when touched to suspected foods or held over an open bottle of wine. This test differs from the CHEMetrics test for sulfites in that the CHEMetrics version will indicate the quantity of sulfites in numerical form, while the dipstick indication is more qualitative. The Sulfitest would be more convenient for someone who wants a quick warning before consuming food or wine in a restaurant. Sulfitest test strips are available from Center Laboratories, EM Industries Inc. (Port Washington, N.Y. 11050), at a cost of $20.00 plus $2.50 for handling, for a color-chart container with 100 dipsticks.

What to Watch Out For

With the CHEMetrics test, if the liquid to be tested is colored, it may be necessary to make a preliminary dilution so that it is as colorless as possible; be sure to note this dilution and consider it when figuring the final result. When placing food in water to make a solution, be sure the water alone does not contain sulfites. Always test wine immediately after opening the container; liquids whose container has been opened can lose some of their sulfur compounds in the air. And cooking, such as with seafoods, may cause a sulfide coating to evaporate.

With Sulfitest strips, certain foods cannot be tested accurately for sulfites because of their color (tomato sauce, red wines), acidity (lemon, lime, and orange drinks tend to show lower sulfite values because of their acidity) or the normal presence of related chemicals (sulfide ions occur naturally in eggs, cabbage and broccoli and can interfere with the test). Follow the directions and precautions carefully.

What the Test Results Can Mean

Detecting sulfites by pretesting suspicious foods and beverages can help prevent severe allergic reactions in susceptible individuals. It can be especially beneficial for asthmatics to learn what, if any, of their foods and drinks contain sulfur compounds. If testing for sulfites does nothing more than make those with allergies more aware of the possible use of these preservatives and antioxidants in what they eat and drink, it can help avoid a great deal of illness. Be sure to tell your physician if you even suspect sulfites as a possible cause of your allergies; this substance is not routinely searched for when skin testing is performed to identify allergies. Your doctor can then test you specifically for sensitivity to these chemicals. Should you confirm or even suspect, the illegal presence of sulfites in food or beverages, be sure to notify your local FDA office for further investigation.

Reliability

The CHEMetrics test is 95 percent accurate. The Sulfitest is considered 70 percent accurate, there have been instances of false-negative results in dried fruits and some wines; when in doubt avoid such foods. False positive tests have occurred with some fish, meat and poultry; such reactions are not dangerous if the food is avoided. The Sulfitest works best with lettuce and potatoes.

DRINKING WATER CONTAMINATION
(Unfortunately, a not uncommon cause of illness)

If any one environmental element is automatically considered "safe"—even more so than the air we breathe—it is publicly supplied drinking water. Yet a recent study has revealed that as many as one out of every five public water systems is contaminated by several of more than 2,000 different chemical waste products; and nearly 200 of these substances are known to be harmful to one's health. When it comes to rural drinking water sources, such as private wells, the chances of pollution are three times greater. Since there are close to 80,000 public water systems in the United States, it can be assumed that at least 16,000 of them are serving up relatively unsafe water.

In addition to **lead** and **radon** (both discussed under Environmental Tests) as extremely dangerous drinking water contaminants, there are more than 200,000 buried gasoline storage tanks that are leaking harmful compounds; as a result of the use of chemicals on farmlands, herbicides, pesticides and fertilizers are picked up by groundwater, which ultimately is consumed; and who really knows what harmful substances drain from landfills into drinking water?

You can learn what is in your drinking water. And of even greater importance, you can do something about contaminated water should you find yourself at risk. Furthermore, by eliminating drinking water contaminants, you may find some vague, heretofore unexplained symptoms (headaches, depression, learning difficulties and even skin problems—to mention but a very, very few) disappearing. In addition, water pollutants are known to cause decreased fertility, and in 1988 three separate studies revealed that women who drank publicly supplied tap water had far more miscarriages and children born with birth defects than women who drank only bottled water.

Although contaminated water sometimes looks bad (colored, cloudy, foaming) or smells and tastes foul, the vast majority of harmful substances can only be detected through careful chemical analysis. Most large cities list drinking water testing laboratories in the yellow pages. And there are certified mail-order laboratories that offer either complete water analysis or testing for only one suspected illness-causing substance, such as lead. A few laboratories include: National Testing Laboratories, Cleveland, Ohio; call [800] 458-3330 for information and costs; WaterTest, Manchester, N.H. 03108; call [800] 426-8378 for information and costs. Sears, Roebuck will supply test bottles and a basic water test that costs $10.00; a relatively complete battery of tests costs $30.00; call [800] 426-9345 for details.

The Ecowater Systems, through its Water Analysis Laboratory, P.O. Box 64420, St. Paul, Minn. 55164, at times offers free basic water testing; they also offer, without charge, an excellent booklet on home water problems and how they may be corrected. In general, costs range from $15.00 to $40.00 to test for specific contaminants such as radon or lead to $180.00 for an analysis to detect close to 100 different potentially dangerous substances. A check for the most common contaminants generally runs from $60.00 to $80.00. Should dangerous substances be detected, most companies also offer advice on how to correct the problem.

When taking a sample of drinking water for testing, it is important to follow the laboratory's directions; most insist that you let the water run for a prolonged period of time (10 minutes or more is not unusual). At the same time, such testing may not reveal problems in the water that first comes out of the tap, such as lead in old pipes within the house, which can accumulate when water is not used for several hours. This is particularly possible if water for cooking is taken from the *hot* tap; minerals and chemicals dissolve much more easily in hot water. This is one of the reasons why water for cooking and eventual drinking should always come from the *cold* tap; another is that heated water tends to be less aerated, causing an unpleasant taste. It can be a good preventive measure to let water intended for consumption run for several minutes before actually using it.

While testing drinking water for the cause of an unexplained illness can be most rewarding (there have been incidents where contaminated water is believed to have caused leukemia as well as liver and kidney disease, and bacterial pollution has been shown to be a common cause of all sorts of stomach and intestinal ailments), there are also relatively inexpensive ways of protecting yourself against a potentially unsafe water supply. The most common device is a filter attached to your cold water faucet (usually, but not necessarily, under the sink). Some filters only eliminate taste and odor problems; others can make water as pure as possible and even eliminate toxic metals, bacteria and parasites.

In general, the best water filters cost from $200.00 to $300.00 as a one-time charge for the plastic or stainless steel case and filtering cartridge, with replacement cartridges—which can last from six months to a year, depending, of course, on your water use—costing about $30.00. One source of detailed information on totally effective filters is the Western Purifier Company (22900 Ventura Blvd., Woodland Hills, Calif. 91364).

Other means of purifying water are distillation units, which boil the water and allow the steam to condense back into a relatively pure supply (some feel that a few chemicals may still be carried over in the steam). But drinking nothing but distilled water can keep the body from obtaining necessary minerals. Home distillation units cost from $200.00 to $300.00 and will only produce from one to four gallons a day. One source is New Medical Techniques (P.O. Box 1356, New Britain, Conn. 06050). Reverse osmosis devices are also said to decrease the amount of sodium in the water, but they usually require an extra water supply and drain and also yield only relatively small amounts of pure water. They cost from $50.00 to $500.00.

Keep in mind that most filters must be changed regularly or they can, themselves, become a breeding ground for disease-causing bacteria. Obviously, bottled pure water from a reliable company is a simple substitute for tap water.

If your drinking water has no taste or odor problems but you are still unsure about your water supply, call your local health department for details on its testing of public water. The Environmental Protection Agency office in your state may also offer similar information. But only by testing your own drinking water, from your tap, will you know just how safe it is.

To be sure, pollution is not limited to the water we drink; poisons have adulterated lakes, rivers and oceans as well. In Japan a few years ago, thousands of people died, and many more were crippled, from eating fish contaminated with mercury.

BODY OBSERVATIONS

The "secret," if there is one, to being a good doctor is nothing more than observation; those who *watched* and learned during medical school days still find that what they see and hear (the patient's medical history) offers the quickest and most accurate clues to diagnosis. While no one expects the potential patient to be as aware as a practicing physician, it is still possible to detect early signs of illness—sufficient to ward off disability—by carefully and regularly observing your body. First, of course, you must observe your body when no illness is evident; then any alteration should become immediately apparent. By paying attention to your skin, nails, hair, various organs such as breasts and testicles, and even whether and how you or someone close to you snores, you may be able to prevent disease; you surely can help maintain your health.

Most bodily observations involve no equipment, entail no cost and require little time. Yet such "tests" are as valuable, and accurate, as searching for some substance in the blood or urine through chemical analysis. True, there are body observations that call for a tool or two—such as an otoscope to see inside the ear, a tuning fork to assess the condition of one's nerves and muscles, a blood pressure measuring device and a spirometer—but these are still really indirect aids to body observation as opposed to direct evaluative apparatus. Your own eyes and ears are still the best test "instruments" in the world.

BODY TEMPERATURE
(A simple test for health monitoring)

Body temperature is a manifestation of the body's metabolism; in actuality it reflects the heat produced by all sorts of body processes: digestion, breathing, hormone production, muscle activity (voluntary muscle movement such as when you move your arms and legs and involuntary muscle activity such as your heart beating) and even the formation of brain chemicals while thinking. When certain body processes (physical exercise, conversion of an excessive amount of food in the intestines, even fear) are occurring that tend to raise your body temperature, you might start to perspire, and as sweat evaporates, it acts as a cooling mechanism to counteract the temperature rise. In a cold environment, especially without adequate protection such as warm clothing, your muscles may start to tremble, and the shivering will help to raise your body temperature.

Body temperature can be considered an indication of how efficiently your body is performing—much as with any other engine or machine. Although when it comes to illness, most people think almost exclusively of elevated body temperature (fever), a lower-than-normal body temperature (hypothermia) can also point to certain diseases and even be life-threatening; more than 500 people die each year from hypothermia. Most often, a normal body temperature does signify good health, albeit there are exceptions (see Figure 2).

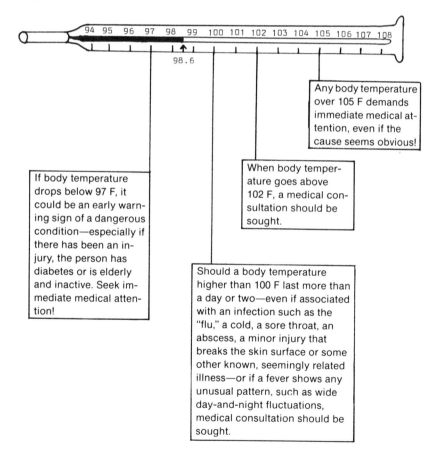

Any body temperature over 105 F demands immediate medical attention, even if the cause seems obvious!

When body temperature goes above 102 F, a medical consultation should be sought.

If body temperature drops below 97 F, it could be an early warning sign of a dangerous condition—especially if there has been an injury, the person has diabetes or is elderly and inactive. Seek immediate medical attention!

Should a body temperature higher than 100 F last more than a day or two—even if associated with an infection such as the "flu," a cold, a sore throat, an abscess, a minor injury that breaks the skin surface or some other known, seemingly related illness—or if a fever shows any unusual pattern, such as wide day-and-night fluctuations, medical consultation should be sought.

Figure 2. Body temperature.

A common cause of fever, not directly resulting from disease and frequently overlooked, is the use of certain drugs. Medicine taken for one purpose can have a secondary action, or side effect, of raising body temperature. Drug fever can be an early warning sign of an impending dangerous drug reaction and warrants immediate medical attention. A few examples of such drugs include: antibiotics, especially penicillin and related drugs, sulfanilamide derivatives and streptomycin; antihistamines; procainamide; nicotinic acid and some other vitamin B_3 derivatives; anticoagulants; iodine and iron compounds; barbiturates; most narcotics, especially cocaine; amphetamine products; a few drugs used to control heart rhythms; anticholinergic medications, including atropine; even aspirin products or several cups of caffeine-containing coffee, tea or cola drinks can indirectly raise body temperature. Your doctor or pharmacist can tell you whether your medicines have this effect.

Basal body temperature is also used to test for ovulation as a means of enhancing the opportunity for pregnancy (see the discussion of basal body temperature in Genitourinary System Tests, **Ovulation Time**).

What Is Usual

Although the figure 98.6 F (37 C) is most often quoted as normal, most doctors take little notice of a body temperature ranging between 98 F (36.7 C) and 99.5 F (37.5 C) when the temperature is measured orally (with the thermometer under the tongue and the mouth closed). A rectally measured temperature may be normal even though it is a ½ degree to 1 degree higher. An axillary measurement (taken with the thermometer held under the armpit and the arm firmly pressed against the side), when normal, is usually ½ to 1 degree lower than an oral temperature.

What You Need

The test requires one of the following types of thermometers:

- Glass, filled with mercury (usually silver-colored) or some other chemical (generally red); they cost from $1.00 to $4.00.
- Electronic, with a sensitive metal tip connected to a measuring device that displays the temperature on a scale or in digital form; they cost from $6.00 to $15.00.
- An aural thermometer, which, when placed at the opening of the ear, reads the body temperature from the eardrum; while good for adults, it is especially useful for young children, since it enables the temperature to be measured during sleep. It should cost less than $30.00.
- A small, flat, plastic-coated circle fever detector that adheres to the skin surface on the forehead (it can be left in place for days for continuous readings and can be reused 10 to 12 times). It immediately shows body

temperature in the form of a digital display in either Celsius or Fahrenheit. One manufacturer also makes a hypothermia model for detecting lower-than-normal body temperature, which can be very valuable for monitoring the elderly. Such devices cost $1.95 each.
• Special glass thermometers that read body temperature as low as 75 F (23.8 C), for use when hypothermia is suspected.

If a thermometer is not available, it is still possible to tell whether someone has an elevated temperature by placing your palm or the back of your hand on your own forehead—assuming your body temperature is normal—and then comparing that with the degree of warmth felt on the patient's forehead.

What to Watch Out For

Always make sure the thermometer reading is below normal before measuring body temperature. With an ordinary glass thermometer, lower the temperature reading to 95 F (35 C) by shaking the thermometer while holding the end opposite the measuring tip or bulb; or you can immerse the tip in cold water for a few minutes.

If you are particularly testing for hypothermia, be sure your thermometer will indicate readings as low as 94 F (34.5 C). A typical thermometer that must first be shaken down has to have its indicator below 94 F before it can be used to test for hypothermia; the temperature reading usually does not drop below the level set by shaking down. If, after you use such a thermometer, it shows no rise above 94 F, immediate medical attention is warranted. For regular monitoring for hypothermia, a special low-reading thermometer should be obtained.

Unless the thermometer's accompanying instructions indicate otherwise, it should be left under the tongue or in the rectum for at least three minutes; if axillary measurements are taken, the thermometer should remain well inside the armpit for at least five minutes.

When oral temperature is measured, the person whose temperature is to be taken should not eat, drink or smoke for at least one-half hour before testing, and the mouth should be kept tightly closed for the entire time the thermometer is in place. Ideally, there should have been no physical activity for at least one hour prior to testing, no matter what technique is employed.

When you record the temperature, it is a good confirmatory measure to record the pulse rate (see Heart and Circulation Tests, **Pulse Measurements**) and the rate of breathing (respiration) as well. Normally, the pulse and breathing rate increase as body temperature rises.

Keep in mind that body temperature tends to be lower in the morning and higher toward evening.

If a high or low body temperature reading does not seem to correspond with the patient's body warmth and other symptoms that usually accompany fever (flushed face, rapid pulse and breathing, lethargy) or hypothermia, first check out the thermometer by measuring your own temperature or by comparing the reading with that of another thermometer. Should there still be some doubt, most doctors and hospitals verify their observations by measuring the temperature of a freshly passed urine sample.

When using plastic fever strips or other skin-surface-type thermometers, be sure that no lamp or even direct sunlight shines on the thermometer's surface; the warmth can cause false-high readings.

What the Test Results Can Mean

If you know, or have good reason to suspect, that an infection exists, evidence of elevated body temperature (fever) is to be expected. Fever above 100 F (37.8 C) warrants medical consultation. In most instances the degree of fever corresponds to the severity of the illness. As treatment is applied, the reduction of body temperature is a reasonable indication of the treatment's efficacy. On the other hand, if, after a prescribed medicine is used for more than 24 hours, there is no lowering of body temperature, this could be a warning that the drug is not effective, and immediate medical attention should be sought.

Should there be evidence of fever without any obvious or reasonable explanation (a recent fall or other injury, exposure to one of the many childhood illnesses or the residual effects of a return from foreign travel—some tropical-type diseases do not reveal themselves until weeks or months after exposure), then that fever could well be an early warning sign of a hidden kidney problem, a complication of liver metabolism or any of a hundred different conditions that warrant medical consultation.

At times fever reflects itself as night sweats—in which one wakes up during the night hot and sweat-soaked. Body temperature measurements may be close to normal during the day. Repeated bouts of night sweats usually come from low-grade infections, but they can also be a cancer warning sign; they warrant a medical consultation.

If a woman develops a fever during the first four weeks of pregnancy, she should immediately notify her doctor; it seems that a high fever in a pregnant woman can cause defects in fetal development.

The pattern of fever during the day and over a period of several days may offer an important clue to a doctor as to the cause of an illness (see Figure 3). The body temperature usually stays below 103 F (39.4 C) when a severe cold or pneumonia is caused by a virus; when the source of the infection is a bacteria or fungus, the fever is almost always higher than 103 F. When the fever seems close to normal every morning and then rises to more than 101 F (38.3 C) each evening, it could suggest brucellosis (sometimes called undulant fever), which can come from drinking raw milk. If a fever

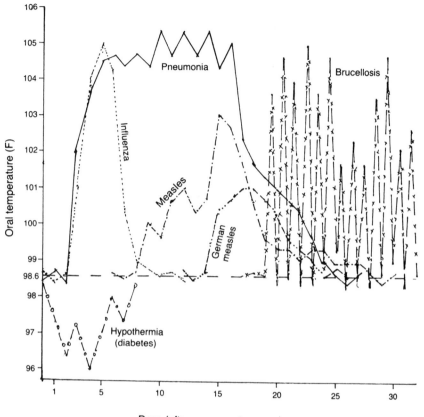

Figure 3. Some examples of disease fever patterns.

pattern stays high for several weeks without any usual dips, it can suggest psittacosis, a pneumonialike disease that can be caught from infected birds, such as pigeons, parrots or parakeets. A fever chart that shows a very high temperature for a day or so, then a sudden drop for 12 hours to 24 hours, followed by another sharp rise, could make your doctor consider a hidden abscess. With malaria a patient can show a high fever for anywhere from two to three days and then return to normal for a few days—depending on which of the four types of malaria he or she has contracted. Since many diseases have distinct fever patterns—especially when fever can be correlated with the pulse and respiration rates—it can be of great value to record these observations for your doctor.

Because it is common for people over the age of 60 to have a normal temperature as low as 97.6 F (36.4 C), it is easy to accidentally miss hypothermia (abnormally low body temperature)—from 95 F to 97 F (35 C to 36.1 C)—which can be extremely dangerous. As we become older, our body metabolism tends to slow down normally, and this, in turn, helps lower body temperature. Hypothermia as an illness may occur following an injury, along with malnutrition or dehydration, as an insulin reaction in patients with diabetes and even as a consequence of alcohol use. It is considered good preventive medicine to measure the body temperature of any elderly person daily—especially if he or she is living alone. People usually shiver and cannot perform some normal tasks when body temperature drops below 96 F (35.5 C). Below 95 F (35 C) there may be slurred speech and dilated pupils. In younger people a body temperature of 97.6 F (36.4 C), especially when it occurs in the morning and does not rise during the day, can be an early sign of thyroid disease. Repeated lower-than-normal body temperatures warrant a medical consultation; a temperature of 97 F or less in an elderly person warrants medical attention.

Reliability

Rectal temperature measurements are considered to be the most accurate (the thermometer should be left in place at least three minutes) but are really only necessary for infants or others who cannot hold a thermometer in the mouth; oral temperature measurements are sufficiently accurate for virtually all purposes. Axillary and skin-surface temperature measurements are the least accurate. Direct-reading thermometers, such as those with digital displays, while easier to read, are no more accurate than ordinary glass thermometers. Fever "patterns" are accurate in pointing to a specific disease about 80 percent of the time. When doctors were evaluated to see whether they could determine whether a patient had a fever by using only their hands, they were right almost 90 percent of the time.

Thyroid functioning. Body temperature measurements may also be used as an indication of thyroid activity—or lack of same. It has been a general medical observation that patients with hypothyroidism (reduced thyroid hormone production) have a lower-than-usual body temperature (except when they have an infection or other fever-producing illness); patients with hyperthyroidism (excessive thyroid hormone production) almost always have a slightly higher-than-usual body temperature.

As a screening test for thyroid function, leave a thermometer, set well below "normal," on a table next to your bed. On awakening, before you perform any activity—even getting out of bed—place the thermometer snugly in your armpit for 10 minutes. *Note:* Normal body temperature when measured under the arm ranges from 97.6 F (36.4 C) to 98 F (36.7 C). A persistent early morning temperature below 97.6 F could well be an early warning sign of hypothyroidism; it warrants a medical consultation.

The test is considered accurate enough for doctors to use to monitor patients for whom they have prescribed thyroid hormone; if the armpit body temperature suddenly goes above normal—with no other obvious explanation—it can mean that the patient is taking too much of the hormone. Keep in mind, however, that starvation or dysfunction of the adrenal or pituitary gland can also cause a decrease in body temperature, but these conditions are usually self-evident.

BREAST SELF-EXAMINATION
(Yet another possibly lifesaving screening test)

Most women who examine their own breasts regularly are able to notice a potential abnormality early enough to avoid drastic treatments; they also become aware that the majority of breast lumps are not cancerous. More specifically, over 98 percent of breast lumps measuring one-half inch or less that are discovered by self-examination do not require any disfiguring surgery. Breasts should be self-examined once a month. If you are menstruating, a few days after the menstrual period is over is the best time, since at other times of the month—especially just before menstruation—the breasts are more apt to be swollen or tender. If you examine your breasts on the same day each month, you are more likely to recognize any change. While there are several techniques for breast self-examination, once you have learned a method satisfactory to you, consistency and regularity are the keys to successful testing. Some women find that bath or shower time is easiest; others prefer lying in bed. In any event, the basic steps (shown in Figure 4) include:

- *Observation:* Stand in front of a mirror with your arms by your side, then with your hands on your hips and your elbows as far back as possible and then with our arms straight up over your head.
- *Palpation:* First while you are standing in front of the mirror and then while lying on your back with one arm (the arm on the same side as the breast being examined) behind your head and using the rib cage for resistance, press the fingertips gently but firmly into the skin under the arm and then into the breast tissue, using a circular motion from the outside in toward the nipple, until the entire breast has been palpated.
- *Squeezing the nipple.* You should observe whether this produces any discharge.

It has been discovered that women whose mothers or sisters have had breast cancer run two to three times greater a risk of contracting this disease than women who have no family history of breast cancer. Also, breast cancer is extremely rare before the age of 35.

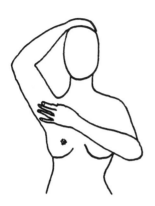

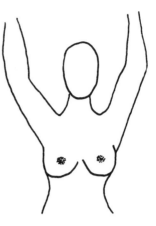

While standing, press the fingertips into the skin under the arm and then in a circular motion over the entire breast (some say that this part of the examination is more sensitive if performed when the skin is wet and soapy).

While in front of a mirror, raise both arms over your head and look for any bulges, dimples or depressions on the skin of the breasts.

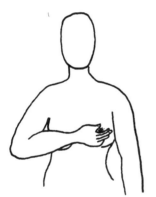

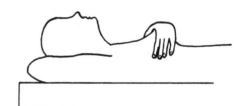

Gently squeeze the nipple to see if there is any sort of discharge or secretion.

While lying down, press the fingertips against the breast, using the underlying rib cage to provide a resistant background.

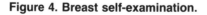

Figure 4. Breast self-examination.

Women who examine their breasts regularly and detect a lump that requires treatment still need major surgery less than half as often as those who never practice self-examination.

A 1988 research project revealed that women who received a one-time classroom-type instruction in breast self-examination became more than twice as competent in detecting lumps. For women who are not quiet sure about their breast self-examination technique, such classes are offered in many medical centers around the country; your local public health department should be able to provide detailed information. For even more specific instructions—including how to differentiate harmless nodules from possible dangerous lumps, there is the MammaCare Learning System (breasts are medically referred to as mammary glands; hence, the name *MammaCare*). There are MammaCare Centers all over the country; call [800] 626-2273 for the one nearest you. Here a woman is given individualized instruction using a breast facsimile selected by a "certified" trainer to most closely resemble the woman's own breast. The model breast becomes part of a practice kit that the woman can take home for review on a monthly basis just prior to self-examination. The cost of the training starts at $35.00, and the kits cost $20.00; the program does eliminate the common apprehension some women have about never being sure just what they are supposed to feel.

It must be kept in mind that most breast lumps are cysts (doctors call them fibrocysts), and about one woman in five will develop one or more of these often-tender cysts between the ages of 20 and 50. These cysts are believed to be related to monthly hormone changes and usually disappear after the menopause. Recent medical advances now offer many treatments that are alternatives to surgery.

Many drugs and some foods are suspected to be the cause of breast cysts. Some women claim their cysts disappear when the avoid certain medicines or eliminate one or more foods or beverages from their diet. Problems have been reported with the following:

- *Foods:* Those containing xanthines or caffeine, such as coffee, tea, cocoa and some cola drinks. Foods (chicken, beef) that contain residual traces of hormones fed to animals may cause breast swelling.
- *Vitamin E:* The excessive use of vitamin E has been followed by breast cysts in some women.
- *Nonprescription medicines:* Those containing caffeine or a form of methylxanthine, such as Anacin, Dexatrim, Dristan, Empirin, Excedrin, Midol, NoDoz; many pain relievers, cold and sinus preparations, and appetite suppressants.
- *Prescription drugs:* especially those containing theophylline, used to treat asthma and other chest conditions, and pain relievers that include methylxanthine products.

• *Hormone:* birth control pills (although some women find that their cysts disappear when they take oral contraceptives); estrogens taken after the menopause.

Your doctor or pharmacist can tell you whether any of the above-mentioned ingredients are found in your medicine.

What Is Usual

When you stand in front of a mirror, you may notice that one breast is slightly different from the other in size, shape or even position (one slightly higher than the other). This can be quite normal, and once you become aware of these differences, they will cause no apprehension. While you are palpating, the tissue should be of the same consistency in all areas (it is not unusual for the tissue in the lower half of the breast to seem a little firmer to the touch than that in the upper half, but it will still be of an even consistency). Upon squeezing the nipple, there should be no discharge.

What You Need

The test primarily requires patience and the willingness to spend 15 minutes one day a month to perform the examination properly. Should you be reluctant, have your sexual partner perform the examination; doctors frequently teach husbands and partners the proper technique.

What to Watch Out For

The major stumbling blocks are fear and apprehension, allowing unfounded suspicions to prevent a proper examination, an unwillingness to acknowledge the finding of what seems to be a lump and an even greater unwillingness to seek professional diagnostic follow-up. If you are not sure of how to perform breast self-examination properly, have your doctor or MammaCare show you and review your technique. Be sure to learn whether any medicine you are using contains any form of methylxanthine (caffeine is but one form).

There are doctors who feel that breast self-examination can cause excessive anxiety in some women, especially those who are unaware that in the event of positive results, noncancerous lumps greatly outnumber dangerous lumps. If you feel unusually apprehensive about such a self-examination, you might better leave the checkups to your doctor.

What the Test Results Can Mean

The suspicion or finding of any lump in the breast warrants further testing by a physician. This could include:

• Simple observation on a monthly basis.
• Mammography (special X-rays); but keep in mind that in a recent survey

an initial mammogram indicated the presence of a tumor in 14,851 out of 268,141 women. However, after careful reevaluation only 1,460 ended up positive; the error rate was greater than 90 percent.
- Thermography (professionally administered heat-detection scanning).
- Ultrasound (similar to mammography but without the dangers of X-rays; this test can differentiate between solid and fluid-filled lumps).
- Aspiration (an office procedure in which the doctor withdraws fluid or tissue for further examination).
- Biopsy (removal of a small piece of the lump for further examination).

Any wrinkling or dimpling of the skin over the breast, a discharge of any kind from the nipple or in fact any change—no matter how subtle—from what had been usual warrants medical attention.

Always keep in mind that 90 percent of all breast lumps are harmless.

Note: A recent psychological survey revealed that women who regularly examine their breasts tend to have higher self-esteem, less anxiety and more comfortable relationships with other people than women who do not; they are also known to take more responsibility for their own health.

Reliability

At present, there are some doctors who feel that breast self-examination is not accurate enough to be recommended; they claim it is only about 40 percent accurate. At the same time, when 80 doctors (including specialists in surgery and women's diseases) were tested to see whether they could determine the presence of lumps in breasts, the family practitioners detected 20 percent more lumps than the obstetricians/gynecologists, whose accuracy matched that of patients. The physicians' failure to detect the lumps was blamed on haste; they averaged less than two minutes to examine both breasts.

Other studies show that 98 percent of breast lumps smaller than one inch in size—and not necessarily cancerous—were discovered by women who spent at least 15 minutes performing breast self-examination. In cases where the lump turned out to be cancerous, women who performed self-examination had a survival rate almost 50 percent greater than those who did not do the home test.

EDEMA
(Water retention as an early warning sign of illness)

Although observation for edema may not at first seem to be a medical test, in point of fact it can be one of the best diagnostic discovery techniques; it is in the same category as skin, personality and weight observation. Edema means water retention—the accumulation of abnormal amounts of tissue fluids under the skin—most commonly in the face or lower extremities, within or around the lungs, around the heart, within the cranium around the brain or in the abdomen. Observing where it is located, how much seems to be present and whether or not it can be "pitted" can help detect its underlying cause. Pitting edema—in which, after the fingertips are pushed into the swollen areas, the hollow impression of the fingers remains as a pit-type depression—usually means that at least 8 to 9 pounds of excess water are present.

Normally, 6 pounds of every 10 pounds of body weight is water, in the form of various tissue fluids. If you eat and drink the way the average person does, you usually take in from two to three quarts of fluid a day, and your body easily rids itself of the same amount, most commonly via urine, feces, sweat and respiration. A properly working body can handle up to eight quarts of water a day without difficulty. But when the body's water-regulating system is altered or interfered with—be it by heart or circulatory troubles (varicose veins), kidney disease, liver disease, lung impairment, hormone imbalance, certain infections, allergies, anemia or, in some people, excessive sodium (see Body Observations, **Salt Measurements**) in the diet—water is retained and usually seeks places of least resistance (particularly the skin around the eyes) or places where gravity aids its storage (the feet and ankles).

Many people equate edema with puffiness, and some types of puffiness just cannot be helped. Hormonal changes with premenstrual tension can cause generalized puffiness regularly, even to the point where the eyeballs swell sufficiently to prevent the wearing of contact lenses. Due to anxiety or other stressful conditions, the body can produce an antidiuretic hormone, which causes retention of sufficient fluid to result in edema. The use of many drugs, especially birth control pills and other hormones, can cause edema as a side effect, as can menopause and pregnancy. Eating meat or poultry that has been fed or injected with hormones to increase the animal's weight can cause a similar weight increase in people due to hormonally induced water retention. Taking large amounts of vitamin E can cause generalized skin and breast swelling; many plastic surgeons will not operate on a patient until the patient has stopped taking any vitamin E for a month prior to surgery. Eating in restaurants where foods often contain large amounts of sodium products (such as flavor enhancers, chemical dips and sprays that act cosmetically to keep lettuce green, keep meat red and eliminate odor from fish) as well as using excessive amounts of table salt can cause a temporary bout of edema. Traveling that entails long periods of uninterrupted sitting, high attitudes or hot, moist climates can bring on edema, most often in the lower extremities. Then there is "idiopathic" edema, which seems to be unexplainable.

Recent surveys indicate that three out of every four patients who consult a physician have some form and degree of edema. It is considered the exception to the rule when a woman between the ages of 12 and 50 does not have several episodes of edema just prior to a menstrual period. And it is estimated that half of all men who visit a doctor will have some edema if it is deliberately searched for. But the evident edema is only the tip of the iceberg; the physical and psychological symptoms that edema can cause are the real problem: headaches, personality changes, difficulty in breathing, fatigue, weakness, palpitations, diarrhea, ulcerations and itching as well as aches, cramps and pains, usually limited to the swollen areas. Edema, then, is not a specific disease but more a reflection of some underlying body re-action and/or pathology; testing for the degree, location and consequences of edema can be helpful in that it permits the identification of early warning signs of impaired body function, disease and psychological disorders.

What Is Usual
Any amount of edema or puffiness is really not normal, but when con-sidered as a temporary, brief, expected response to certain body functions or environmental factors—menstruation, prolonged sitting, tight clothing (especially garters), climate change, drug use, stress or a sudden, extremely high intake of sodium—it is not always abnormal. A small amount of facial edema, especially around the eyes, usually occurs after lying down for a long time. Water retention that amounts to a weight gain of no more than one to two pounds in a day, lasting no more than a day or two, may also be a physiological response to some environmental precipitating factor and still not be abnormal.

What You Need
The test requires a critical eye and a commitment to honest observation, a willingness to admit puffiness and a good scale for daily weight checks.

See Body Observations, Salt Measurements, for a device to measure the amount of salt (sodium) in your foods and beverages.

What to Watch Out For
Because so much edema comes from excessive salt, you should not attempt to fool yourself or unknowingly be fooled about your diet. If you are hy-persensitive to sodium, it only takes 1,000 milligrams (mg), or less than half a teaspoon of salt to cause temporary edema. One medium-size dill pickle contains 2,000 mg of sodium (about 10 times the amount you need all day); eight ounces of most canned vegetables, two four-inch round pancakes from a commercial mix, two hot dogs, four slices of bologna, one cup of bran, a cup of sauerkraut and just two teaspoons of baking powder all contain 1,000 mg of sodium. Then again, one hamburger or piece of fried chicken from an animal that has been fed hormones can act on the body as if it contained well over 1,000 mg of sodium. Check with your doctor or pharmacist to see

whether any drugs you are taking contain large amounts of sodium (antacids, aspirinlike products) or whether they contain hormones that could cause water retention. Asthmatics taking steroid drugs usually have some edema from their medicine.

What the Test Results Can Mean

If there is no ready explanation for edema with a weight gain of more than two pounds, no matter where it appears, and especially if it lasts for more than a day, a medical consultation is warranted. As a rule of thumb, severe ankle edema usually comes from heart problems; profuse facial edema most often reflects kidney disease; and abdominal edema is usually associated with liver disease. Pitting edema warrants medical attention even if you think you know the reason for it; this type of edema usually indicates far too much water retention to have come either from extraneous or environmental causes or as an expected reaction to body activities and functions. An edema that develops slowly, over a period of days, often accompanied by a slight fever, can indicate a parasitic infestation—especially trichinosis (or filariasis, if you have traveled to one of the tropical countries where elephantiasis is endemic), but it can also signal a nutritional disorder or a vitamin B_1 deficiency. Persistent puffiness of the face, especially the eyelids, and hands can be an early warning sign of thyroid disease. Obvious edema that cannot be easily explained, especially if it lasts for more than two days, warrants a medical consultation.

Reliability

Unexplainable edema (not due to diet, drugs, etc.) is considered 70 percent accurate as an indication of some underlying disease.

FINGERNAIL OBSERVATIONS
("Look at my nails")

Careful scrutiny of the fingernails can often help identify disease conditions in other parts of the body. Nail changes alone are not necessarily a diagnostic sign for a specific disease, but they can provide useful clues in pointing to problems. Badly bitten nails suggest a psychological difficulty, perhaps chronic anxiety or depression; longitudinal ridges in the plate part of the nail are often seen in older people with impaired circulation.

Note: Nail problems are caused more often by nail cosmetics than by disease. For instance, nail glues, nail colorings and artificial nail coverings can be irritating to the normal nail bed. If such products are used, avoidance may lead to relief of a nail problem.

What Is Usual

The nail plate, which is the horny (hard) transparent surface that we usually call the nail, should lie smoothly and convexly (slightly arced) over the normally light pink nail bed. The sides of the nail plate are normally buried in folds of skin called nail folds and cuticle. The cuticle and nail beds should appear smooth and not irregular, with no redness or swelling. The "white" semicircle (lunula) should rise out of the cuticle to about ⅛ to ¼ of the nail length.

What You Need

This test requires your powers of observation, applied regularly and systematically, in order to notice something new or different about the appearance of your nails.

What to Watch Out For

Do not ignore the possible implications of changes in the state of your nails. Color changes or changes in the shape or texture of the nail not attributable to a known trauma or cosmetic should be checked with your doctor. There should be no clublike swellings at the fingertips.

What the Test Results Can Mean

The nail plate should not be raised above the nail bed, nor should it become translucent or change color or shape. Randomly scattered small white spots are usually due to insignificant bruises, but transverse white lines are seen with arsenic poisoning, infectious fevers such as malaria, and kidney problems. Yellow nail plates are sometimes seen with bronchiectasis and sinus infections. Clubbing at the fingertips has been associated with pulmonary (lung) and cardiac (heart) conditions.

A fungus infection is one of the most common nail diseases. The same fungus infection that is found in hair (ringworm) or in the mouth or vagina (monilia or candidiasis) can cause a loss of the nail plate's luster, followed by discoloration and easy breakage. The specific diagnosis requires a laboratory examination of nail scrapings.

The nail *bed* should not show small hemorrhages or abnormal redness, which can suggest many disorders, including endocarditis and lupus. Paired white transverse lines are seen with low serum albumin. The nail bed may appear white with a pink edge in liver disease (cirrhosis). Other color changes in the bed (not due to injury) warrant medical consultation.

The lunula can take on a reddish color in heart failure and some skin and connective tissue disorders; it has a bluish appearance with liver problems (hepatolenticular degeneration, Wilson's disease) and in people who are constantly exposed to silver salts, such as in photography. Opaque white nails could indicate a thyroid disorder.

Reliability

In general, nail abnormalities are primarily nonspecific early warning signs of a generalized disease. Most doctors consider unusual nail signs to be about 70 percent accurate in revealing an underlying condition.

HAIR OBSERVATIONS
(Hair as an indication of illness)

Hair observations include:

- Presence or absence of hair.
- Location (whether hair is present in appropriate or inappropriate areas).
- Areas of baldness (male or female patterns).
- Texture.
- Whether or not hair can be pulled out of the scalp easily.
- Shape and structure of hair roots (anagen-telogen test).

Through such observations, many cases of hair loss, as well as certain underlying disease conditions, can sometimes be explained.

Hair usually grows in three stages: The anagen stage, which lasts anywhere from six months to six years, is newly formed, growing hair; the catagen stage is the point at which hair stops growing temporarily but could start again; and the telogen stage is that in which hair stops growing completely and is most susceptible to falling out—either from physical actions such as brushing, from rough cosmetic treatments or because a new hair has started growing in the same place (follicle). When hair first grows, especially in children, it is usually fine and silky, without a surrounding capsule or sheath. In later life, after hair has been growing a while, it becomes more coarse and curly; it also acquires color and a surrounding capsule that gives it more body and firmness. Later in life, hair may lose its pigmentation and become gray, white or colorless.

An abnormally large growth of hair, especially in areas of the body where it would not be usual, is called hirsutism; the word most often refers to hair growth on the upper lip, chin, chest and lower abdomen of women. In contrast, loss of hair, or baldness, in body areas where hair normally should be found is called alopecia. Either of these conditions can be, but is not always, a significant signal of something's being wrong.

Hair growth, hair loss and hair pattern distribution can also be affected by drugs as well as by disease. Large doses of aspirin or vitamin A, many drugs used to treat tumors, anesthetics, anticoagulent medicines, drugs used to lower blood cholesterol levels and certain hormones can cause hair loss; the sudden stopping of birth control pills has been known to produce temporary baldness in women. In contrast, other drugs such as male hormones and some diuretic preparations can cause excessive hair growth—usually in inapporpriate areas. X-rays—especially to the face, head or neck—can cause hair loss. An emotional stress or anxiety is a known cause of a type of alopecia that is usually reversible once the underlying reason for the mental anguish is eliminated. A "normal" temporary hair loss can occur for two weeks to six weeks after having a baby or following an injury.

Anagen-telogen (hair-pull) test. To perform the anagen-telogen test, sometimes called the hair-pull test, count out 10 adjacent hairs, preferably on top of the scalp, and pull at them gently; no more than 2 should come out easily, and these should look like "club," or telogen, hairs; when examined under a pocket microscope, the root at the end of these hairs should be of a ball or pea shape (clublike), with little or no surrounding capsule. The second part of the test is to count out 20 adjacent hairs and, with a firm grip near the scalp, pluck all of them out; no more than 4 should be telogen hairs, while the others should be anagen hairs, with the root structure at the end of the hairs more elongated, showing a definite capsule or sheath around it—somewhat resembling a spear (see Figure 5).

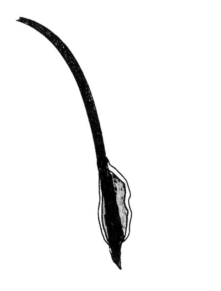

Anagen root (growing hair)   Telogen root (resting hair)

Figure 5. Hair strands and their roots after being plucked from the scalp—the anagen-telogen distinction.

What Is Usual

Most people, quite aware of normal hair distribution, easily notice the unusual presence or absence of hair, with hair growth being especially obvious on inappropriate areas. Depending on certain inherited traits, one can have a great deal more hair than would seem usual but still not have hirsutism; baldness, too, may be a genetic trait, and such tendencies must always be considered before a "different" hair pattern is labeled as abnormal. As to texture and color, most body and scalp hair should have some firmness and pigment; it should not all be fine and colorless.

What You Need

Mostly, the test requires your powers of careful observation, combined with knowledge of your family background with respect to hair proclivity and baldness, along with a pocket light microscope from 10-power to 30-power, which costs from $7.95 to $30.00

What to Watch Out For

You should not erroneously assume that unusual amounts of hair and seemingly inappropriate distribution are always signs of something's being wrong; it could be natural for you, or it could also be idiopathic, meaning that while a specific diagnosis cannot be made, the cause is most apt to be genetic. If you are suffering from dandruff (seborrheic dermatitis), acne, or a bacterial or fungus infection of the scalp, or if you have been applying any sort of chemical to the scalp (dyes, permanent wave solutions, excessive heat or even unusual hair tonics), you must clear up the underlying condition or avoid the chemicals for several months before you can use your hair for specific test purposes. If you suffer from trichotillomania (a condition in which a person constantly pulls hair out in either small or large amounts), this alone, while not really a hair condition, warrants a medical consultation before proper hair testing can be performed.

What the Test Results Can Mean

Hirsutism, or excessive hair, especially in the wrong places on a woman, such as the chest or chin, can signal a tumor, usually in the adrenal gland, the ovary or the pituitary gland. Growth of a woman's pubic hair up to the navel (umbilicus), as is expected in men (a woman's pubic hair usually stops growing in a straight line across the lower abdomen well below the navel) is another example. Hyperactive glands without tumors can also cause hirsutism. Any sudden, profuse or out-of-place hair growth warrants a medical consultation.

Baldness, or hair loss, is most often hereditary, as is the age at which it becomes noticeable. Inherited male-pattern baldness usually starts with a receding hairline at the forehead and proceeds along the top of the head;

hair along the sides, behind the ears and in the eyebrows rarely falls out. Female hair loss occurs over the entire scalp (including the sides) but is more apt to involve thinning rather than total hair loss, as with men; it can also be a normal consequence of aging or the aftereffect of traumatic hair treatment. Patchy, thinning hair loss that occurs in a few separated areas and is unrelated to drug use is most often associated with a scalp infection; when the patches show complete loss of hair, leaving distinct circular areas of baldness, it could be an inherited trait or the result of an emotional problem, but it could also be the consequence of thyroid or parathyroid disease, old infections (syphilis, fungus), exposure to a toxic metal, anemia or psoriasis. Any unexplainable loss of hair warrants a medical consultation.

If the anagen-telogen test shows more than 3 telogen-root hairs out of 10, it most likely reflects a drug effect, a recent illness, pregnancy or emotional stress, and the hair will often regrow once the underlying condition is resolved. If all the hairs show anagen-type roots, or if hairs that seem to fall out on their own are of the anagen type, and drugs cannot be blamed, a medical consultation is warranted to search for the underlying cause. If the hairs show a large variation in diameter and color, it could indicate a male hormone deficiency.

Reliability
Abnormal hair observations, not related to drugs or heredity, are considered about 70 percent accurate as an indication of an underlying disease.

Mineral analysis. It is believed that as hair is formed in its follicle, it includes, as part of its protein substance, a trace of the minerals that are circulating in the bloodstream. Later, as hair grows, it can also include on its surface evidence of minerals in the environment (cadmium, **lead** [see Environmental Tests], mercury) or residue from substances used on or in contact with the hair (hair dyes, shampoo, swimming pool chemicals). Thus, knowing the rate of growth of hair and exactly how far from the skin surface a hair sample was obtained may offer an additional clue as to when toxic exposure, if present, took place (on the average, scalp hair will grow approximately one-half inch from the skin surface in four to six weeks). Some doctors feel that hair analysis can reflect exposure to toxic metals that took place months ago, whereas blood and urine testing usually show only the minerals present at the time of testing.

Although the actual analysis of minerals in and on hair is not performed at home, the collection of the hair sample for testing is. Some laboratories request that hair samples be sent to them by a doctor, but there are hair analysis laboratories that will test samples submitted directly by individuals. At the present time, hair analysis is considered useful as an aid in screening for the possibility of poisoning from toxic heavy metals: aluminum, arsenic, beryllium, cadmium, lead and mercury. Heroin, morphine and other opiate drugs, marijuana, PCP and even Quaaludes can be detected in hair for months after they were last used; hair testing can also pinpoint how much of these substances was used and when. A recent analysis of Napoleon's hair claims to show that there is no doubt the emperor was murdered by arsenic. As for measuring the status of substances related to nutritional needs, hair analysis is still considered to be in the experimental stage.

Although hair from anywhere on the body can be tested for its mineral content, most hair analysis laboratories prefer hair from the nape, or back, of the neck (midway between the ears). The hair should be cut off close to the scalp; this location also helps preclude obvious public evidence of hair loss. You will need about one-half gram (one tablespoon to two tablespoons) of hair, and this usually amounts to a scalp area that could be covered by a nickel. Some laboratories provide a makeshift paper balance-beam scale to help you determine the necessary amount when they send directions and cost information. If, however, that hair has been exposed to chemicals such as permanent wave lotions, bleach, dyes, conditioning or dandruff shampoos, or detergent soaps, or if it has been subjected to physical stress from hair dryers, sunlight, swimming, and so on, some of these factors, while interfering with chemical analysis, can be taken into account beforehand and allowed for in the analysis. In most such instances, however, pubic hair or other body hair becomes a better source for testing.

Hair analysis has been used to screen children for poisoning by lead and other heavy metals, especially when there is a sudden falling off of learning abilities (see Mental Ability and Personality Tests, **Mental Ability**). It can also be of value where symptoms of depression, lethargy, irritability, hallucinations and inappropriate behavior cannot be explained by usual diagnostic studies; many of these symptoms can be the first reflection of lead or mercury intoxication. Cadmium poisoning, while related to cigarette smoking as well as to industrial exposure, is also known to cause high blood pressure when the metal accumulates in the kidneys; the first hint of cadmium toxicity could come from hair mineral analysis. As for the hair's toxic mineral content, today's environment is such that a bare trace of such minerals might be expected (less than 1 part per million [ppm] or 2 ppm), and while this is still not normal, it can be considered usual.

While there are many laboratories throughout the country that perform hair analysis, only a few are "certified" by state health departments and/or the federal Centers for Disease Control; your city or county health department can tell you which laboratories are so licensed. If your doctor does not regularly use a particular laboratory, some are listed in the yellow pages of most telephone directories. In general, the cost is from $20.00 to $30.00 for a mineral analysis. Some reports simply identify the amount of metal detected, while others include a comprehensive subjective interpretation of the findings.

Any hair mineral analysis that shows abnormal levels of toxic minerals should first be repeated—preferably at a different laboratory. Consistently reported high levels of toxic metals in hair—especially in children who show possibly related symptoms—warrant a medical consultation and confirmation by other, more specific, tests. As to accuracy, in one instance, when hair was taken from one individual, divided into two equal test samples and sent to two different hair analysis laboratories, almost totally opposite results came back. At present, hair mineral analysis is not considered a proven, definitive test in clinical medicine.

SALT MEASUREMENTS
(Does the salt in your diet really affect you?)

It would be hard to imagine that there is anyone who is not aware of the purported relationship between the sodium in salt (salt is a compound called sodium chloride, or NaCl) and high blood pressure. At the same time, scientific evidence linking the two is not absolutely conclusive for everyone. Still, many medical authorities now advise just about everyone to lessen his or her intake of table salt as well as sodium from other sources. Common sources of sodium are as follows:

- The sprinkling of salt over food is a major culprit; studies have shown that the "typical" amount added in this way is from 100 mg (milligrams) to 150 mg of sodium for each food item; one teaspoon, or about 5 grams (5,000 mg), of salt contains approximately 2,200 mg of sodium.
- Eight ounces of tap water contains from 15 mg to 75 mg of sodium (an average based on mineral analysis of drinking water from all over the country); chemically softened water that uses salt for recharging can contain from 50 mg to 200 mg for every eight ounces, depending on the initial water hardness. Water with an initial hardness of 20.0 grains per gallon will require the addition of 150 mg of sodium for each quart of softened water; 40 grains of hardness will require the addition of 300 mg of sodium, and so on. Your water company can tell you the hardness of the water you use.
- Flavor enhancers—such as monosodium glutamate (MSG), disodium inosinate and disodium guanylate—are a source of sodium; food antioxidants, such as sodium metabisulphite and sodium bicarbonate, in which foods are dipped or with which they are sprayed to keep a fresh color and disguise spoilage and odors, can add another 100 mg to 1,000 mg of sodium to fresh, packaged or processed foods. Such ingredients usually, but not always, are listed on the labels of prepared foods, but their presence is rarely revealed in restaurant foods.

- Most condiments are salt-based: Ketchup averages 200 mg of sodium per tablespoon; mustard has 900 mg per tablespoon (French-style contains even more); and soy sauce has 1,050 mg per tablespoon.
- Most canned and commercial food contains much more salt than would usually be used at home: A 10½-ounce can of Campbell's chicken noodle soup contains 2,573 mg of sodium (Campbell's now offers low-sodium soups); a 3½-ounce portion of canned tuna fish in oil averages 800 mg; and a slice of commercial bread can have 150 mg of sodium.
- Most "fast-food" meals also include from 2,000 mg to 4,000 mg of sodium (a small hamburger on a bun with all the trimmings has 1,000 mg).
- Many medicines contain sodium: There are 521 mg of sodium in one dose of Alka-Seltzer; a daily dose of some forms of penicillin tablets can contain 1,000 mg; and if vitamin C is made of sodium ascorbate instead of ascorbic acid, its sodium content is almost equal to that of table salt.

Sodium is a normal body and blood electrolyte (molecules of bicarbonates and atoms of chlorides and potassium are the other major electrolytes) and is absolutely essential to maintain the body's cell functioning, water metabolism and acid-base balance. An excess of sodium in the body tends to cause water to be held in the blood and tissues until the kidneys normally eliminate it. But it does seem that some people are more susceptible than others to the water-retaining powers of sodium. It is suspected that any overload of fluid in the blood can raise blood pressure in those who have an unusual sensitivity (possibly inherited) to sodium. Others may react to excess body fluids with **edema** (see Body Observations), and it is now thought that edema around the brain provokes headaches and premenstrual tension (sodium is not the only cause of water retention; cortisone products and female hormones, either naturally produced or taken as medicine, can do the same thing).

It is estimated that the "average" person on a "typical" diet takes in about 6 grams (6,000 mg, or ⅕ of an ounce) of sodium a day, equivalent to two to three teaspoons of salt. It is then eliminated from the body, not only by the kidneys but also by sweating (through exercise, fever or sitting in a sauna), bowel movements (especially with diarrhea) and vomiting. Present public health recommendations suggest reducing one's daily salt intake to less than 2,000 mg (the body supposedly uses only about 200 mg a day), but many studies have shown that unless sodium intake is less than 500 mg a day, there is little or no effect on blood pressure in susceptible people; even a moderately reduced-sodium diet can help lessen edema, however.

Blood pressure effects. One way of estimating your reactions to salt and other sodium products is to take your **blood pressure** (see Heart and Circulation Tests) and observe your body for edema after purposely eating the equivalent of two teaspoons of table salt. *Note:* If you know you are salt-sensitive, have high blood pressure or are being treated for any illness, do not perform this test unless you have your doctor's permission.

First, take your blood pressure after fasting for at least four hours; also examine your body for any edema. Then drink a solution of two teaspoons of salt dissolved in eight ounces of water, or eat enough salty foods to equal that amount (for example, four pickles; three to four ounces of regular, not low-salt, smoked salmon; eight slices of bacon). Then measure your blood pressure every 15 minutes for the next two hours (be sure to sit quietly for at least 5 minutes before taking any blood pressure measurement) and observe your body—especially your feet and ankles, hands and under your eyes—for edema. Keep a record of all foods, body observations and times.

What Is Usual

No one really knows how much sodium is absolutely essential to life; it is thought, however, that it is unnecessary to ingest over 200 mg per day and that the excess is automatically eliminated from the body. Insofar as taste discrimination goes, it is said that much depends on foods first tasted as an infant, cultural practices, where one eats and physical activity. Several years ago when the Campbell Soup Company reduced the sodium content of many of its foods, especially its canned soups, sales dropped to the point where additional sodium had to be put back in order for the company to stay competitive; consumers missed the "salty" flavor.

After eating a large amount of salt, there should be no sustained elevation of blood pressure (it may rise 5 mm [millimeters] to 10 mm in the first half-hour but should return to its original reading within two hours); no edema should be observed.

What You Need

In part, the test requires an innate ability to perceive the flavor of salt. But even if you think your ability to discern a salty flavor is unexcelled (see Brain and Nervous System Tests, **Taste Function**), it is virtually impossible to determine through taste alone just how much sodium you regularly eat. In one medical study people were asked to discriminate between chicken soup containing varying amounts of sodium products (salt, MSG, etc.); even those who thought they had the lowest threshold for salt discrimination and needed the least amount succumbed to selecting the soup with the most sodium as the best-tasting. And although some food companies are now showing the sodium content on their labels, you still need a bit of mathematical agility to translate that number into reality:

- Even when itemized, the amount of sodium is usually noted on a per-serving or per-portion basis, with the serving or portion size being determined by the company; you must then decide how much you eat in relation to the manufacturer's suggested portion (some people do not dilute canned soups as much as the directions suggest and therefore take in much more sodium than what is listed as the per-portion amount).

- In some instances sodium is labeled as to its amount in each 100 grams (a bit over 3½ ounces); you must then calculate your sodium intake in terms of the exact amount of that food that you eat.
- With most fresh foods you will just have to hazard a reasonable guess (one large stalk of celery usually contains 60 mg to 70 mg of sodium; half of an average-size avocado contains 350 mg; most meats average 10 mg for each ounce, while fish averages 50 mg an ounce; and there are about 60 mg in an egg).
- Pickled or cured products are, of course, made primarily with salt and usually contain from 400 mg to 500 mg per ounce; corned beef has about 270 mg per ounce, bacon over 500 mg per ounce and smoked fish up to 2,000 mg per ounce.

You will, of course, need a blood pressure measuring device if you want to observe your body's response to salt intake. Many mail-order companies that carry scientific equipment sell meters that give the sodium content of foods and liquids; they cost about $100.00.

A pocket-sized device to measure the amount of salt (sodium) in foods and beverages, called a Salt Sensor, is available. It sells for $29.95; details from Smartek Inc. (3317 S.W. 11th Ave, Fort Lauderdale, FL 33315).

What to Watch Out For

You may have a tendency, deliberately or unconsciously, to exclude from your reckoning the salt that you cannot easily calculate or measure, the salt that you shake on food, the sodium that is hidden in fresh pastries from the bakery, in ice cream and other fresh dairy products, and in whatever you eat away from home. But most of all, if you do want to avoid sodium, study the labels on foods and learn to decipher euphemisms for sodium ingredients that masquerade as something else: flavor enhancers, "natural flavor," and so forth. And keep in mind that the amount of sodium in packaged foods can change periodically; years ago the Campbell Soup Company increased the sodium content of some of its foods from 10 percent to 40 percent.

You may also be surprised to learn that some foods labeled "low-salt," "low-sodium" or "no salt added" may still contain large amounts of sodium. This labeling is legal if the ingredients themselves naturally contain large amounts of sodium; only salt added during processing must be indicated on the label.

And watch out for low-sodium products that use potassium as a substitute; too much potassium can be harmful, especially when you are taking certain medicines. Check with your doctor before you start using products that would increase your potassium intake beyond the amount that occurs naturally in foods in your diet.

What the Test Results Can Mean

If you are unusually sensitive to sodium, the results of sodium measurements might allow you to reduce your sodium intake, which could be an advantage in your fight to prevent high blood pressure or assist your doctor in treating it. Less sodium in your diet might help you avoid heart disease and strokes as well. In general, cutting the amount of salt in the diet can also help reduce edema and its related symptoms.

An awareness of an evident blood pressure sensitivity to salt could enable you to prevent the early development of hypertension and its consequences.

And it is very important to know that not everyone should reduce his or her intake of sodium. People with kidney disease and certain forms of adrenal disease; some patients with diabetes or malnutrition; those running a high fever, especially if it is accompanied by vomiting and diarrhea; and those who exercise or otherwise perspire profusely may be worse off with inadequate salt in the diet. Thus, it is well worth a medical consultation prior to experimenting with reducing salt in your diet. If your doctor indicates that a low-sodium diet might be helpful, then even a relatively expensive salt meter could be considered low-cost therapy.

Recent research has begun to focus on the chloride portion of salt as a possible cause of hypertension. Although not as yet proved to be directly involved, chloride does add to the indictment of excessive table salt in the diet as a cause of high blood pressure in susceptible individuals. In some persons excess sodium without chloride did not raise blood pressure. Some doctors now believe that calcium is also part of the hypertension mechanism and that if calcium replaces sodium in the body's cells, blood pressure is less likely to be high.

Reliability

When blood pressure is obviously sensitive to salt, there is an 80 percent chance that hypertension will develop—if it has not already—by the age of 40. Taking particular note of one's salt and sodium intake, and reducing same, is said to offer a 70 percent chance of avoiding some forms of hypertension.

The Salt Sensor was 95 percent accurate in detecting high sodium foods and beverages.

SINUS TRANSILLUMINATION
(A possible clue to toothaches, headaches and pains)

Sinus problems are extremely common; moreover, an infected sinus can cause pains imitating dental disease, eye problems and headaches as well as chills and fever imitating serious body infections. Confirmation of a stuffed-up sinus can save time, aggravation and money by eliminating unnecessary visits to the dentist, the eye doctor and other medical specialists. While X-rays will, at times, show occluded (blocked) sinuses, transillumination can often offer sufficient information to point out the pain-causing pathology, without radiation exposure.

Go into a darkened room and stand in front of a mirror. Place the tip of a bright flashlight inside the mouth so that no light can be seen from around the lips when the mouth is closed. It then becomes quite easy to see whether one or both maxillary sinuses (those on either side of the nose just behind the cheeks and under the eyes) are clear or cloudy (infected or congested; see Figure 6). When the light is placed just under the center of the bony ridge above each eye, the frontal sinuses (see Figure 7) can also be checked for congestion. There are other sinuses in back of the nose, and while these cannot be checked by transillumination, they are far less frequently involved in sinusitis conditions. A bright light can also be placed in the center of each cheek, under the eyes, and the transilluminated maxillary sinuses can be viewed by looking at each side of the palate (the roof of the mouth). Sinusitis can follow an upper respiratory infection (cold, flu) and seems much more prevalent in people with allergies. If, of course, your nose feels stuffed up

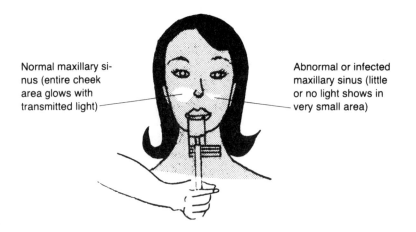

Normal maxillary si-
nus (entire cheek
area glows with
transmitted light)

Abnormal or infected
maxillary sinus (little
or no light shows in
very small area)

Figure 6. Sinus transillumination of the maxilary sinuses (the light is completely inside the mouth).

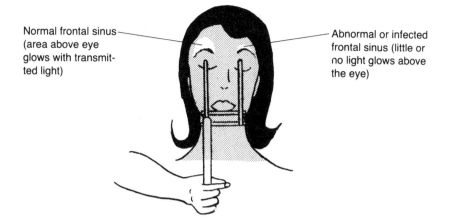

Normal frontal sinus (area above eye glows with transmitted light)

Abnormal or infected frontal sinus (little or no light glows above the eye)

Figure 7. Sinus transillumination of the frontal sinuses using a twin transilluminator (the light is placed under the bony ridge just above the eye).

and a yellowish-colored mucus is produced when you attempt to blow your nose, together with pain and/or redness over the sinus area, these signs tend to confirm sinus problems.

What Is Usual
The transmitted light should be clearly visible over each sinus area and should be of equal intensity on both sides. Cloudiness, a noticeable reduction in the amount of light transmitted through one or more sinuses or a difference in the amount of light transmitted when two sinuses are compared with each other usually indicates congestion. If you are not sure of just how much light should be visible, try the test on someone who has clear, open sinuses.

What You Need
The test requires a penlight-type flashlight with a very bright tip—one in which only the tip glows when it is lighted. A professional penlight made for such purposes costs from $3.00 to $12.00. A special twin transilluminator is available with an adjustable light control and twin shielded lights, adjustable for cheek and eye width (they come together for mouth insertion); it costs from $15.00 to $20.00. These lights can also be used for transillumination of the testicles.

What to Watch Out For
Be sure the light does not show either around the tip when placed against the skin or outside the mouth when the lips are tightly closed. Be sure the room is dark enough to allow transillumination to show clearly.

What the Test Results Can Mean

The cause of unexplained tooth, eye, head or face pains, when accompanied by a sinus that cannot be transilluminated, may be corroborated by trying nasal decongestant nose drops or sprays to see whether shrinkage and drainage of the sinus brings relief. Oral decongestants, which work though the bloodstream, may sometimes give better results than nose drops. A few drops of decongestant on a cotton-tipped stick (Q-tip) inserted gently upward in the nose for one minute is the most effective way of opening and draining sinuses. If no relief is obtained within a few hours, and the pains persist or fever develops, a medical consultation is warranted.

Reliability

Transillumination revealing a congested sinus is considered 90 percent accurate; the stuffed-up sinus itself, however, may not always be the specific cause of tooth or head discomfort.

Nasal mucus clearance time. Some people do seem unusually susceptible to sinus infections. Normally, particles such as allergens, bacteria and dust, when breathed in through the nose, are quickly transported to the back of the throat by sinus secretions and tiny hairs throughout the naval cavity. However, it has been observed that there are some people with extremely slow mucus clearance systems. One way to test your ability to rid the nose of irritating substances is to place a tiny particle of soluble saccharin about one-half inch inside the lower part of the nose and note how long it takes before you notice a sweet taste after swallowing every half-minute. Usually, it takes from 5 minutes to 15 minutes before the sweet taste is observed. Should it take more than 15 minutes, it could indicate an intranasal problem such as nasal polyps, a deviated septum, the residue of drug damage or chronic sinus disease; if you also have discomfort, a medical consultation is warranted.

SKIN OBSERVATIONS
(The skin is the largest organ of the body; use scrutiny of it as an all-encompassing test.)

Although *eczema* is the name given to any number of skin conditions characterized by redness, itching, scaling or rash, it is not a specific medical diagnosis. Beyond eczema, there are a few specific skin observations that can provide early warning signs of underlying disease, and their prompt discovery and interpretation could help prevent subsequent disability. As an example: Persistent, pale-yellow-tinted, dry skin, especially when accompanied by a puffy face—particularly around the eyes—and swollen hands (see Body Observations, **Edema**) can be the first indication of thyroid disease.

While there are many ways to describe skin changes, it will suffice to consider three basic characteristics:

- *Color:* The presence or absence of pigment (which usually does not include generalized redness) should be noted.
- *Physical structure:* Some abnormalities include macules, which are lesions, usually colored, that are not raised above the skin's surface (they cannot be felt as bumps when touched); papules which are areas raised above the skin's surface (tiny "bumps," somewhat like a mosquito bite, can be felt); skin plaques, which are large papules; vesicles or bullae, which are blisterlike lesions containing fluid (when infected, they are called pustules).
- *Blanchability:* You should observe whether or not the skin's color disappears when pressure is applied—usually by a fingertip.

The skin lesions mentioned above should also be distinguished from hives, or urticaria, which differs from eczema in that it is an allergic rather than an inflammatory reaction, characterized by red, pink, or sometimes pale swollen patches that arise suddenly and are rarely permanent. Because drugs can also cause a variety of skin conditions, often precipitated or exaggerated by sunlight, they must always be considered; antibiotics, aspirin and aspirin-like medications, birth control pills, food colorings, diuretics and even some vitamins are very common causes of skin rashes.

Diet can also be related to skin lesions. There have been several reports that a diet high in polyunsaturated fats is associated with several different cancers—malignant melanoma in particular. Should one or two reddish pimples happen to erupt on your nose or face one morning, try to recall whether you had eaten any beef in the last day or two. The female hormones used to fatten cattle can cause an acnelike reaction in some people—even those well past the acne age.

Pigmented blemishes are most often various shades of blue, blue-red or brown (see Figure 8). Dark "black-and-blue" spots (called ecchymosis) commonly follow an injury, but if they appear anywhere on the body without evident provocation, they can be an indication of bleeding disorders (petechia) or liver disease (see Heart and Circulation Tests, **Capillary Fragility**). If pressure is applied to these small dots, they will not turn pale or white (blanch), as do most skin lesions of no medical significance. A venous "star" appears most often on the legs; its center is a blue or purplish area about the size of a rice grain that has thin, wavy lines radiating outward one inch to two inches from it. They do not blanch when pressed and usually suggest the development of varicose veins. In contrast, a spider angioma is more reddish and smaller than a venous star and will blanch, or momentarily disappear, when pressure is applied. These usually are limited to the upper part of the body and are a normal consequence of aging, although some doctors feel they reflect liver problems.

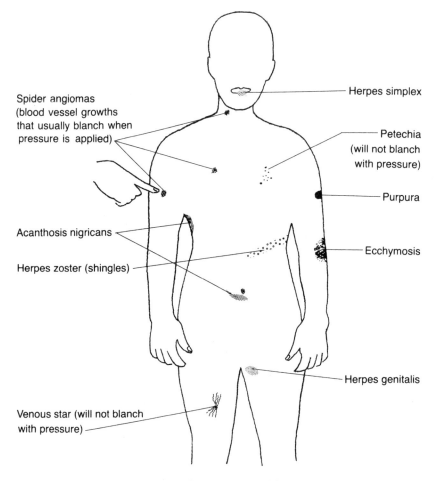

Figure 8. Skin abnormalities.

The sudden appearance of brown pigmentation, especially on exposed surfaces, can be the first indication of an adrenal gland disorder (Addison's disease); it can also come from anemia, cancer and several other connective tissue conditions. Many women taking birth control pills also develop areas of brown pigmentation that appear most often over the cheekbones and around the nipples.

Tiny clusters or blisters appearing around the mouth, commonly called "cold sores," are usually caused by a herpes virus. It is believed that once the virus establishes itself in the body (usually in the nerves), it remains for a lifetime and can be reactivated by upper respiratory infections, sunlight, stress and steroid (cortisone) drugs. The same form of the herpes virus or a different, second, form can also cause blisters to appear on and around the genitalia, and it has been reported that 25 million Americans now have genital herpes, while half a million more men and women between the ages of 18 and 35 are contracting the disease every year. It is considered the fastest-growing sexually transmitted disease in the United States. And a third form of this virus can cause blisterlike lesions around the torso, following the distribution path of a nerve from the spinal cord to the skin (herpes zoster, or "shingles").

In the past, skin tags (little flaps of normal- to slightly darker-than-normal-colored skin that are medically called pedicles, and are usually less than one-quarter inch in diameter) were thought to be related to polyps and even cancer in the large intestine. The most recent research, however, shows the association to be only 50 percent, and observing these tags must no longer be considered a definitive sign of an underlying problem.

What Is Usual
The skin should be clear, have good turgor (firmness and elasticity) and be free of blemishes—other than those known since birth (birthmarks). Rashes, itching, blisters, dryness, scales and any sudden appearance of one or more lesions on the skin are not normal, albeit they may either be attributed to a drug or contact with an allergen or appear subsequent to trauma.

What You Need
The test just requires your powers of observation, applied regularly and systematically, in order to notice something new or different about the appearance of your skin.

What to Watch Out For
You must beware of ignoring a skin lesion; it may take one medical consultation to identify it, but assurance that a lesion is not serious is well worth the peace of mind that it brings. Do not fail to consider the possible effects of any medicine you are taking; check with your doctor or pharmacist to find out which of your drugs can cause skin reactions.

What the Test Results Can Mean
Any pigmented, new skin lesion, especially one that does not blanch when pressed, warrants a medical consultation. Any brown-pigmented macular (flat) or papular (raised) lesion that seems to become darker or blacker warrants immediate medical attention.

Many doctors feel that cancers inside the body can reflect their existence through skin lesions. Dermatomyositis looks like a profuse, reddish macular rash that is almost always accompanied by weakness of the muscles—usually, but not always, directly under the rash; the muscle weakness may be much more extensive than the obvious skin lesions, or there may be a profuse rash all over the body with only one or two muscles affected, but muscle weakness must exist to make a diagnosis of dermatomyositis. Suspicion of this lesion warrants a medical consultation. Once the diagnosis has been made, it is known that up to 50 percent of adults with this skin-muscle condition also have cancer—most commonly in the gastrointestinal tract or lung.

Acanthosis nigricans is a brown- to black-pigmented papular thickening of the skin, most often under the armpits, in the groin and on the abdomen around the umbilicus, or navel—especially if the skin in that area tends to fold or flop over itself. Most people who have these lesions tend to describe them as "dirty skin" that cannot be cleaned. There are doctors who feel that at least half of all people who develop this skin condition also have internal cancer—most commonly in the gastrointestinal tract; suspicion of this condition warrants a medical consultation.

Herpeslike blisters, especially on or around the genitalia, warrant medical attention to ascertain the diagnosis—both to protect others from catching the disease and because, if the condition is found in a pregnant woman, it can cause brain damage and death in newborns. And herpes-type lesions have all too frequently been associated with cancer of the cervix and lymph cell cancers such as leukemia.

Ichthyosis—dry, rough, scaling skin (somewhat like fish scales), usually on the trunk or outer surfaces of the extremities—can be a reflection of some internal disease. If it appears suddenly, it warrants medical attention.

If you have been camping out in the woods or wilderness, and there were ticks in the area, any sudden appearance of petechia, purpura, macules or papules warrants medical attention; it can be the first indication of Rocky Mountain spotted fever or Lyme disease. If isolated papules and/or vesicles appear, check yourself for insect bites.

Skin conditions that do not fit into any of the patterns described warrant medical consultation unless you are already aware of the cause (allergies, bacterial or fungus infections, psoriasis, etc.). The sudden disappearance of skin pigmentation, most commonly called a secondary leukoderma, is usually a consequence of a previous skin disease such as psoriasis, but it can also come from thyroid disease, diabetes, certain cancers and old infections such as syphilis and leprosy. It can also be the result of exposure to certain industrial chemicals. It warrants a medical consultation.

Reliability

Skin reflections of disease are considered 75 percent accurate in men; for some unknown reason the accuracy rate is lower in women. The medical profession is still divided on whether certain types of skin manifestations indicate an internal cancer.

SKIN INFESTATIONS

Common causes of insect skin infestations that are difficult to see with the naked eye include fleas, lice and scabies (bedbugs, ticks, spiders, etc., are usually large enough to be easily recognized). Once the causative insect has been identified, proper treatment can follow. The primary problem with insect bites, however, is that the red, usually swollen spots are often mistaken for other, far more serious conditions such as blood problems (for example, purpura; see Heart and Circulation Tests, **Capillary Fragility** test), infectious diseases, allergy and eczema. Flea bites are much more common than is generally believed. And if insect bites do persist and then get infected, the condition can become dangerous and quite difficult to treat.

SKIN INFESTATIONS—FLEA BITES
(Helping to find the cause of skin rashes, welts and itching)

Fleas live mostly on animals, and while household pets may be carriers, fleas are found primarily on rats, birds, chickens and especially in sandy soil such as at beaches. They obtain their nourishment by burrowing under the skin and sucking blood and are not particular—dog fleas will relish people as much as animals. They can live for seven months or more around the house. Fleas also carry and transmit diseases such as plague, typhus and even tapeworms. Although flea bites are usually more common on the lower legs, feet and exposed areas of the arms, they can occur anywhere on the body.

What Is Usual
No evidence of fleas or flea bites is normal. But if fleas do exist, they can be identified through a magnifying glass; the particular features of this insect are the absence of wings and legs that are unusually large and long in proportion to the size of the body (see Figure 9). If you suspect that your pet has fleas, check to see whether the animal's brushed hair or loose fur contains tiny, mostly black specks (usually, it will if fleas are the problem). Drop a bit of water on these dark spots; if they are flea-bite residue, the water will show the pink tinge of blood. Flea eggs are white and about the size of a small grain of salt; they are more likely to be found in bedding, upholstery, carpets and even cracks in the floor.

What You Need
You need to keep in mind the possibility that fleas may be present and have the willingness to admit same and search for them. A good magnifying glass would be useful, or a 30-power battery-operated light scope (microscope), which costs from $7.95 to $30.00, would be even better.

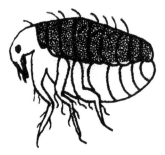

Figure 9. The flea.

What to Watch Out For

Flea bites can persist for weeks and will seem much more severe (and less like flea bites) in people who are unusually allergic. Do not be fooled if the skin shows only one or two bites; they could still be flea bites.

What the Test Results Can Mean

If you specifically identify fleas, and no infection is evident, ointments containing antihistamines or cortisone products may offer relief while you eliminate the source, through thorough washing, vacuuming and disinfection of pets, infested individuals, clothing and furniture. If the bites persist after a day or two of locally applied treatment, medical attention may be required to remove the embedded fleas. A medical consultation may be warranted to obtain oral antihistaminic or analgesic medicine if the discomfort persists. Should flea bites occur while you are camping out in the woods or other remote location, be on the alert for a fever, rash, bronchitis or swelling under the armpit or in the groin developing anywhere from 2 days to 10 days after you were bitten; this could be the first sign of plague. In fact, flea bites associated with such environmental exposure warrant medical attention to obtain preventive treatment. If spots that appear to be flea bites persist, and no fleas or other insects are identified, medical attention is warranted.

Reliability

Flea identification is easy and at least 90 percent accurate.

SKIN INFESTATIONS—PEDICULOSIS (LICE)
(Looking for lice to help explain the cause of some skin rashes and bites)

Pediculosis means "a skin infestation of lice." It is the second of the three common parasites that can cause uncomfortable skin problems that are quite similar in appearance. When statistics on lousiness were last tabulated, in 1976, more than 6 million cases of head lice infestation were uncovered in the United States, and the rate had been doubling every three years; it is now estimated that at any given time 20 million Americans are lousy. The condition is so common that any single issue of different pharmacists' trade magazines contains several full-page advertisements telling of the profit to be made by selling pediculicides, and surveys show that pharmacists supply these lice-killing medications for 2 out of every 3 cases. In Japanese bath houses, lice are so common that louse-killing medications are given free to all patrons.

Head lice (shown in Figure 10) are but one form of the condition; there are also body lice (better known as "cooties") and pubic lice (better known as "crabs"). Body lice and head lice look similar, but the body louse is a bit

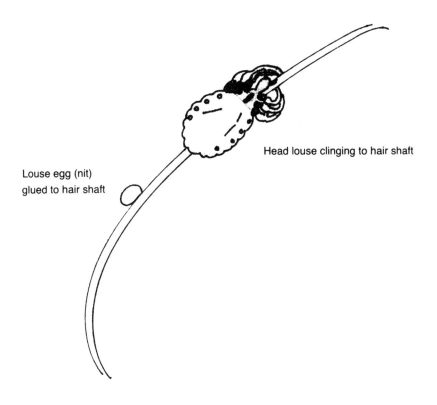

Head louse clinging to hair shaft

Louse egg (nit)
glued to hair shaft

Figure 10. Pediculosis (lice infestation)—head louse.

bigger; all females are larger than males. Crab lice are shorter and fatter and really do resemble a crab (see Figure 11); they are found mostly in the pubic hair around the genitalia and in the eyebrows. Pubic lice in the eyebrows, and especially when they infest the eyelashes, are often misdiagnosed as conjunctivitis or infection of the eyelids; the usual antibiotic ointment used to treat conjunctivitis will not kill the lice, and lice-killing lotions are not recommended for use near the eyes. Any suspicion of lice infestation in hair adjacent to the eyes warrants medical attention. In addition, one should consider the possibility that children who manifest this condition have been sexually abused; the Public Health Service has designated pubic lice as a sexually transmitted disease. And in spite of what you may have heard, pubic lice *can* be caught from a contaminated toilet seat. Lice can also be picked up from theater seats—even the most expensive ones—from trying on clothing in stores, from checking a coat or hat in a common cloakroom and from a night in a hotel.

More often, though, pediculosis is transmitted by direct contact with someone already harboring the lice, such as schoolchildren or people who rarely change their clothes; in dormitories, barracks, camps, public transportation and queuing; and from people who share combs, brushes and clothing. As with fleas and scabies, lice are difficult to see with the naked eye, even where intense itching occurs. Usually, the first real indication of pediculosis, after a period of constant scratching, is the spotting of a nit or

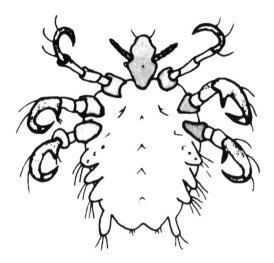

Figure 11. Pediculosis (lice infestation)—pubic louse (also called crab louse or simply "crabs"; it is found mostly in pubic hair and, inexplicably, in eyebrows).

several nits (shown in Figure 10). The nits are hard, tiny, whitish gray tufts on hair strands that resemble pussy willows but are much smaller; they are the eggs, which hatch in from three to five days. The lice themselves can usually be identified through a good magnifying glass. Although lice can carry and transmit the germ that causes typhus—a serious generalized infection that can be fatal—the primary problem they cause is skin infection, which occurs when the underlying sores are scratched and the lice feces get beneath the skin; this can also cause lymph node pain and swelling.

What Is Usual
No evidence of lice or nits is normal. If present, however, the nits are usually quite obvious to the naked eye; when profuse, they give the impression of dappled hair. The lice may even be seen in combs or brushes after combing or brushing the hair. They may also be found in the seams of clothing, especially underwear.

What You Need
First, you need a willingness to consider the possibility of lice infestation. A good magnifying glass is useful, or a 30-power battery-operated pocket light scope (microscope), which costs from $7.95 to $30.00, is much better.

Special disposable combs that can isolate the lice and their nits, and make identification easier, are also available at most pharmacies. These combs have beveled teeth that prevent scalp injury, and some also contain a built-in magnifier and replaceable teeth so that family members cannot reinfest each other. They cost from $1.00 to $3.00.

What to Watch Out For
Mostly, you should be alert for other people with obvious nits. As with so many skin conditions, pediculosis can imitate flea bites, scabies or eczema.

What the Test Results Can Mean
A specific finding of identifiable lice can be treated by several over-the-counter and prescription medications. Many of these preparations can also cause a skin reaction and must be used exactly as the directions say. They should not be used on people with known allergies until after a discussion with a doctor. If no identifiable parasite is detected and the rash or evident skin bites persist, medical attention is warranted. Sprays are available to treat inanimate objects only (garments, bedding, furniture).

Note: There is recent evidence that excessive use of nonprescription treatments for lice, and even some prescription products, can cause nerve toxicity and blood problems; check with your doctor before applying such a medication.

Reliability

Louse identification is fairly easy and at least 90 percent accurate.

SKIN INFESTATIONS—SCABIES
(Detecting mites to help find one cause of skin bites and rashes)

Scabies is a dermatological condition that has always been considered one of the most difficult to diagnose because the red eruption that is produced looks like so many other skin problems: flea bites and pediculosis, in particular, but it can also resemble an allergy, eczema, measles and mosquito bites—to name but a few. This skin infestation alone is reported to account for nearly 4 percent of patient visits to dermatologists in the United States. Although it occurs most often in the 15 to 45 age group, it is also found in institutions where close contact is unavoidable.

The cause of the observable skin abnormalities is the biting of, and burrowing under the skin by, an insect called an itch mite (scientifically known as *Sarcoptes scabiei;* specifically, it is an arachnid, or member of the spider family, having eight legs instead of six). The male only bites; the female both bites and burrows under the skin to lay her eggs. And it is the burrowing, most often in a corkscrew fashion, that can sometimes be a clue to the diagnosis. The parasites themselves usually cannot be seen with the naked eye other than as white or gray specks.

The burrows cause itching, more frequently at night, and are most commonly found along the side of the fingers (see Figure 12), on the palm side of the wrist, the elbows, the nipple area, the skin around the testicles (scrotum), alongside the penis and on the buttocks. The affinity these insects seem to have for the genital area has caused the Public Health Service to designate the condition as a sexually transmitted disease (as it has done with pubic lice, or pediculosis); indeed, it has been reported that from 60 percent to 80 percent of scabies cases come about by direct sexual transmission or by sleeping in the same bed with someone already harboring the mite.

In Europe scabies are identified by the *burrow ink test,* which is performed as follows: The underside of an old-fashioned fountain pen point that has been filled with washable ink is rubbed over the raised bite area—usually where itching occurs. The excess ink is then wiped off with an alcohol-soaked gauze pad. If a scabies burrow is there, the ink will fill it and easily reveal its presence as a zig-zag line just under the skin starting at the bite.

But the primary problem is that the classic signs of the disease—the short, spiral burrows—are not always seen unless searched for deliberately. Failure to diagnose the infestation early enough can lead to serious overall skin infections and skin ulcers.

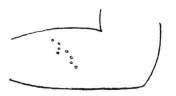

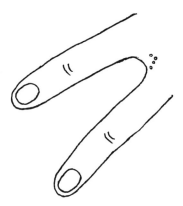

Most commonly found in the forearm
and in between the fingers, usually
in a corkscrew pattern

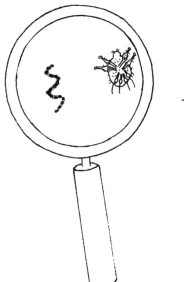

The scabies mite

Figure 12. Scabies infestation.

What Is Usual

Obviously, no evidence of an infestation is normal, but if scabies are present,
the corkscrew burrows are the definitive clue. If you take a sharp, sterilized
tweezer point (or needle or pin), dip the point into a drop of mineral oil
and probe the end of the burrow, and then look at the point through a

strong magnifying glass or through a pocket microscope, you should be able to see the eight-legged creature or some of its dark, reddish-colored feces.

What You Need
The test requires a good magnifying glass of at least 4-power strength (that is, it magnifies 4 times), which costs from $1.00 to $10.00, or a battery-operated pocket light scope (microscope), usually 30-power (it magnifies 30 times), which costs from $7.95 to $30.00.

What to Watch Out For
Be sure the pointed object you use to probe the burrow is meticulously clean; you can hold it in the flame of a match for a second or two and then let it cool or hold it in rubbing alcohol for a few seconds. Do not poke too hard into the end of the burrow—that is, not hard enough to draw blood. Actually, the scabies mite will cling to the mineral oil if it is merely touched.

What the Test Results Can Mean
If scabies is evident, the condition is quite easy to treat (the entire family should be treated at the same time). Even if there is no reason to suspect sexual transmission, it is important to try to locate the source to avoid reinfestation; schoolchildren have been known to bring the mites home. Discovery of the mites usually calls for nothing more than a medical consultation to obtain an effective scabicide. Should sexual transmission be possible, the medical consultation should include tests for other sexually transmitted diseases. Failure to detect the mites or their burrows (and failure to identify flea bites or pediculosis) in the presence of any skin problem warrants medical attention—especially in very young children.

Note: There is recent evidence that excessive use of nonprescription products, as well as some prescription treatments, for lice and/or scabies can cause nerve toxicity and blood problems; check with your doctor before applying such a medication.

Reliability
While mites are not as easy to identify as fleas or lice, it is felt that 80 percent of mite infestations can be detected by direct observation. The burrow ink test is considered 90 percent accurate.

Chigger bites. Another mite, called the chigger or red bug, can also cause a skin infestation similar to scabies, although it is not as common. It is sometimes called "grocer's itch" or "grain itch" because it seems to occur more frequently in those who handle certain vegetables and plants. These mites do not burrow under the skin, as do scabies; they attach themselves with sucking claws that rarely draw blood (instead, they feed off skin cells). They can carry typhus and other dangerous diseases. After they bite, they generally drop off the skin, but the itching (usually worse at night in bed) can last for two weeks. When present on the skin, while biting, they look like tiny red dots; sometimes they are surrounded by swollen skin. One "test" for this condition is to apply clear nail polish to the irritation; if it is a chigger bite, the polish usually kills the chigger and gives instant relief of itching. Suspicion of chigger bites warrants a medical consultation because of the possibility of other, related infections.

TESTICLE SELF-EXAMINATION
(A screening test for one of the most curable cancers in men)

The testicles are egg-shaped glands that lie in the scrotum, the skin-covered sac that hangs between a man's legs, just below the penis. The two testes are the male gonads, which produce sperm and testosterone; they correspond to the egg- and estrogen-producing ovaries in a woman. Normally, they are in place at the time of birth, although in 1 or 2 of every 100 boys, they may not descend from the groin area until two or three weeks after birth. They generally do not become active until after 12 years of age. Only one testicle is needed for normal sexual functioning. The size of the testicle seems to correlate with its functioning; the largest ones not only yield more sperm but produce sperm that are more active and more normally shaped. Larger testicles also produce greater quantities of testosterone.

The testicles are subject to infections, varicose veins, hernias, edema, cysts and tumors. Regular examination of the scrotum and testicles is comparable to regular self-examination of the breasts in women; the earlier any seeming abnormality is discovered, the better the prognosis. While testicular cancer is the most common cancer of young men, it is also one of the few cancers that, when detected early, has a high rate of cure with drugs. White men have the highest incidence of testicular cancer, blacks the lowest, with most occurring at approximately 30 years of age (about 7 per 100,000 white men).

To perform this examination, start by standing in front of a mirror and observing the size and symmetry of each testicle in the scrotum. Then, with one foot resting on an elevated surface, apply the thumb and fingertips to the scrotal sac opposite the raised leg (see Figure 13). Gently roll each testicle between the thumb and fingers until all surfaces have been inspected. Next, in a darkened room, place the tip of a lighted flashlight behind, and in the center of, each testicle and note the amount and dispersion of the light shining around the testicle through the scrotal sac (see Figure 14).

What Is Usual
When a man is standing in front of a mirror, both testicles in the scrotum should appear egg-shaped and the same size, although it is common for the

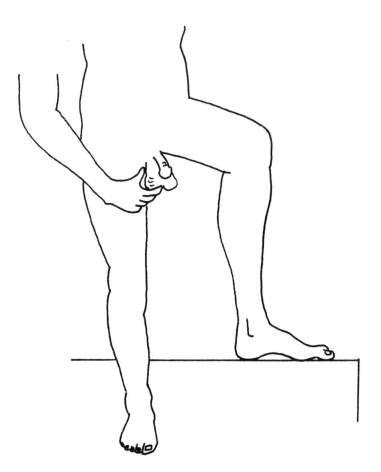

Figure 13. Testicle examination (when examining a testicle, it is best to raise the opposite foot off the floor).

left testicle to be slightly lower than the right. The evident surface of each testicle should appear smooth, with no bumps, nodules or bulges showing. When palpated (examined by touch), each testicle should be almost two inches long, very smooth on the surface, with a firm, spongelike consistency. Above the testicle a cordlike structure (the spermatic cord, containing the epididymus and vas deferens, which carry sperm to the penis) is felt going into the groin area. It is not unusual for the testicle and cord to be quite sensitive to palpation, especially when this examination is performed for the first time. With a bright light behind the scrotum and each testicle, the testicle itself should appear as a smooth, oval, dark shadow surrounded by an even, red glow. As the light is moved about the scrotum, no other shadows or irregularity in the testicle's shape should be seen.

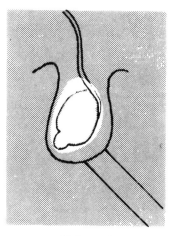

Usual

Not usual

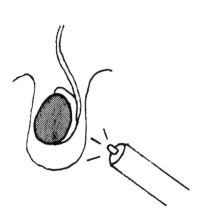

In a darkened room, with the light behind the testicle, there should be an even, uninterrupted glow around the testicle

Figure 14. Testicle transillumination.

What You Need

The test requires a penlight-type flashlight with a small bulb or a small, bright light source; an area that can be darkened; and a low stool (or a few books) upon which to rest one foot. The twin transilluminator, described in the **Sinus Transillumination** test (see Body Observations), will also work for this test.

If the size of your testicles is of great concern, and you feel embarrassed to bring this to your doctor's attention, you can obtain an orchidometer for size measurements (*orchio* is the Greek word for testicle) from most medical supply houses for a few dollars. You can even make your own by cutting an elliptical (oval or egg-shaped) circle out of cardboard, with a length diameter of 1½ inches and a width diameter of 1 inch.

What to Watch Out For

Do not try to examine your testicles if you are in a cold environment; low temperatures cause the scrotum to shrink in size and can hinder a proper examination. Do not be too delicate when palpating, or small nodules might be overlooked; but if the spermatic cord seems unusually tender, it could indicate the beginning of an infection called epididymitis, and immediate medical attention is warranted. Do not attempt a testicle examination if you have been exposed to someone with mumps or think you might have the disease.

What the Test Results Can Mean

If, after your first testicle examination, you can have your own observations confirmed by your doctor, and the results indicate normal testicles, you can achieve great peace of mind by performing this test monthly and uncovering no possible abnormalities. If, prior to palpation, you have a "heavy" feeling in your scrotum, even without any evident enlargement or lumps, a medical consultation is warranted. Should one scrotal side appear larger and somewhat pear-shaped, but still allow the transmission of light, it could be the start of a hydrocele, or excessive fluid surrounding the testicle, a slow-developing condition that warrants a medical consultation. A somewhat similar condition that feels like worms around the testicle and usually does not allow light transmission could be the beginning of varicose veins from the spermatic cord; it, too, warrants a medical consultation. If either or both testicles feel, or measure, smaller than 1½ inches long, this could reflect an inherited condition but may also reflect a hormone dysfunction. Should you have edema (water retention) elsewhere in your body, such as around your ankles, it is not uncommon for the scrotal sac to swell up with fluid as well. The average-size testicle of an adult, including the stretched scrotum over it, and without any swelling from some other cause, should not fit through the 1½-inch by 1-inch oval cutout mentioned earlier. If it does, it warrants a medical consultation. Most of all, you should be on the lookout for any hard, especially painless, node or bump that mars the usually smooth surface of the testicle, and particularly a lump—no matter how tiny—that does not allow light transmission. Such a test result warrants immediate medical attention.

If you know that you had one or both testicles undescended at birth, even if they later descended by themselves or were surgically repaired, you should be aware of the statistics that indicate you have a 40 times greater chance of developing testicular cancer than men born with descended testicles. Men with such a medical history should be even more careful to perform testicle observations monthly starting at 15 years of age.

Reliability
While any irregularity or swelling of the testicle is not likely to be cancer, 90 percent of the time it justifies medical attention. Testicle size is an accurate measure of functioning 80 percent of the time.

WEIGHT MEASUREMENTS
(An accessible clue to underlying disease and a possible indication of longevity)

Involuntary weight loss of only a few pounds rarely seems sufficient reason for a medical consultation; in many instances the loss of a few pounds either goes unnoticed or, at times, is even appreciated. But in medicine there is a maxim that any unexplainable weight loss of more than 5 percent of one's usual body weight within a one-month time period is assumed to come from some hidden disease until proved otherwise. Studies have shown that should a 100-pound woman lose more than 5 pounds or a 150-pound man lose 8 pounds in a month or less, assuming usual diet and activities, the most common cause of this sudden weight loss, if not from deliberate dieting, is cancer. Secondary causes of enigmatic weight loss include: stomach ulcers, infections, obstructive lung diseases, heart or circulation problems, nerve pathology, hormone dysfunction and emotional problems, such as depression. Recent studies have revealed that about 50 percent of patients admitted to hospitals are malnourished, and regular physician observations failed to recognize the problem.

On the other hand, persistent weight gain is not as common an indicator of disease; it may be genetic, or it could reflect thyroid gland or other metabolic disorders, but most often weight gain comes from eating too much and exercising too little. Surprisingly, obese and overweight do not mean the same thing. Obese means having an excess of body fat, while overweight means having a greater body weight than that shown on standard height-weight tables. A football player may be overweight because of an excess of muscle tissue, but he is not obese. Obesity, or too much body fat in proportion to the size of one's body, can become a medical problem.

While fat deposition and distribution are related to age, they are controlled primarily by body hormones. Women usually store fat in their breasts, buttocks, hips and thighs. Men, on the other hand, most often store excess fat in and around the stomach area. Obesity as a consequence of thyroid or adrenal disease or diabetes tends to show up more in the face, neck and upper torso.

Standard weight tables are usually correlated to one's age, sex and inherited body build as well as height. Body build is generally a reference to the size of one's skeletal frame and is most often described as small, medium or large. The tables indicating so-called normal, or desirable, weights have been derived primarily from insurance company morbidity (sickness) and mortality (death) statistics and are purported to represent the ideal weight for healthy individuals. Times do change, though, and while it was once believed that weighing 10 percent more or less than the ideal stipulated by the standard tables was unhealthy, most doctors now feel that weight alone does not pose any significant risk unless there is a variation of 20 percent or more from "normal."

A revised set of weight–height–body build tables has been published based on new information from the Life Insurance Medical Directors of the United States and Canada. The updated tables, reflecting the first changes since 1959, show ideal weights to be 5 percent to 15 percent higher than the figures recommended nearly 30 years ago. But even these new figures have already incurred opposition from several medical experts; however, keep in mind the words of one insurance actuary: "Such a chart simply advises people that if they keep to this weight, they'll have the best chance of the greatest longevity."

Two things are evident from the revised height and weight tables: The supposedly "ideal" weights are higher than once proclaimed, and people with slightly higher weights seem to live longer. In essence, these weight statistics reflect nothing more than insurance company findings that best suit the companies' purposes; they do not offer any assurance that matching the stipulated weights will prevent illness. Of interest, the old tables assumed that a man's clothing with shoes weighed seven pounds and a woman's clothing came to four pounds. The new tables include only five pounds of clothing for a man and three pounds for a woman. Another sign of changing times: Heights for men used to include a one-inch heel, while women were granted a two-inch consideration. Today, both men and women are only allowed a one-inch heel height for shoes. But no matter what the tables show, if you are extremely over- or underweight, it warrants a medical consultation.

Anthropometric measurements. While weight–height–body build observations are fine for generalized health screening, there are more specific parameters for measuring the amount of body fat and muscle (protein) in relation to one's size and weight. These include skinfold thickness along with extremity circumference and diameter measurements; when considered together with comparisons to standard weight tables, these observations are called anthropometrics. Anthropometric measurements not only can help reveal the cause of obesity (be it disease or gluttony), but they can also help assess nutritional

status—malnutrition, malabsorption of food, improper or inadequate metabolism—and identify the possible cause of previously unexplained symptoms such as anemia or depression.

Skinfold thickness. When the skin is "pinched" and pulled away from the
body, it forms a fold, whose thickness can be measured with a caliper (shown
in Figure 15). The distance between the two skin surfaces when pulled away
from any underlying muscle is considered a reasonable estimation of body
fat; the amount of fat under the skin approximates the amount of fat
throughout the rest of the body. While just about any skin surface can be
used for skinfold thickness measurements, the two most common areas are

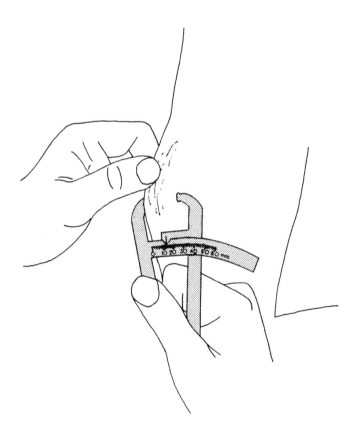

**Figure 15. Using skinfold calipers (pinching the skin away from the un-
derlying muscle and measuring its thickness; in this instance, 14 mm).**

the subscapular (just below the bottom edge of the large shoulder blade bone on either side of the back) and the triceps (the skin over the large posterior upper arm muscle, which straightens out the forearm).

When performing the triceps skinfold thickness test, it is important to make the measurements at a standard location each time so that future measurements will always be comparable to the original one. To measure the triceps skinfold, place the upper arm at your side with the elbow bent, so that the lower arm is parallel to the floor. Measure the distance between the bony projection at the top of the shoulder and the point of the elbow, preferably in centimeters (a cloth measuring tape works best). Mark the point midway between the two bony protrusions. With the arm hanging loosely straight down at the side, at the marked point, pinch the skin and underlying fat together on the back of the arm between the thumb and index finger so that it is pulled away from the muscle. Place the jaws of a skinfold caliper around the pinched skin and muscle according to the particular caliper's directions and measure the thickness of the fold. It is suggested that three different measurements be made a few moments apart and that the average of the three readings be recorded. This is considered a reasonable estimate of an individual's body fat reserves.

Body fat analyzer. A more precise measurement of body fat is thought to be obtained by using the Futrex-5000 Body Composition Analyzer. The device, similar to a flashlight, is touched to the biceps muscle of the arm and offers an instant total body fat percentage; it can also determine relative fat distribution anyplace on the body. Based on computer technology, it also provides a printout of findings and automatically takes age and sex into consideration. While used by some physicians as an aid to determining susceptibility to certain diseases, it is also used at home by individuals and groups as a means of evaluating fitness and athletic performance.

The Futrex-5000 is available from medical supply stores or from Futrex Inc. (P.O. Box 2398, Gaithersburg, Md. 20879); its present price is $1,990.00.

Of particular interest is the recent observation (made possible by the fact that more precise body fat measurements are now more easily obtainable) that the sympathetic and parasympathetic nervous systems (see Heart and Circulation Tests, **Cold Pressor and Finger Wrinkle** tests) seem less active as the body fat percentage increases. Whether this reduced activity, in turn, is a cause of obesity is still under study.

Extremity (midarm) circumference. Using the same point marked on the upper arm for the triceps skinfold thickness, measure the midarm circumference, or the distance around the arm—again, preferably in centimeters.

Midarm muscle circumference. There is a formula for estimating the body's muscle mass, or protein reserve, as opposed to fat mass. It requires you to convert your measurements to centimeters (cm) unless your tape measure is so marked (1 inch = 2.54 cm; ¼ inch = 0.635 cm). Multiply the triceps skinfold thickness in cm by 3.14 and then subtract the result from the midarm circumference measurement in cm. As an example, if the midarm circumference measured 32 cm (12½ inches) and the triceps skinfold thickness measured 12 mm (1.2 cm) by the calipers, midarm muscle circumference would be:

$$32 - (1.2 \times 3.14) = 32 - 3.77 = 28.2 \text{ cm}$$

By following the changes in weight along with arm fat and muscle measurements over a period of time, it is sometimes possible to discern the cause of weight loss or gain, especially when related to specific metabolic or digestive maladies. Such tests can also help distinguish between deliberate overeating, avoidance of food or an underlying disease.

Heatstroke sensitivity. People differ in their susceptibility to heat exhaustion or heatstroke—especially when engaged in strenuous physical activities. One particular weight observation can help you find out how sensitive you might be to the effects of heat. Wearing as little clothing as proper, weigh yourself before and after engaging in your usual sport or exercise for the usual amount of time. The activity itself should be performed with the clothes you normally wear while being physically active. If you find that you lose body water by sweating to the extent of more than 3 percent of your body weight, you are probably more sensitive than most people; if you lose more than 5 percent, you run a much greater risk of heatstroke and should be very careful, especially if your activities require clothing that causes increased sweating. And it seems the more muscular you are, the more susceptible you are to heatstroke.

What Is Usual

The figures and measurements offered in Figure 16 are compilations of several tables showing "ideal" weights; they are not meant to be absolute, since there is at this time no general agreement as to what normal weight should be. If your weight—according to your age, body build (see Figure 17), height and sex—lies within the range of 20 percent more or less than the suggested figure, it can be considered usual. For example, the ideal weight of a 45-year-old, 68-inch-high, medium-body-framed man is listed as 150 pounds, but any weight between 120 pounds and 180 pounds could still be considered within normal limits.

At birth the usual weight of a child is from 6 pounds to 9 pounds (average 7½ pounds), and the usual length is from 19 inches to 21 inches (average 20 inches); the height-weight difference between boys and girls at that time is negligible. The rule of thumb is that a baby's weight doubles in six months,

Figure 16. Height-weight tables (in inches and pounds).

Height	Men Age Group			Height	Women Age Group		
	18–35	36–55	Over 55		18–35	36–55	Over 55
62	125	130	130	58	100	105	110
63	129	134	133	59	103	109	110
64	132	138	138	60	105	112	115
65	135	141	141	61	108	116	117
66	138	145	144	62	111	119	120
67	140	148	147	63	114	123	123
68	145	150	148	64	118	126	126
69	149	154	150	65	121	130	130
70	154	160	155	66	125	135	134
71	158	165	161	67	130	138	137
72	162	169	163	68	134	140	139
73	165	175	164	69	138	143	142
74	170	180	172	70	142	146	145

*With indoor clothing but without shoes. Weights listed are for a medium body skeletal frame (using body skeletal frame guide—Figure 17). Those with a small frame, deduct 7 percent; those with a large frame, add 7 percent.

triples at 1 year of age, and then the child adds 5 pounds a year until the age of 5. Growth in the first year averages about 10 inches; 5 inches during the second year; 4 inches during the third year; 3 inches during the fourth; and 2 inches through the fifth. From the age of 5 through adolescence, weight depends on inherited growth characteristics, such as height and body build, sexual development, eating habits and physical activity. The "average" boy or girl at 5 years of age is 42 inches tall and weighs 40 pounds; by 10 years both the boy and the girl have usually grown to 53 inches and weigh 70 pounds. By 18 years of age, the "average" boy has grown to 68 inches and weighs 143 pounds; the "average" girl is 64 inches tall and weighs 122 pounds.

During adulthood it is believed that men continue to gain weight until they reach their early 40s, while women seem to gain weight until their early 50s. Weight should stay the same until the 70s, and then it usually decreases.

As for anthropometric measurements (see Figure 18), the "usual" range for the triceps skinfold thickness and midarm muscle circumference is within 10 percent of the charted figures. The midarm circumference measurement can vary by 20 percent and still be usual. Much depends on whether the measurements are used to detect obesity or assess the nutritional status. In general, the triceps skinfold should not be greater than 20 mm in men and not over 30 mm in women.

Figure 17. Body skeletal frame guide.

Find the two bony protrusions on either side of the wrist and, just below those points (toward the hand), measure the circumference around the wrist with a cloth measuring tape. Use the smallest measurement possible. Compare your wrist to your height, as shown below, as a reasonable indication of the size of your body build.

Height	Wrist Circumference	Skeletal Frame
Under 62 inches	Less than 14 cm From 14 cm to 14.5 cm Greater than 14.5 cm	Small Medium Large
From 62 inches to 65 inches	Less than 15 cm From 15 cm to 16 cm Greater than 16 cm	Small Medium Large
Over 65 inches	Less than 16 cm From 16 cm to 16.5 cm Greater than 16.5 cm	Small Medium Large

What You Need

Weight observations require a good scale—one that is accurate and easy to read. Many inexpensive scales can vary more than a pound with each use. Spring scales should have a manual zero adjustment and show weight in quarter-pounds; dial-reading scales cost from $8.00 to $20.00 where the reading is at floor level and $25.00 and up for those that show weight at waist level (this can be important if it is difficult to see around the abdomen). Digital display readout scales cost from $20.00 to $100.00, depending on where the display is located and whether or not the scale has a built-in "memory" that shows the previous weight for several members of a family. Digital scales should show weight in 0.2 pounds. Balance-beam scales (like the ones used in most doctors' offices) are considered the most accurate, should precision be desired, and cost from $60.00 to $200.00, depending on whether they use sets of weights on a bar or a digital display to show the result; some may include a telescoping height-measurement bar. It is a good idea to check your scale at least once a month by weighing an item whose weight is known, such as a 25-pound bag of kitty litter, a large box of laundry detergent or something similar.

Figure 18. Anthropometric upper arm measurements.

Age	Midarm Circumference (in cm)		Triceps Skinfold (in mm)*		Midarm Muscle Circumference (in cm)	
	Men	Women	Men	Women	Men	Women
18–19	30.1	26.2	8.5	17.5	27.4	20.7
20–24	31.0	26.5	10.0	18.0	27.9	20.8
25–34	32.0	27.8	12.0	21.0	28.2	21.2
35–44	32.7	29.2	12.0	23.0	28.9	22.0
45–54	32.1	30.3	11.0	25.0	28.7	22.5
55–64	31.7	30.2	11.0	25.0	28.3	22.4
65–74	30.7	29.9	11.0	23.0	27.2	22.7
(Should be greater than)	26.3	25.7	8.5	14.9	22.8	20.5

*If the skin behind the upper arm is pinched between the fingers, instead of using skinfold calipers, the thickness should not be greater than 12 mm (½ inch) in men and 25 mm (1 inch) in women; to convert mm to cm, multiply by 10.

It is usual for women to have 50 percent more stored body fat than men; women average 22 percent body fat, while men average only 15 percent.

Skinfold calipers range in cost from free to $150.00, depending on their sensitivity. For home testing, inexpensive plastic models are quite adequate. If you buy the book *Coaches' Guide to Nutrition and Weight Control*, by Dr. Patricia Eisenman and Dennis Johnson, at a cost of $9.95 (published by Human Kinetics Publishers Inc., Box 5076, Champaign, Ill. 61820), you will also receive a coupon redeemable for a free skinfold caliper along with detailed instructions for measuring body fat. One pharmaceutical company gives doctors plastic calipers at no charge, and your doctor may pass one on to you. Many mail-order houses now sell the SlimGuide calipers for $20.00. Automotive and tool calipers, which sell for from $7.00 to $70.00, will work just as well, as will drawing calipers, which cost $4.00 to $5.00, along with a ruler marked in millimeters (mm). Precise skinfold calipers include the Lange and the Harpenden; they cost from $100.00 to $150.00 and take into account skin tension, the amount of pressure applied to the instrument and even the slope of the skin surface.

What to Watch Out For

For consistency you should weigh yourself at the same time every day, preferably after awakening and having emptied your bladder. Ideally, you should wear the same garment each time. If you want to check your scales with those in your doctor's office or in a commercial establishment, be sure to wear the identical clothes each time and make the comparison within an hour's time; it is not unusual for body weight to vary one to two pounds up or down during a 24-hour period.

Do not weigh yourself after a loss of body water as from exercise or diuretic pills; temporarily induced water loss usually returns within hours, and you would only be fooling yourself. The same applies to any drastic change in your diet; eating a large quantity of salty products (delicatessen food, pretzels, potato chips, etc.) can cause excess water to be retained in your body for hours. Many women taking birth control pills or other hormones tend to gain weight (hold water) during the first two or three weeks of their menstrual cycle. It is also possible to gain several pounds after a severe emotional upset; that weight can last for up to a day or two after resolution of the problem. Be honest with yourself; if you know the cause of weight gain or loss, do not try to hide it from yourself or your doctor.

What the Test Results Can Mean

If you are more than 20 percent over or under the ideal weight suggested, a medical consultation is warranted. Even if you know you have been eating too much, or too little, such a discrepancy warrants investigation as to the reason why. The connection between obesity and arthritis, atherosclerosis and high blood pressure, and diabetes is fairly well established, and it can make many other disabilities much worse than they would otherwise be. Obesity can be the cause, as well as the consequence, of many emotional and social problems.

An equal number of disease conditions are related to being underweight. For one thing, individuals who are underweight because of malnutrition usually have very poor immunity to many other seemingly unrelated conditions, especially infections. They also fail to heal normally following an injury or surgery; they show an increase in clotting time (see Blood Tests, **Bleeding and Clotting Time**), making them more susceptible to strokes; and they almost always suffer from some form of anemia. As with being overweight, being underweight also causes, and results from, emotional problems; depression, irritability and memory problems seem to go hand in hand with malnutrition. In general, however, it is now believed that maintaining a body weight of 10 percent below so-called usual numbers may lead to increased longevity.

Any sudden weight loss in a short period of time warrants medical attention. In women of childbearing age, the loss of fatty tissue can be accompanied by a loss of estrogens, or female hormones; a good portion of estrogen is stored in fatty tissue. The consequences can be menstrual irregularities— even the failure to menstruate for months at a time—and an inability to become pregnant.

Any unusual distribution of obviously excessive fat, especially when concentrated in only one or two areas, warrants a medical consultation. While obesity is not a true disease in itself, it can be an early warning sign of some other body problem. It also increases the body's work load (try carrying a 10-pound box of detergent around for a few hours). And keep in mind that edema, which rarely has anything to do with fat deposition, can also cause a marked increase in body weight; repeated bouts of edema warrant a medical consultation.

If your upper arm measurements show an excess of muscle tissue over fat (increased midarm muscle circumference over decreased triceps skinfold thickness) and your weight is much greater than predicted, it could mean that your increased weight is normal for you, especially if you are an athlete or into physical fitness. If the arm measurements are reversed, however, and you are overweight, a medical consultation is warranted to rule out a hormone disorder. Should your triceps skinfold measurement be greater than usual without obesity, it also warrants a medical consultation. As you become older, and are less physically active, however, it is not unusual to show a bit more fat than muscle tissue.

Upper arm measurements that are well below usual values, no matter what your weight, warrant a medical consultation; they can be the first signs of protein malnutrition (conditions called marasmus and kwashiorkor). In elderly people anthropometric measurements that are below usual values can be clues to why certain drugs are not working as they should; they can also explain some bowel problems and prevent unnecessary surgery. In many instances the proper interpretation of upper arm measurements can indicate some simple, easily correctable vitamin or mineral deficiency that can eliminate a great many uncomfortable symptoms.

Understanding the difference between overweight and obesity as well as the problems of being underweight or undernourished—and seeking professional help for any unusual weight observations—is considered one of the best ways of practicing preventive medicine.

Reliability

A better understanding of weight and body fat percentage is now becoming formalized; as such, its true accuracy as an indicator of health has not been precisely established. Some people within their normal weight limits and having a low body fat percentage may still not be physically fit—in the athletic sense of the term. Obesity, as opposed to being overweight, does seem to be a 75 percent accurate indication of an increased susceptibility to heart disease and high blood pressure. Skinfold measurements, when performed precisely, are about 80 percent accurate as a gauge of body fat; they are much more accurate than weight observations alone. Midarm circumference measurements have proved to be 75 percent accurate in predicting serious illness due to malnutrition.

URINE TESTS

When it comes to the simplest, relatively least expensive way to monitor one's personal health—especially to help detect some incipient or latent disease—urinalysis probably offers more generalized health information than any other home test. Many urine tests require nothing more than observation; no devices or chemicals need be purchased. Yet the information that you can obtain can be as valuable as that provided by the most sophisticated professional laboratory. Where some apparatus is needed—most likely a chemically coated plastic dipstick (shown in Figure 19)—it is available at pharmacies under various brand names, and the cost averages from $0.06 to $0.30, depending mostly on the number of tests the dipstick offers; dipsticks run from a single analysis up to 11 different observations on one dipstick:

A few of the potential disorders that can be revealed by urine testing include:

- Kidney, bladder, prostate and urethral diseases, especially infections
- Drug use, drug abuse and poisonings
- Certain genetic, or inherited, conditions
- Hormone activity
- Liver and gallbladder functioning
- Metabolism of carbohydrates, fats and proteins
- Vitamin and mineral absorption and utilization
- Bone activity, including susceptibility to osteoporosis
- Blood production and utilization
- Parasite infestation

OBTAINING A URINE SAMPLE

For most urine tests all you need is a clean, dry container, preferably made of clear glass, with a capacity of at least 16 ounces (one pint). The opening of the container should be wide enough to allow urination into the container without difficulty. For the tests described in this book, the container need not be sterilized unless your physician specifically requests this extra step—primarily when testing urine for specific bacteria. Most "dipstick" tests can

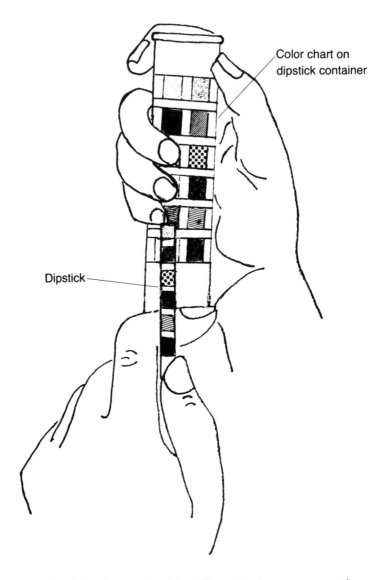

Figure 19. Dipstick urine testing (six different test measurements).

be performed by simply holding the stick in the urine stream for one second; no container is necessary.

The clean-catch specimen. At times, a clean-catch specimen is preferred, such as when testing for blood or infections in women in general, especially during menstruation, and in uncircumcised men. A man simply pulls back the foreskin of the penis and wipes the tip with warm soapy water followed by a clear water rinse. A woman should spread the lips of the vaginal opening and wash the urethral opening with warm, soapy water followed by a clear water rinse. The urine should then be passed immediately (see Figure 20). Many doctors suggest that an initial, small amount of urine be passed and discarded and that the urine for testing be taken from "midstream," discarding the last portion as well as the very first.

While urine passed at any time of the day is usually satisfactory for testing, most doctors and professional laboratories consider the first morning specimen upon awakening to be the best for generalized testing.

Because urine is the end product of almost all catabolic functions in the body (that is, the functions that generate the waste products of metabolism that the body must eliminate), outside of the many other strictly visual Body Observations (skin, weight, breasts, testicles, etc.), it is the ideal way to begin technical home testing for health maintenance.

URINE OBSERVATIONS

There are five simple observations of urine that can offer a wealth of health information. Regular attention to the clarity, color, odor and volume of urine, along with noting how often one feels the need to urinate, can offer early warning signs of some bodily dysfunction or latent disease. As with all do-it-yourself medical tests, a change in what has been usual is in no way diagnostic; it could, however, be the first clue to some developing disorder where prompt professional medical attention could not only allow a simple, inexpensive and possibly painless cure but also prevent a subsequent disability.

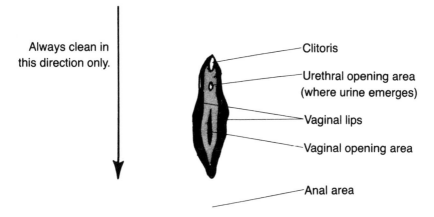

Figure 20. Female genital area.

For the health-conscious, urine observations can be the first step in a system of regular "checkups," putting the initial responsibility where it properly belongs—in the hands of the patient. For those who, wrongfully, have delegated total liability for their health to a doctor, it could mean taking the first step into the health milieu by starting to practice preventive medicine— becoming a participatory patient.

URINE OBSERVATIONS: COLOR
(An obvious, but effective, urine observation)

The color of urine can reflect many different conditions—from illness to drug use (there are more than 100 commonly used drugs that alter urine color). Exposure to industrial chemicals can also be identified by a change in urine color. While it can be something of a shock to notice an abrupt difference in the color of your urine, it can also be an early warning sign of some impending disease. Then again, it can also be nothing more than a consequence of your diet; and it can be quite a relief to learn that your reddish-colored urine is caused not by blood but by your having eaten beets.

What Is Usual
Most of the time urine color ranges from light yellow to dark amber. The yellow color of urine comes primarily from bile—the same bile secreted by the liver; the more bile, the more yellow to amber-colored the urine. The greater the volume of urine (see Urine Tests, **Urine Volume**), usually along with a lessened amount of dissolved material (dilution), the more apt it is to be lighter or paler in color (see Urine Tests, **Clinical Analysis: Specific Gravity**). After strenuous exercise, excessive sweating or a greatly reduced fluid intake, urine usually assumes a darker color.

What You Need
The test requires a clear glass container and good color perception.

What to Watch Out For
Do not forget to take into consideration any drug you are using; check with your doctor or pharmacist to see whether your medicine does affect urine color. Menstruating women may show pink or red-colored urine.

What the Test Results Can Mean
Pink to red, peach, brown or brown-black-colored urine, without a definite food or drug explanation, should first be considered to contain blood (red blood cells and hemoglobin). The urine blood test (see Urine Tests, **Clinical Analysis: Blood**) can help verify the presence of blood. If the test for blood

is positive, immediate medical attention should be sought. Red-orange, pink or red urine can also be due to:

• Foods such as beets, blackberries and rhubarb.
• Food coloring.
• Laxatives such as Ex-Lax, Dorbane, Modane and Senekot.
• Drugs, especially some tranquilizers such as Thorazine, Mellaril and Haldol—to name but a very few; some analgesics such as Pyridium.
• Porphyrins; this can mean liver disease, exposure to toxic chemicals or drug abuse, and if no other explanation is obvious, a medical consultation is warranted.

A vivid yellow-orange color not subsequent to exercise or some other explainable cause of concentrated urine (dehydration) can be due to:

• Anemia
• Thyroid disease
• Decreased kidney function
• Foods such as carrots
• Drugs such as the sulfa medications, cascara laxatives and warfarin products

The chances of kidney disease are such that a repeated vivid yellow or yellow-orange-colored urine warrants medical consultation.

Urine color of green to blue-green could result from:

• An infection due to a particular bacteria.
• Liver or gallbladder trouble (see Urine Tests, **Clinical Analysis: Bilirubin** and **Clinical Analysis: Urobilinogin**).
• Use of drugs such as Indocin and Robaxin for treating arthritis, gout and muscle pain; antidepressants such as Elavil.
• Excessive ingestion of certain vegetables; Chloret tablets.

Black or very dark urine could suggest the presence of melanin (a pigment of skin cancer), or it could reflect old blood that remained in the bladder. Poisoning from napthalene, a moth repellent, can also cause black urine. Such a finding warrants medical consultation.

And then, if urine seems consistently colorless, especially when accompanied by excessive volume, it could be an early sign of diabetcs (see Urine Tests, **Urine Observations; Volume** and **Clinical Analysis: Glucose**).

Note: Some doctors suggest that for the color test only, the urine be left standing for an hour or two after observing the original color; at times the urine will later darken to a red-brown or black color when certain inherited or metabolic illnesses are present, especially those that cause arthritic pains.

Reliability

If not due to drugs, foods or exercise, an abnormal color change in urine is considered to be a 90 percent accurate indication of some bodily dysfunction.

URINE OBSERVATIONS: ODOR
(A somewhat unusual clue to illness)

While it is easy to imagine a reluctance to test the aroma of urine, it should be kept in mind that long before the era of advanced medical technology, doctors not only routinely noted the scent of urine but tasted it as well as a means of diagnosis. And even today there are some doctors who ask their patients to eat asparagus, drink two glasses of water and urinate every half-hour, making a note of how long it takes before the vegetable's characteristic odor appears in the urine as a rough measure of kidney function. Many other foods and drugs affect the aromatic nature of urine but with insufficient consistency to indicate any diagnostic coincidence.

What Is Usual

Urine should have some odor, but it is usually not disagreeable; some people describe it as "spicy." If urine is left standing for a prolonged period of time, it usually acquires an ammonialike odor.

What You Need

To check the odor of urine, you should have a clean, dry container and normal smell function (see Brain and Nervous System Tests, **Smell Function**).

What to Watch Out For

A container having any residual soap or detergent odors can disguise urine odors.

What the Test Results Can Mean

A sweet or fruity odor can mean:

- Diabetes (see Urine Tests, **Clinical Analysis: Glucose** and **Clinical Analysis: Ketones**); if you are eating few, or no, carbohydrates, the consequent production of acetone in urine can cause a similar odor.
- A maple syrup odor, usually in the urine of infants, points to an inherited disorder actually called maple syrup disease.

A sour or otherwise unusual odor coming from an infant's urine can be an early warning signal of several other genetic metabolic disorders.

An ammonialike or disagreeable odor in fresh urine hints at a urinary tract infection (see Urine Tests, **Clinical Analysis: Nitrite** and **Clinical Analysis: Leukocytes**).

There are some people who constantly complain of having urine with a "foul" odor. While there are diseases such as cancer that can cause this problem, doctors now have drugs that can, in many instances, relieve the complaint if it is not attributable to any underlying disease. However, any unusual urine odor warrants a medical consultation.

Reliability
An abnormal urine odor is about 60 percent accurate as an indicator of disease.

URINE OBSERVATIONS: TURBIDITY
(Cloudy urine is rarely normal urine)

Turbidity, or cloudiness, is an indication that urine contains some substance that should not be present. Cloudy or milky urine most often comes from an excess of certain minerals, particularly phosphates, but many other substances can contribute to turbidity: Pus, blood, bacteria, parasites, proteins and even fats can, at times, be found in urine.

What Is Usual
Urine should be clear, especially immediately after urination. If a urine sample is left standing for a prolonged period of time, it may appear cloudy without this being unusual.

What You Need
A clear glass container is all that is required to perform the test.

What to Watch Out For
Do not use a container that might have any residue of soap or detergent. If you are a woman with a vaginal discharge, it could make clear urine appear turbid. A man's urine may appear cloudy after sexual activity.

What the Test Results Can Mean
Continuously cloudy urine warrants a medical consultation. It could be an early warning signal of kidney stones, or it could indicate a urinary tract infection; if the urine nitrite and leukocyte tests are also positive (see Urine Tests, **Clinical Analysis: Nitrite** and **Clinical Analysis: Leukocytes**), medical attention is indicated. Some rare causes of turbidity include diabetes,

filariasis (a parasitic invasion of the body), a lymph system problem, a sexually transmitted disease or a tumor somewhere within the body.

Reliability
Cloudy urine is considered to be a 75 percent accurate indication of some underlying problem, but it is not specific as to the cause.

URINE OBSERVATIONS: TWO/THREE-GLASS TEST
(An aid to identifying the location of a urinary tract problem)

When, while urinating, the urine is voided into separate containers, the very first portion of urine (about an ounce) that is voided into the first glass carries with it any substances that lay within the urethra—that segment of the urinary system that starts at the bladder and ends at the point where the urine leaves the body. It can contain material from an infectious process in the urethra (see Urine Tests, **Clinical Analysis: Nitrite**) such as gonorrhea or chlamydia, as well as white blood cells (see Urine Tests, **Clinical Analysis: Leukocytes**), which usually appear in response to an infectious process. The major portion of urine is then voided into a second glass and consists of what has been stored in the bladder. A variation of this test is when, just prior to the termination of urination, the last remaining bit of urine is voided into a third glass in order to help confirm, or reveal, a beginning bladder infection or, in men, a prostate problem. An optional refinement of the three-glass test, in men, is to stop urination just prior to emptying the bladder completely and have the prostate examined (see Genitourinary System Tests, **Prostate Observations**); the third glass could then reflect prostatic involvement. Thus, by observing the urine's turbidity (cloudiness) and color (see Urine Tests, **Urine Observations: Turbidity** and **Urine Observations: Color**) in the two (or three) containers, it is sometimes possible to pinpoint the specific location of a urinary tract problem.

What Is Usual
The urine in the two (or three) containers should be clear and even sparkling. The color should be light yellow (straw-colored), and there should be no turbidity (see Figure 21).

What You Need
To perform the test, you should have two (or three) clear glass containers, one of which should be capable of holding at least one pint. Although this test can be performed at any time of the day, the first morning specimen is best. Void a small quantity of urine into the first container, and then, if the two-glass test is being performed, void all the rest into the large container.

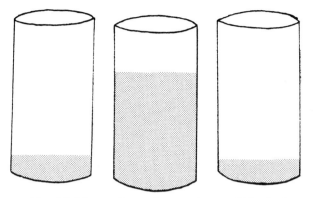

Usual (all two or three glasses clear and identical)

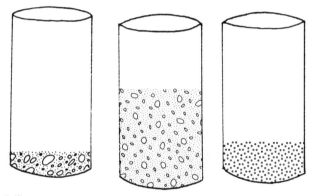

Abnormal (first container most cloudy, decreasing in next one or two; usually from a urethral infection)

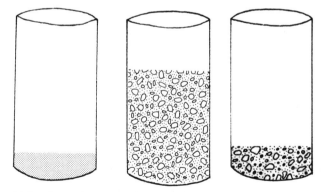

Abnormal (cloudiness increases in second or third container; usually from kidney, bladder or prostate infection)

Figure 21. Two- (or three-) glass urine test.

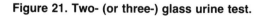

If the three-glass test is to be conducted, the last bit of urine should be voided into the third container.

What to Watch Out For
Any contamination in the glass containers might cause cloudiness in the urine. Do not massage or apply pressure to the penis during urination.

What the Test Results Can Mean
In the two-glass test, if the small amount of urine collected in the first container is cloudy and the second portion less cloudy, it usually signifies a urethral infection, possibly a sexually transmitted disease; it warrants medical attention. Should the first container show clear urine and the second show cloudy urine, there is the possibility of a bladder or kidney infection; it warrants medical consultation. The possibility of a urinary tract infection can also be confirmed by other Urine Tests (see **Clinical Analysis: Leukocytes, Clinical Analysis: Nitrite** and **Clinical Analysis: Protein**). Should both containers appear equally cloudy, and should the other urine tests indicate a possible infection, medical attention should be sought. When the third glass is tested, it should always be clear (or clearer than the other two); otherwise, medical consultation is indicated.

Each of the two or three containers can also be tested for blood (see Urine Tests, **Clinical Analysis: Blood**); a positive result in one of the glasses warrants medical attention and may indicate which area of the genitourinary system is involved (see Figure 22).

Reliability
This test is considered to be 80 percent accurate in helping to localize where a urinary tract problem lies. It is especially valuable in detecting sexually transmitted diseases.

URINE OBSERVATIONS: VOLUME
(As a disease indicator, the quantity of urine can be as valuable as its quality)

How much urine an individual passes in a 24-hour period can be as important an observation as any chemical reaction. Many diseases first manifest their presence by either increasing or decreasing the amount of urine; alterations in one's nutritional state can also affect urine volume. And nocturia, or the need to urinate frequently during the night, can be an early warning sign of several disorders.

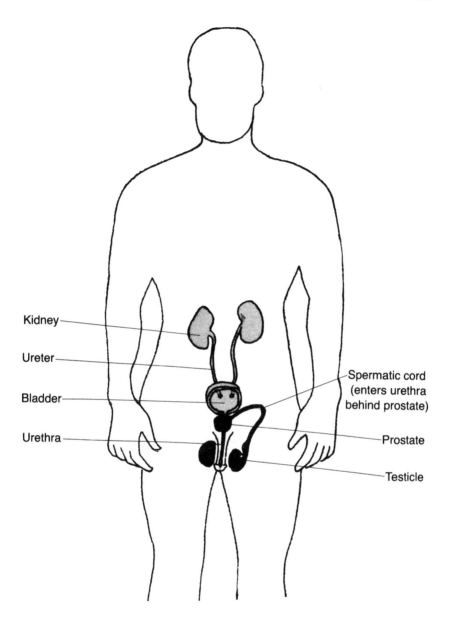

Figure 22. Male genitourinary system.

(The female urinary system is similar; the urethra is shorter and, obviously, there is no prostate, spermatic cord or testicle.)

What Is Usual

The average person, on a fairly typical diet of food and drink, usually passes (voids) from one quart to two quarts of urine within a 24-hour period. It is common to void from 6 ounces to 8 ounces of urine at a time, with the exception being the first morning specimen upon awakening, which averages 10 ounces to 12 ounces. It is not unusual for a woman to have a decreased amount of urine for several days prior to menstruation (believed to be due to hormonal water retention) and to have an increased volume for a few days after menstruation begins.

When volume is compared with the urine's specific gravity (see Urine Tests, **Clinical Analysis: Specific Gravity**), the gravity number should be high with a small volume and low with a large volume.

What You Need

The test is performed using a wide-mouth container with ounce markings on the side (an easy-to-use, inexpensive urine-collection device is a Pyrex one-quart kitchen measuring cup).

What to Watch Out For

In testing for urine volume, keep the following points in mind:

- Be sure to take into account the amount and kinds of fluid drunk prior to, and during, the time you measure your urine volume; a large quantity of liquid taken in can cause a corresponding increase in urine output, and even small amounts of alcoholic beverages, coffee and tea can disproportionately increase urine volume.
- Cold weather can cause an increase in urine output (the kidneys handle the body fluid that is usually lost through perspiration), while warm weather or prolonged physical activity can reduce urine output.
- Do not attempt to measure urine volume if you are taking any form of diuretic drug, are using salt substitutes or are under a doctor's care until you have discussed the test with your doctor.

What the Test Results Can Mean

If, after all the factors that can normally cause increased or decreased urination have been taken into account, the 24-hour urine volume is repeatedly greater than two quarts a day, it could mean:

- Diabetes mellitus—the kind of diabetes that comes from an inability to metabolize carbohydrates; sometimes called sugar diabetes.
- Diabetes insipidus—the kind of diabetes that comes from the inadequate production of a brain hormone; sometimes called water diabetes.
- Kidney disease (there is a form of diabetes caused directly by the kidneys).

- A reflection of several different hormone imbalances.
- Some form of metabolic disorder.
- An indirect consequence of a psychological problem, usually accompanied by increased fluid intake.
- Kidney stones in the bladder, which could cause frequent urination during the day, but not at night.

If the 24-hour urine volume is less than 16 ounces (one pint), it could mean:

- Kidney disease
- Heart disease
- A urinary tract obstruction
- An intestinal obstruction
- A reflection of a hormone imbalance
- A reaction to a stressful situation, primarily emotional

Repeated increases in urine volume or the need to urinate more often (especially during the night) warrants medical consultation. An increase in the frequency of urination without an increase in the volume, or urine volume that does not correspond with the urine's expected specific gravity, also warrants a medical consultation. An unexplainable decrease in urine volume requires immediate medical attention; passing less than 8 ounces of urine a day should be considered a medical emergency.

Reliability
Abnormalities in urine volume are considered to be 80 percent accurate as an early warning sign of disease.

CLINICAL ANALYSIS: BILIRUBIN
(An early warning sign of liver disease)

Bilirubin is formed from the hemoglobin in red blood cells after they break down at the end of their usual life span (four months). It is a gold-colored pigment that normally colors bile and is excreted primarily by the bowel, which helps gives feces their dark color. Usually, the urine color will range from a very dark yellow to brown if abnormal amounts of bilirubin are present, especially if the urine sample forms a yellow foam when shaken. Many different antibiotics, hormones, tranquilizers, diuretics, laxatives and pain relievers can cause a positive urine bilirubin test, as can prolonged alcoholism. The yellow color of jaundice seen in the eyes and skin is usually caused by excessive amounts of bilirubin in the blood, and in fact, the test for bilirubin is most often performed when some form of liver disease is suspected, since urine can test positive for bilirubin before the rest of the body shows evidence of liver damage. While the test can also reflect some forms of anemia, when this is suspected, the urine urobilinogen test (see Urine Tests, **Clinical Analysis: Urobilinogen**) should also be performed.

What Is Usual
No trace of bilirubin should be detected in the urine.

What You Need
Any one of several different dipstick testing strips can be used to check for the presence of bilirubin; most multiple-test dipsticks incorporate this test. They cost from $0.10 to $0.30 per test, depending on the quantity purchased.

What to Watch Out For
The urine must be fresh and kept from prolonged exposure to light. If urine is more than 30 minutes old, do not use it to perform this test. The best time to test urine for bilirubin is late in the day, when excretion is at its peak. Because so many drugs can interfere with the test, check with your doctor or pharmacist to ascertain whether any medicine you are taking will affect the test. A urinary tract infection or taking vitamin C can cause a false-negative result (see Urine Tests, **Clinical Analysis: Leukocytes** and **Clinical Analysis: Nitrite**). The test strips must be fresh, and because the color change is so slight, excellent color vision is essential.

What the Test Results Can Mean
Any indication of bilirubin in the urine, even without symptoms, warrants a medical consultation. If there are related symptoms (fever, jaundice, lethargy), medical attention should be sought. A positive test can be an early warning signal of hepatitis, and immediate medical attention can help ward off cirrhosis of the liver. The presence of some other conditions—such as gallstones, cancer and even thyroid disease—may be signaled by a positive urine bilirubin test. And although drug use may cause a positive test, the test could also reflect liver damage from drugs or alcohol. Following a blood transfusion, or any suspected exposure to infectious hepatitis, many doctors advise a weekly home urine bilirubin test as the best means of detecting potential liver problems early.

Reliability
As with many urine tests, the home dipstick method is identical to the way the test is performed in doctors' offices and commercial laboratories. All brands of dipsticks are equally sensitive. For bilirubin a positive test can be considered 95 percent accurate when extraneous causes such as drugs are eliminated.

CLINICAL ANALYSIS: BLOOD
(A test primarily for occult [hidden] blood, called hematuria)

First of all, should a substance that even seems to be blood appear in the urine, even if some drug or food is suspected as the cause, a medical consultation is warranted. In most instances, however, when real blood is present in the urine, it is "occult" (not visible to the eye). The test for urine blood detects both hemoglobin and red blood cells, so that it can reflect old as well as new bleeding somewhere in the urinary tract, even blood cells that are abnormally passed through the kidneys; a positive test does not reveal the cause or source of the bleeding. However, when the test is performed along with the two-/three-glass urine test (see Urine Tests, **Urine Observations: Two-/Three-Glass Test),** it can offer a clue as to just what part of the urinary tract is bleeding.

Many drugs—such as pain relievers (nonsteroidal antiinflammatory drugs, or NSAIDs), certain tranquilizers, some antihistamines and a few antibiotics (such as penicillin and especially the sulfas)—can irritate the kidneys to the point where occult blood will be detected in urine. Anticoagulant drugs that are purposely used to prolong bleeding (see Blood Tests, **Bleeding and Clotting Time**) often cause a positive urine blood test, and this can be an early warning sign of a dangerous overdose of the drug. Excessive exertion and physical exercise, especially marathon running or prolonged jogging, can cause a positive test, but this is rarely considered a sign of disease. Obviously, menstruation, and even hemorrhoids, can cause a false-positive test result.

What Is Usual
No indication of blood should be detected in the urine. Even if there seems to be a logical explanation for a positive test, such as a drug or exercise, that positive finding still warrants a medical consultation to rule out an underlying disease.

What You Need
One of the dipstick-type tests is easiest to use. There is a Hemastix strip that tests only for blood and costs about $0.08 per test, depending on the quantity purchased. Most multiple-test strips include blood detection as one of the tests, and they cost from $0.10 to $0.30 per test strip, depending on the number of different tests included and the quantity purchased.

What to Watch Out For
If urine contains a large amount of vitamin C (see Urine Tests, **Clinical Analysis: Vitamin C**), the test may show a false-negative result (blood is present but will not be detected because of the vitamin C effect); if you are taking vitamin C, be sure to test your urine for this first. Some bacteria that

can cause urinary tract infections can also cause a false-positive test result even though no blood is present; a urine nitrite test (see Urine Tests, **Clinical Analysis: Nitrite**) may help reveal this error. Red-tinged urine caused by the presence of blood must also be differentiated from red-colored urine caused by certain foods and drugs (see Urine Tests, **Urine Observations: Color**).

What the Test Results Can Mean

A sudden positive urine blood test warrants medical attention, if only to eliminate any extraneous cause. Although one out of every five runners shows hematuria after exertion, all traces of blood should disappear after 24 hours of rest. Blood in the urine can indicate a great many diseases: several kinds of anemia (sickle-cell, in particular), liver disease, immunological conditions such as lupus erythematosis and some inherited illnesses. Bodily injuries, burns, shock, and many drugs and poisons can cause urinary tract bleeding. A very common cause is kidney stones, especially in children, and there is usually an increase in urine calcium (see Urine Tests, **Clinical Analysis: Calcium**) at the same time. Any infection in the urinary tract, including the prostate gland, may cause urinary bleeding, but other infections such as malaria and pneumonia can also be to blame. Even high **blood pressure** (see Heart and Circulation Tests) can cause a positive test. Many doctors feel that regular urine testing for blood can help detect cancer in its earliest stage (see Mouth, Throat and Gastrointestinal Tests, **Occult Blood [Feces]**).

At the same time, it is important to keep in mind that close to 5 percent of the population will test positive for blood in the urine but will show no specific cause nor have any related illness. It is also possible for relatives of patients with hematuria to test positive for hematuria without having any disease; the condition is considered familial but warrants a medical follow-up. Still, many doctors now feel that drugs may be the most common cause of a positive test.

Reliability

All dipsticks, regardless of brand name, are considered 90 percent accurate in detecting blood in the urine—even to the extent of only two red blood cells in one drop of urine. However, even when the test is positive, the true cause of blood in the urine can be professionally diagnosed only about 75 percent of the time.

CLINICAL ANALYSIS: CALCIUM
(An indication of how the body uses calcium)

The amount of calcium that can be detected in the urine is a fairly reliable indication of how much calcium you eat and absorb (it is one process to ingest calcium, but quite another to digest it) and how well calcium is metabolized and utilized by the body. A test for urine calcium can also reflect calcium's interaction with phosphorus compounds (excessive phosphates, as in soft drinks, can interfere with calcium metabolism) and, as such, can be a screening device to help detect various hormone disorders, particularly of the parathyroid and thyroid glands. Dietary calcium is necessary to maintain muscle contractions, nerve transmissions, cell structure and blood clotting and to prevent vitamin D deficiency or toxicity. Testing for calcium in the urine, using the Sulkowitch test (named after the American physician who devised the chemical reagent), can also aid in the detection of certain cancers, kidney disease and susceptibility to osteoporosis (a demineralization or rarefaction of bone substance—particularly in women past the menopause— that can cause stooped posture of the spine and very easy breakage of bones). Excessive calcium in the diet has been blamed for kidney stones. In Israel, where some drinking water contains very large amounts of calcium, the incidence of calcium-related kidney stones is great enough to be a serious public health problem.

It is easy to test your urine for its calcium content; you can also measure how your body reacts to calcium in your diet. When equal amounts of urine and Sulkowitch reagent, usually a teaspoon of each, are mixed in a clear glass tube, the reagent causes the urine to become cloudy, depending on how much calcium is present. No cloudiness is reported as 0; slight cloudiness is 1+; heavier cloudiness that still allows you to read the printed words of a book or newspaper through it is 2+; cloudiness that will not allow you to see or read through it is 3+ or 4+, depending on its intensity. This is the same way physicians and laboratories report their findings.

What Is Usual

Normally, the body excretes sufficient calcium in the urine to cause some cloudiness, a 1+ or 2+ reaction. After food or medicine containing large amounts of calcium is consumed, the cloudiness should increase to a 3+ or 4+ reaction. Omitting calcium from the diet for a day should cause a 0 or 1+ reaction the day after. The first morning specimen of urine is more likely to show the least amount of calcium; a test specimen passed an hour or two after you eat a typical meal is apt to show the most calcium. Always note the time of day and relationship to eating when reporting the test results to your doctor.

Note: Some doctors tell their patients to eat a specific diet that contains a measured amount of calcium prior to performing this test at home; you might want to consult your physician about this.

What You Need

Many doctors will give you a test tube and a supply of Sulkowitch reagent, along with instructions, to perform the test at home. Chemical supply companies sell the reagent for approximately $14.00 a pint, which is enough for 100 tests.

What to Watch Out For
In performing a urine calcium test, keep the following in mind:

- It is always good to check your urine for protein before performing the Sulkowitch test (see Urine Tests, **Clinical Analysis: Protein**); protein in the urine can imitate the cloudiness of calcium.
- Take into account the amount of calcium in your diet, or in pills, in considering the significance of the result.
- Keep in mind that other nutrients such as sodium, magnesium and phosphates can affect the amount of calcium in the urine, and check with your doctor or pharmacist to see whether any medicine you are taking contains any interfering substances. Antacids, diuretics, vitamins (large doses of vitamin D can cause an increase in urinary calcium), laxatives, and some antibiotics and steroid preparations can alter calcium excretion. Birth control pills can cause a decrease in urinary calcium regardless of diet.
- The reagent is a mixture of two dilute acids; do not let the reagent touch anything—especially clothes, furniture or your skin—and keep it well away from children.

What the Test Results Can Mean
If, after several tests while on a typical diet, your urine shows either too little (0) or too much (3+ or 4+) calcium, it warrants a medical consultation. Abnormal calcium excretion can reflect a wide variety of illnesses. Then again, lying in bed all day or excessive "resting" can also increase calcium excretion. While no evidence of urine calcium usually reflects an inadequate intake of the mineral, it can suggest intestinal problems, hormone imbalance, kidney disease or some nutritional deficiency as well. It can also come from excessive ingestion of soft drinks that contain phosphates. If, after first avoiding calcium-containing foods and after then taking a large dose of calcium, your urinary calcium does not show any change, this could be an early warning sign of osteoporosis and warrants medical attention. Some doctors have their pregnant patients test for urinary calcium weekly; a sudden decrease can be a early warning sign of a pregnancy problem.

Note: One out of every 20 people will regularly show an excessive amount of calcium in the urine; in most instances this is an inherited trait and does not reflect disease.

Reliability
Urinary calcium measurements are about 90 percent accurate in determining the body's reaction to ingested calcium. Abnormal urinary calcium tests

are about 80 percent accurate as a reflection of disease. At the present time there is no very accurate test for susceptibility to osteoporosis, and urinary calcium testing is as good as anything available.

CLINICAL ANALYSIS: DRUG ABUSE IDENTIFICATION
(Detecting dangerous drugs before it is too late)

Have you ever taken a drug that seemed to cause an unusual side effect such as extreme weakness, hallucination, an inability to think clearly, profuse sweating or slurred speech? Have you ever come across a strange pill, capsule or powder in your home and wondered what the substance was? Should you suspect the possibility of dangerous street drugs such as barbiturates, cocaine, Dilaudid, heroin, marijuana, PCP (angel dust), Preludin or Quaaludes, to name but a very few, you can now find out anonymously what the unknown drug is. Here is what to do:

1. Wrap the sample securely in foil or plastic and place it in an envelope.
2. Identify each sample with a random five-digit number (for instance 58294). Enclose a note giving the number and any details about the sample (such as what it is believed to be and whether you suspect a particular substance), the effects of the drug (if someone has used it), and the city and state or the country from which it was obtained.
3. Enclose $25.00 for each sample, preferably in the form of a money order.
4. Enclose a self-addressed, stamped envelope if you wish to receive the results by mail.
5. Mail the sample to: SP LAB (5426 NW 79 Ave., Miami, Fl. 33166).
6. After about 20 days call (305) 757-2566 or, outside Dade County, Florida residents may call (800) 432-8255 toll free. Be ready to give the random five-digit number you assigned in order to obtain the test results.
7. Before submitting a sample, it is suggested that you call to verify the mailing address and the appropriateness of your sample for analysis. Note that SP LAB tests only for active drug ingredients and that inactive fillers, cuts and other pharmacologically inert substances will not be identified.

The laboratory will test your submitted sample only for the presence of different drugs; however, many street drugs also contain adulterants and diluting agents that can be a greater hazard than the drug itself. The lab will only tell you the name of the drug but will not tell you its quantity or strength without a court order. The laboratory is licensed to test drugs anonymously by the Federal Drug Enforcement Administration on the condition that it pass on to the agency the results of each test and where the envelope containing the drug sample was postmarked. This provides the agency with generalized information about what kinds of drugs are being offered and used and where.

There are other drug-detection screenings that can easily be performed at home. Your doctor can give you a KDI QUIK TEST (*KDI* stands for Keystone Diagnostics Inc., in Columbia, Md.; [800] 331-3505); this home test will screen urine for cocaine, crack, morphine/heroin, PCP, amphetamines, methadone, codeine and librium in less than three minutes. A positive reaction requires more sophisticated testing to identify the specific drug, but as a first indication of the possible presence of, or freedom from, drug abuse, the test can be quite valuable. It costs the doctor $6.50 per test kit. A separate KDI QUIK TEST is available for marijuana screening. Other companies make drug abuse screening tests, and your doctor may have a preference for a different one based on his or her experience.

Keep in mind that alcohol is, at times, considered a drug of abuse (see Breath and Lung Tests, **Breath Alcohol**), especially when used along with other drugs such as tranquilizers and sedatives (see Urine Tests, **Clinical Analysis: Phenylketonuria Screening**).

Behavioral observations. Yet another "test" to detect the possible abuse of illegal drugs—as well as alcohol, antidepressants, sedatives, stimulants and tranquilizers—is careful observation. While even unbiased impressions are not definitive, certain behavioral and social changes in an individual that are not readily explainable may warrant more specific drug identification screening:

- Increased absence from school or work, especially without an excuse or more so with an implausible one.
- A sudden, unexplained decrease in performance at school or work.
- Changes in personal appearance, attire or cleanliness.
- Changes in customary attitude, behavior or mood, especially if bizarre and without provocation.
- Changes toward family members, such as an unwillingness to assume usual responsibilities or share experiences.
- An unusual tolerance of and tendency to defend drugs and drug users.

What Is Usual
The only usual finding is the specific identity of a previously unknown drug. However, the National Institute on Drug Abuse says it is not unusual for at least 30 percent of the population to be using marijuana regularly and for up to 10 percent to be using other drugs of abuse; in such people a positive test would be usual.

What to Watch Out For

When mailing a sample, do not send in vitamins, food or herb samples; do not request insecticide or herbicide analysis; do not send in blood, urine or other body excretions or secretions. Be sure the drug effect that you experienced or observed was not due to the use of alcohol alone or to the use of alcohol in combination with a drug.

Keep in mind that simply being in a room where marijuana is smoked can cause a positive urine test for that drug in a nonuser for several weeks after exposure. Eating certain foods, such as poppy seeds (on a cake), can cause a false-positive test for morphine and other opiate drugs. And many relatively safe drugs can cause false-positive reactions. Benedryl can give a false-positive PCP result; certain diet aids as well as cold and asthma remedies— and even some nose drops—can mimic cocaine and amphetamine abuse.

What the Test Results Can Mean

The sooner illicit drug use is discovered, the easier it is to treat and the more successful the treatment is apt to be. Of interest, one laboratory reports that more than half of all drug samples submitted to it for anonymous analysis contain drugs other than those alleged. Actually confirming the use of a dangerous street drug warrants medical attention for the user.

Reliability

In general, nonspecific drug screening, as opposed to quite expensive testing (from $100.00 to more than $1000.00) to identify a specific drug, is not too accurate. Positive results should only be considered as preliminary and must always be confirmed. While there have been reports of errors in up to 40 percent of all forms of drug-screening tests, when you stop and think that about 50 million such tests are performed each year, even a 1 percent error rate could be tragic, because it would translate into half a million false results. And even the costly, more specific tests are not 100 percent accurate. While much depends on the care and precision of the laboratory, a great deal also depends on the population being tested; in a group of people where half use illegal drugs, the accuracy will be better than where drug use is rare.

When illegal drugs are used, they vary considerably in how long they will remain in the body and give a positive test result. Marijuana has been known to last for three weeks after only one use. Barbiturates and PCP can last up to a week, cocaine and tranquilizers for three days, and amphetamines up to a half-day after a single use.

Note: Food and Drug Administration (FDA) regulations now require every drug-screening test kit to include a list of all substances that can interfere with the test's accuracy.

CLINICAL ANALYSIS: GLUCOSE
(A way of detecting one form of sugar in the urine)

Although urine may contain traces of several kinds of sugar (glucose, fructose, galactose, etc.), the usual test for sugar in the urine is the one specifically for glucose (also see Blood Tests, **Glucose**). Normal carbohydrate metabolism is such that most people rarely have a positive test for glucose in their urine. If glucose is repeatedly detected, it usually means that the amount of glucose in the blood is elevated—most commonly due to diabetes (but urine glucose levels alone are not to be considered a reliable indicator of blood glucose levels). When blood and urine glucose tests are performed together, they can indicate how high blood glucose levels must go before the kidneys filter the glucose from the blood into the urine.

While urine specimens can be tested at any time of the day, for this particular test most doctors prefer the second morning specimen (after discarding the first one upon awakening), since it better reflects blood sugar levels. A first morning specimen tends to be an accumulation of all urine filtered by the kidneys during the night and is therefore less indicative of diet and metabolism.

As with so many tests, there are a number of non-disease-related factors that can cause a positive urine glucose test, but the test should become negative once the factor or factors are eliminated. Positive results can occur under the following circumstances:

- After eating extremely large amounts of refined sugar or sugar-containing foods.
- After taking large doses of vitamin C.
- After extreme physical exertion.
- During and immediately after extreme anxiety or emotional upset.
- With the use of many different drugs: adrenalin and related medicines used to treat allergies, certain digitalis preparations, some aspirin-containing products, most steroid (cortisonelike) drugs, most diuretics, a few forms of penicillin and some other antibiotics, barbiturates and drug abuse with narcotics such as morphine.
- Pregnancy.

Note: Patients who know they have diabetes should follow their doctors' advice only regarding urine glucose testing; this is just one of several screening tests for urine glucose and not a specific test for diabetes.

What Is Usual

No glucose should be detected in urine (nondisease exceptions have been cited above). It was once believed that it took a blood glucose level of 180 milligrams (mg) per 100 milliliters (ml) or more before blood sugar would pass through the kidneys into the urine and that a combination of an elevated blood glucose level plus a positive urine glucose test automatically meant diabetes. Recent research has shown, however, that some "normal" people may have blood sugar levels anywhere from 140 mg to 240 mg per 100 ml before they "spill" sugar into the urine; several other tests, such as the blood glucose tolerance test (see the discussion of glucose tolerance in Blood Tests, **Glucose**), are now required before a diagnosis of diabetes can be made. In the past, 100 mg in 3½ ounces, or 100 ml (1 deciliter [dl]), of urine was considered a "trace"; now, 50 mg per dl is officially a "trace," or positive result.

What You Need
The test is performed with a dipstick-type testing strip that includes glucose (many people find that the Diastix is the easiest to read; these test strips limit their findings to glucose determinations and cost from $5.00 to $6.00 for a bottle of 50 strips). TES-TAPE comes as a continuous roll of test paper (much like a Scotch Tape dispenser) and costs $3.50 for a minimum of 100 tests; many doctors feel that this is the most accurate paper-type test because it is the least affected by drugs. Multiple-test dipsticks usually contain glucose as one of the tests on the strip and cost from $0.10 to $0.30, depending on the quantity purchased and the number of different tests on the dipstick.

What to Watch Out For
In performing urine glucose testing, keep the following points in mind:

- Many urine glucose tests depend on timed measurements, the directions for which must be followed exactly to avoid false results; the time is not the same for all the tests.
- Be sure that the test strips are not old and that they are in good working order.
- Do not attempt color-change interpretation unless you have normal color vision.
- If you are taking large doses of vitamin C, an excess of this vitamin in the urine can cause a false test result (see Urine Tests, **Clinical Analysis: Vitamin C**); do not take vitamin C for three days prior to testing for urine glucose.
- Be sure to take into account any medicine you are using (even one you bought without a prescription); a recent study showed that one out of three inaccurate urine glucose tests were the result of ignoring a drug or forgetting to take it into account.
- There are some doctors who feel that these dipsticks may be cut in half (to save money). This is not recommended for urine dipsticks, since the glucose-detecting pad contains a measured amount of reagent that determines the test's specificity.

What the Test Results Can Mean

Urine glucose tests that are positive for two or three days in a row warrant medical consultation, even if there is a possible extraneous cause, if only to rule out a disease process. In most instances repeated positive glucose reactions indicate diabetes, especially if there is a family history of the disease. But because a positive urine glucose test could mean some other hormone disorder—faulty glucose metabolism can reflect adrenal, pituitary or thyroid gland disorders—as well as the latent consequences of an old heart attack, little strokes, liver disease or even an old brain injury, a diagnosis of diabetes is not absolute until confirmed by additional professional testing. Some infectious diseases, such as pancreatitis, may also cause a positive glucose test.

Reliability

Although different brands of dipsticks vary with respect to how much glucose must be present before they show a positive result, all are better than 90 percent accurate and are quite adequate for screening purposes.

CLINICAL ANALYSIS: KETONES
(A test that can indicate abnormal carbohydrate and/or fat metabolism)

Urinary ketones, sometimes called ketone bodies, are composed primarily of two different acids and acetone. They can reflect the metabolism (utilization) of fat and fatty acids in the body. When insufficient carbohydrates are available to supply energy, the liver usually starts converting fat to energy as an alternative, and this is reflected by the presence of ketones in the urine (a condition called ketonuria). Because people with diabetes have problems with carbohydrate metabolism, they are most apt to show ketones in the urine. There are, however, other circumstances that provoke ketonuria:

- An inadequate food intake, usually over several days, or even severe vomiting can cause the body to produce excess ketones.
- Dehydration as well as inadequate intake, or loss, of water.
- Conditions that interfere with proper digestion.
- Diseases that cause a high fever.
- Alcoholism.
- The use of certain medicines that can cause a false-positive reaction (some drugs used to treat the symptoms of Parkinson's disease, some urinary pain relievers, some aspirinlike products and a few sleeping preparations); an excess of vitamin C.

• A diet that omits virtually all carbohydrates (the Atkins diet utilizes urine ketone measurements as an indicator of adherence).
• Certain genetic disorders.

This test is primarily one for known diabetics to use as an additional means of following the course of their disease.

What Is Usual
Ketone bodies should not be detected in the urine.

What You Need
The test can be performed using any one of the dipstick strips that test specifically for ketones, such as Chemstrip K or Ketostix, or the Acetest tablet test, which cost approximately $8.00 per 100 strips or 50 tablets. Most other multiple-test strips include ketones as part of the battery; their prices range from $0.10 to $0.30, depending on the quantity purchased and the number of different tests on the dipstick. A new reagent test strip that allows more precise measurements of ketones, especially in smaller amounts, is called the Ames Keto-Diastix 5 (it also measures glucose in the urine more precisely). It is particularly valuable for diabetic patients who are especially prone to producing ketones during periods of stress or illness. The cost is $12.25 for 100 strips.

What to Watch Out For
The following are some guidelines for testing urine to detect the presence of ketones:

• Do not test a urine specimen that has been left standing for more than 30 minutes; it can produce a false-negative reaction.
• The color comparison chart for ketone testing is not easy to read; it is suggested that two people evaluate the color change.
• The ketone testing chemicals in the strips may fail to change color if they have been exposed to air even for short periods of time; be sure the test strips are fresh and have been properly stored (this caution is more for patients with diabetes who test for ketones as an advance warning against the possibility of diabetic coma). Close the container tightly immediately after withdrawing a dipstick. When kept properly (not exposed to air or moisture), all brands are equally effective. If exposed to air for prolonged periods, such as while testing, they lose all effectiveness.

What the Test Results Can Mean
A positive ketone test in a patient with diabetes is sufficient warning to seek immediate medical attention. A persistent positive ketone test in someone

without evident diabetes or a known dietary alteration warrants medical consultation.

Many doctors have their pregnant patients test their urine weekly; a positive ketone test can be an early warning sign of a disorder in the fetus.

Reliability

Although some doctors feel that the Ames tests are the least sensitive, all are at least 95 percent accurate and are therefore sufficiently sensitive for home testing.

CLINICAL ANALYSIS: LEUKOCYTES
(A possible indication of a urinary tract infection)

A leukocyte is a white blood cell, of which there are many types; they are particularly important in helping to fight infections. When there is an infection or inflammation in the body, the amount of leukocytes usually increases at the site of the infection. Thus, any noticeable increase in leukocytes in the urine usually indicates an infection called pyuria somewhere in the urinary tract (kidneys, ureters, bladder, urethra, plus the prostate in men). The test helps confirm the results of the urine nitrite test (see Urine Tests, **Clinical Analysis: Nitrite**) as an indication of a urinary tract infection.

What Is Usual

It is normal to find a few leukocytes in urine, and women seem to have more leukocytes than men, but these should never amount to more than a trace when tested by a dipstick color indicator.

What You Need

Obtain a dipstick-type test strip such as the Chemstrip L, which costs approximately $10.00 per 100 strips. Some multiple-test dipsticks include the leukocyte test and the urine nitrite test. They cost from $0.10 to $0.30 per test, depending on the quantity purchased and the number of different tests on the dipstick.

Note: Most doctors suggest using a midstream urine specimen for this test. One exception is testing the first ounce of urine (called a first-catch specimen) when a sexually transmitted disease is suspected, since such conditions usually affect the urethra first (see Urine Tests, **Urine Observations: Two-/ Three-Glass Test**).

What to Watch Out For

Because the color change is so slight between a positive and negative result, good color vision is required. When using the Chemstrip L, it may be necessary to leave the dipstick in the urine for 15 minutes before a color change appears.

What the Test Results Can Mean

A positive test, especially one confirmed by a positive urine nitrite test, is sufficient to warrant medical consultation. If the positive tests are accompanied by any symptoms of a urinary tract infection, immediate medical attention should be sought. If a first-catch specimen is positive, even if there are no symptoms, medical attention is warranted.

Reliability

When this test is positive, there is a 90 percent chance that a urinary tract infection exists. It is considered accurate enough for professional use and is usually the primary test performed in hospitals, doctors' offices and commercial laboratories.

CLINICAL ANALYSIS: NITRITE
(Primarily an indication of a urinary tract infection)

A urinary tract infection is now the second most frequently diagnosed infection in medicine; it is estimated that 8 million Americans (7 million of them women) will have this condition at any given time. It has also been reported that 30 million women will suffer pain or discomfort during urination every year and that a urinary tract infection is the cause of 80 percent of this problem. By learning to test your urine for nitrite on a regular basis, before symptoms occur, it is possible to detect this infection early enough to avoid pain as well as extensive and expensive treatment and to prevent kidney complications. Once symptoms develop (burning, frequency of urination, low abdominal cramps, etc.), a medical consultation is warranted.

Urine nitrite testing offers a reasonably accurate means of indicating the possibility of a urinary tract infection. It does not, however, ascertain the source or location of the infection; it could be in the kidneys, the ureters (the tiny tubes that carry urine from the kidneys to the bladder) or the bladder itself. At times the test can hint at an infection of the prostate or urethra (the tube that carries urine from the bladder to the outside). The test result depends on obtaining urine that has stayed in the bladder for several hours, allowing bacteria, if present, to act on dietary nitrates and change them to nitrites; thus, the first morning specimen is best for testing. Because not all types of bacteria affect urine in the same way, the test is not an absolute one. When urinary tract infection is suspected, however, the test can help confirm the suspicions, and when used in conjunction with the urine leukocyte test (see Urine Tests, **Clinical Analysis: Leukocytes**), the accuracy and significance of the test are increased.

The technique for collecting the urine is important; obtaining a clean-catch specimen (see the discussion of the clean-catch specimen in Urine Tests, **Obtaining a Urine Sample**), with all the attendant cleansing that this requires, also helps ensure greater accuracy.

When patients are susceptible to repeated urinary tract infections, many doctors have those patients test their urine weekly (or even every other day). Should the results be positive, the patients then take a prescribed dose of whatever medicine the doctor prefers; this can abort a full-blown infection and prevent the many uncomfortable symptoms that usually accompany the condition. The test is also employed to follow the success or failure of a particular treatment for a urinary tract infection.

What Is Usual
Normally, urine is sterile; thus, the urine nitrite test results should be negative (show no evidence of nitrite that would be produced by urinary bacteria).

If the total urine specimen is tested, as opposed to a clean-catch specimen, the test may be slightly positive due to the possibility of bacteria at the entrance to the urethra.

What You Need
The test can be performed using a dipstick-type testing strip that includes the nitrite test; the N-Uristix is the least expensive, at approximately $14.00 for 100 test strips, and this strip also includes the urine glucose and protein tests (see Urine Tests, **Clinical Analysis: Glucose** and **Clinical Analysis: Protein**). Other multiple-test dipsticks that include the nitrite test cost from $0.10 to $0.30 per strip, depending on the quantity purchased and the number of different tests on the dipstick.

A Microstix-Nitrite kit is also available; it includes three nitrite test dipsticks and three urine-collection cups and costs $6.55. The kit, which the manufacturer claims will detect 90 percent of all urinary tract infections, allows for three consecutive days of urine self-testing.

What to Watch Out For
The urine sample to be tested should have been in the bladder for at least four hours prior to testing. Also keep the following points in mind:

- If you are taking large amounts of vitamin C and there is an excess of the vitamin in your urine (see Urine Tests, **Clinical Analysis: Vitamin C**), the nitrite test may show a false-negative result.
- Urine that shows a very high result on the specific gravity test (see Urine

Tests, **Clinical Analysis: Specific Gravity**) may also show a false-negative result when tested for nitrites.

• If the urine specimen has been kept standing for more than 30 minutes before testing, a false-positive test may be observed.

• Some drugs that can cause a red color in urine can also cause a false-positive nitrite test.

What the Test Results Can Mean

A positive test usually indicates an infection somewhere in the urinary tract, but it is possible to have an infection and still show a negative test, depending on the causative bacteria. Your doctor can supply you with a special dipstick test called the Microstix-3, which requires a 24-hour incubation period; it can confirm your suspicions and also help identify the bacteria. Two consecutive positive nitrite tests, especially if confirmed by the urine leukocyte test and the **Two-/Three-Glass Test** (discussed under Urine Tests), warrant medical attention. A urinary tract infection can spread back up to the kidneys and become a very serious illness. When used to detect the possibility of a urinary tract infection in infants and children, a positive test and a medical consultation can help prevent complications in later life.

Reliability

This test is considered 90 percent accurate when performed properly. Hospitals and doctors and commercial laboratories use this same test first when a urinary tract infection is suspected. But a negative result does not automatically rule out an infection.

CLINICAL ANALYSIS: pH
(Primarily a reflection of body metabolism)

The pH of urine is an indication of its acidity or alkalinity; pH is usually expressed in terms of a numerical value, with 7 being neutral (that is, neither acid nor alkaline). Less than 7 is acid; greater than 7 is alkaline. Virtually every body activity—the quantity of fluids taken in, the metabolism of food, the amount of physical exertion and even one's emotional state—can alter the degree of acidity of urine.

The kind of foods one eats also influences urinary pH; large amounts of meat or fish in the diet, some fruits such as prunes and cranberries, or even a prolonged lack of food will usually cause an acid reaction. In contrast, eating most citrus fruits (which seem "acid"), along with most vegetables, will cause the urine to be alkaline. Dairy foods seem to prevent acidity in urine.

Some drugs can also alter urinary pH; vitamin C, ammonium chloride used as a diuretic and certain urinary antiseptics may make urine more acid, while antacids such as bicarbonates may make urine alkaline. There are several drugs, especially those used to treat urinary tract infections, that need either an acid or an alkaline urine in order to work more efficiently. Urine ph can also help reflect whether many different body functions are normal. It is possible to help prevent kidney stones by controlling the pH of the urine.

What Is Usual
Urine usually has a pH of about 6; it is slightly acid most of the time. Its pH can normally range from 4.5 to 8, however, depending not only on diet but also on the time of day; it is usually more acid on awakening and more alkaline right after a meal. A good sign of normal kidney function is a pH that varies from 5 to 8 during a 24-hour period.

What You Need
The simplest and least expensive way to test urine pH is with litmus paper. While 100 separate acid and alkaline test strips cost about $0.80, the result will only reveal acidity or alkalinity qualitatively; the strips do not indicate specific numerical values. The test can also be performed with inexpensive chemicals such as those used to test swimming pool water, but these are usually difficult to work with and can be messy. The easiest way of obtaining numerical values for urine pH is by using multiple-test dipstick strips that also measure other urine values. The least expensive of these include pH measurements along with glucose and protein testing. One is called Chemstrip 3; another is called Combistix. They cost from $12.00 to $15.00 for 100 test strips. Test strips that measure up to 10 different urine values, including pH, cost about $0.10 to $0.30 per test, depending on the quantity purchased and the number of different tests on the dipstick.

What to Watch Out For
The following cautions apply when performing pH testing:

- Always keep in mind, in performing this test, that many different foods and drugs can alter urine pH.
- If you are taking drugs, ask your doctor or pharmacist about the possible effect they may have on urine pH.
- Be sure the container used to collect the urine is clean and dry and has no soap or detergent residue that can affect pH.
- Follow the test strip's directions carefully; some dipsticks require a specific waiting period before the test value is read.
- Urine left standing for any length of time allows the growth of contam-

inating bacteria and may show a false-alkaline reaction; it may also give off an ammonia odor.

- When using multiple-test dipsticks, be careful not to let urine from an adjacent test pad contact the pH pad. The adjacent pad could contain test chemicals that alter pH.

What the Test Results Can Mean

If you find that you show a strongly acid pH all the time, it could be from a metabolic condition such as diabetes, but it could also mean kidney trouble, heart or circulatory disease, a lung condition that interferes with proper transfer of oxygen from the lungs to the bloodsteam or an infection somewhere in the body. Prolonged bed rest and starvation can also cause an acid urine.

If you show an alkaline pH regularly, it could reflect stomach or intestinal difficulties, various hormone disorders, some nerve diseases and the possibility of anemia. Urinary tract infections may cause a persistent acid or alkaline urine, depending on the instigating bacteria. A vegetarian diet can also cause a persistent alkaline urine.

Urine that is consistently either alkaline or more than slightly acid warrants a medical consultation.

Reliability

While about 90 percent accurate in determining pH, the test by itself is not significant because the results can mean so many different things. Usually, it is performed along with other related urine tests selected by the doctor for a specific purpose, such as determining the composition of a kidney stone.

CLINICAL ANALYSIS: PHENYLKETONURIA SCREENING
(Primarily a screening test for a genetic disorder; secondarily a test for the abuse of selected drugs or poisoning)

Phenylketonuria (PKU) is an inherited metabolic disorder in which the body cannot properly metabolize phenylalanine, a protein amino acid, because of a genetic deficiency of a particular enzyme. Phenylalanine is found in a variety of foods, especially those high in protein such as milk products; it is rare, or present only in small amounts, in fruits and vegetables. The consequence of an excessive amount of phenylalanine in the body can be mental retardation in about 90 percent of enzyme deficiency cases when phenylketonuria is undetected and untreated. And recently, certain forms of congenital heart disease have been attributed to PKU. The disorder seems to occur once in every 10,000 births and is most common among people from Northern Ireland and western Scotland; in the United States approximately 300 infants are born each year with PKU. Throughout most of the United States, the blood or urine of newborn infants is required to be tested for phenylketonuria. But because of the increasingly common practice of home deliveries and mothers' leaving the hospital a day or so after giving birth, the chances of missing the condition have increased. The test cannot be properly performed until sufficient milk protein in the newborn's diet has had the opportunity to be digested—a minimum of 24 hours (many experts say two weeks) after the infant has had its first meal of formula or milk. Breast-fed infants must be tested again one month later.

The urine dipstick test for phenylpyruvic acid (a by-product of phenylalanine) is only a screening test for PKU; it does not offer a definitive diagnosis. The test, however, can provide a valuable warning signal for pregnant women (large amounts of phenylalanine in the urine of a mother-to-be reflect a condition that can damage the fetus), for relatives of patients with phenylketonuria and for infants who have unexplained convulsions or severe diaper rash, albeit they once tested negative for PKU. Many doctors recommend that every newborn be tested at home once a week until the infant is 6 weeks of age, in order to identify any infant in whom PKU might have been missed during required hospital testing. The test is also performed to help parents evaluate the efficacy of dietary treatment for the disease.

Although this test is primarily intended for PKU screening, it has also been found to be of value in:

- Detecting the abuse of certain tranquilizers (phenothiazine preparations such as Compazine, Phenergan, Sparine, Stelazine, Temaril, Thorazine and Vesprin).
- Detecting salicylate poisoning or abuse (aspirin is one form of salicylate).

What Is Usual
No trace of phenylpyruvic acid should be detected in the urine when the dipstick is pressed against a freshly wet diaper or dipped into collected urine. A very small amount of dietary phenylalanine seems necessary for normal growth, but children differ markedly as to how much they can eat, and properly metabolize, without showing symptoms of phenylketonuria.

What You Need
You should obtain a dipstick-type test strip called Phenistix; these strips cost from $7.00 to $8.00 for a bottle of 50.

What to Watch Out For
In performing this test, keep the following points in mind:

- Only freshly voided urine should be tested.
- Do not perform the test on disposable diapers; many have been manufactured with chemicals that can cause both false-positive and false-negative reactions.
- If the urine has a greenish color also check the urine for bilirubin (see Urine Tests, **Clinical Analysis: Bilirubin.**)

What the Test Results Can Mean

A positive test warrants immediate medical attention, even though false-positive results are frequent; blood phenylalanine measurements must be performed to confirm the diagnosis. The sooner a definitive diagnosis is made, the sooner dietary treatment can begin; early treatment can prevent mental retardation.

Negative tests should be repeated up to 6 weeks of age; a negative test in an infant with any suspicion of retardation, convulsions or eczema (severe rash) should not be considered definitive, and immediate medical attention is warranted.

Note: People who cannot metabolize phenylalanine should not use the artificial sweetener (sugar substitute) called aspartame (one brand name is NutraSweet; another is Equal), since they contain phenylalanine.

Although the test can be performed on mothers-to-be who were once treated, or are still being treated, for phenylketonuria, it is necessary to have blood phenylalanine levels tested as soon as pregnancy is contemplated as well as early in and throughout the pregnancy. Elevated blood phenylalanine levels in a pregnant woman can harm the fetus by causing mental retardation; an excess of the amino acid can also cause congenital heart disease and other birth defects.

Drug abuse. A positive test (color change) unrelated to phenylketonuria screening should make one think of an excessive use of certain tranquilizers or aspirin and other salicylates. Children and the elderly, because of their metabolism, are much more susceptible to salicylate poisoning—especially if they have access to any of the hundreds of products containing aspirin, salicylates, salicylamide or salsalates. Some of the symptoms and signs of salicylate poisoning include: multiple black-and-blue bruises, confusion, disorientation, drowsiness, nausea and vomiting, ringing in the ears, difficulty in breathing, muscle twitchings, inappropriate sweating and a flushed face, a rapid heart rate and low blood pressure; at times such a condition could be mistaken for drunkenness. Usually, the Phenistix turns brownish yellow with moderate salicylate poisoning and purple with a more severe overdose; any color change warrants medical attention (see Urine Tests, **Clinical Analysis: Drug Abuse Identification**).

Reliability
Unfortunately, because phenylketonuria is rare, a great number of false-positive tests occurs; for every real positive result, it is estimated that there are 100 false-positive results—making the screening test alone only about 1 percent accurate. Still, it is better to follow up on a false-positive result in order to help prevent PKU. It must also be noted that not all children with a confirmed positive test have mental retardation.

CLINICAL ANALYSIS: PREGNANCY
(More than just a means of detecting pregnancy; also a means of preventing some birth defects)

Usually, once each month, halfway between menstrual periods, a fertile woman gives off an egg (ovum) from one of her ovaries. This is called **ovulation time** (see Genitourinary System Tests). The egg then starts its travels through the Fallopian tube to the uterus. If, during its passage, the egg meets a sperm, it may become fertilized. If fertilized, it may then attach itself to the wall of the uterus through contact with specially formed cells that eventually become the placenta, and pregnancy occurs. Once the fertilized egg has been implanted in the uterus, those specially formed cells start giving off a hormone called human chorionic gonadotropin (HCG). And it is the detection of this hormone in urine that is the basis for the pregnancy test. As pregnancy progresses, the amount of the hormone increases for the first two months; the usual home-type tests can now detect the hormone at the time that the missed menstrual period should have occurred (certain intricate laboratory assays can pick up traces of the hormone within a week after conception, or prior to when the menstrual period would have begun).

Pregnancy tests not only are performed to confirm an existing pregnancy but also are, or should be, performed before a woman of childbearing age who could be pregnant has X-ray examinations (see Environmental Tests, **Radiation Monitoring**) or takes drugs—even some drugs that do not require a prescription. Only in this way can she avoid any adverse effects that radiation and medication might have on the fetus.

When the pregnancy test is performed prior to the use of a new drug, as a means of avoiding any risk to the fetus, you can also ask your doctor or pharmacist to tell you the *pregnancy category* of the drug. The FDA has assigned use-in-pregnancy ratings for drugs to indicate whether they could damage an unborn child if taken by a mother-to-be. These ratings are shown in Figure 23.

Several relatively rapid screening tests for pregnancy are available from pharmacies and from some supermarkets as well as from doctors directly. The home tests contain HCG, usually attached to human or sheep red blood

Figure 23. The FDA's drug use-in-pregnancy rating scale.

Category	Meaning
A	There is no evident risk based on studies.
B	Animal studies show some risk; human studies show no risk.
C	There is the possibility of risk to the fetus; no adequate studies have been made.
D	There is definite evidence of risk to the fetus.
X	The medication is definitely contraindicated; its risks outweigh any possible benefits.

cells, and HCG antiserum from either humans, sheep or rabbits. The antiserum neutralizes most potentially interfering substances in the urine, and if a woman has been secreting her own HCG, she will also be manufacturing HCG antibodies. When HCG and HCG antibodies are present, they will combine with the blood cells and reveal their presence. One form of pregnancy test uses agglutination, forming a precipitation of granules at the bottom of a test tube when positive. This is easily seen as a ring of particles settling in the form of sediment. If no HCG is present, the blood cells remain in suspension, and no ring or clumping of particles is seen (see Figure 24). Some of the newer home tests use a dipstick technique; others are based on a color change in a test tube. Each home test comes with explicit, easy-to-follow directions. Always use the first morning urine specimen for testing.

A great many drugs can cause a false-positive pregnancy test, and this must be kept in mind. A few examples include:

- Tranquilizers such as barbiturates, Compazine, Librium, Phenergan (also used as an antihistaminic or antiallergy medication), Stelazine, Thorazine and Valium.
- Antibiotics such as penicillin, streptomycin and some sulfa preparations.
- Pain relievers such as codeine, Darvon, Demerol, methadone and morphine.
- Hormones such as cortisone preparations, estrogens, insulin, progesterone and thyroid.
- Caffeine in excessive amounts.

A few of the special pregnancy tests supplied by doctors, however, will not show a false-positive reaction from drugs.

It is also possible to have a false-positive urine pregnancy test if your diet has included raw milk and after you receive certain vaccines for immunization; both can cause the formation of specific antibodies that react with the pregnancy test.

A urine specimen that contains bacteria, blood or protein or has a high specific gravity may show a false-positive result (see Urine Tests, **Clinical**

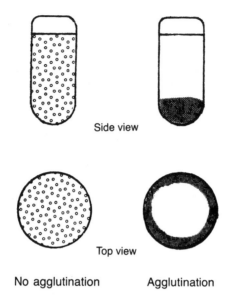

Side view

Top view

No agglutination   Agglutination

Figure 24. Agglutination, such as might be seen in certain urine pregnancy tests.

Analysis: Nitrite, Clinical Analysis: Blood, Clinical Analysis: Protein and **Clinical Analysis: Specific Gravity.**) A urine specimen that has a very low specific gravity may not contain enough HCG to show up on the test.

What Is Usual
It is usual to have a positive test in the presence of pregnancy and a negative test where pregnancy does not exist. Some women in the menopause may show a false-positive result with certain types of pregnancy tests. Because so many drugs can cause a false-positive test, these must be taken into consideration before concluding that pregnancy actually exists. A negative test should be repeated one week later if there is any suspicion or fear of pregnancy.

What You Need
Home pregnancy test kits vary in price, claimed sensitivity, ease of use and time required. There does not seem to be one "best" test at this time. Most take from 15 minutes to 30 minutes. Pregnancy tests supplied by doctors can show results in 90 seconds if pregnancy exists, even before the next menstrual period is due. They cost the doctor from $1.00 to $2.00 per test.

What to Watch Out For
The following are some cautions for at-home pregnancy testing:

- Do not test urine that is more than one hour old; although many tests allow refrigeration of urine if there is to be a delay in testing, the older a urine specimen is, the less accurate the test.
- Do not place the tube in the sun or near any source of heat; it could cause a false result.
- Do not attempt the test if the liquid in the tube is cloudy; the store will usually replace the test without charge.
- Be sure to follow the test's directions for interpreting the result; a positive result may look quite different with each different brand of test.
- If you have any doubt about the color or condition of your urine before you start the test, perform urine blood, nitrite, protein and specific gravity tests (pregnancy tests supplied by doctors usually overcome the interfering effects not only of these substances but of most drugs as well; do not test yourself for pregnancy if your urine tests positive for blood, nitrite or protein or shows a low specific gravity.

What the Test Results Can Mean

A negative pregnancy test, especially after a missed menstrual period, may mean that the test was performed too early to match the sensitivity of the particular brand of test; repeat the test one week later. If still negative, in the face of a missed menstrual period, a medical consultation is warranted.

A positive pregnancy test most often means pregnancy; medical attention is warranted. It is never too early in pregnancy to start professional prenatal care. A positive test can, however, also come from many other conditions: infections such as hepatitis have been known to cause a positive result; various tumors of the ovary and uterus can cause a positive test; even menstrual irregularities may cause a positive test, albeit false. Thus, a positive pregnancy test warrants medical attention—if only to determine the cause should it be a false-positive result.

Reliability

When properly performed, home pregnancy tests are 95 percent accurate. There can be a difference in the sensitivity of the various brands of tests; some detect much smaller amounts of HCG and could detect pregnancy at an earlier point. Because home pregnancy tests are constantly being improved, consult your doctor for the latest information. Failure to follow the instructions is the prime cause of inaccuracy. There have, however, been incidents of manufacturing defects, so if in doubt, and if privacy is important, perform the test again with a different brand. Furthermore, if you "feel" pregnant, especially if you have been pregnant before, seek medical attention. There have been cases of miscarriages following false-negative tests and abortions have been erroneously performed on pregnant women who showed repeated negative pregnancy test results.

CLINICAL ANALYSIS: PROTEIN
(A generalized screening test for several latent diseases)

While urine testing is considered the best, easiest-to-perform home test for health evaluation, the urine test for protein is probably the most valuable single urine examination. It is the best overall screening test for kidney disease as well and can also offer an early warning sign of heart and artery problems; liver, nerve and thyroid dysfunction; and even hidden cancers and viral disease. As blood flows through the kidneys, a very tiny amount of protein is normally filtered out into the urine, but in such a minute quantity that it is usually not detectable through routine testing. Normal protein products in the blood consist primarily of albumins and globulins. Albumins help keep a proper chemical-to-plasma balance in the blood; they also attach themselves to hormones, enzymes, vitamins and drugs and carry them throughout the body to provide nutrition for cells and assist in their metabolic functions. Globulins form and help transport immune substances throughout the body to fight off infections and other diseases.

The use of many different drugs (in particular, those for high blood pressure and for joint pains), certain foods (such as an excessive intake of protein) and irritants such as mustard, exposure to chemical poisons, strenuous physical exercise, being chilled, and even extreme anxiety or discomfort can temporarily cause a positive protein test reaction, and all these nondisease factors must be taken into account when testing urine for protein.

What Is Usual
Although some doctors dismiss an occasional trace of detectable protein in the urine, the general consensus is that unless there is a good explanation for its presence (exercise, cold, the use of certain antibiotics or some sleeping medicines, etc.), there should never be any measurable protein in the urine. And if protein should be detected, it should only be observed temporarily; it should not persist. There is a condition known as orthostatic albuminuria, in which a few people show protein in the urine whenever they are standing for a period of time—such as when playing golf—but the protein should be completely absent when the urine is tested after the individual has been lying down for a few hours. For home testing, however, it is best to consider urine as ideally being totally protein-free.

What You Need
The easiest way to test for urine protein is with a dipstick-type plastic strip. Strips that test only for protein are available as Albustix, for about $9.00 per 100 test strips. Combistix GP strips, which test for both glucose and protein, sell for about the same price. Most multiple-test dipsticks include protein as one component and cost about $0.10 to $0.30 per test, depending on the quantity purchased and the number of different tests on the dipstick.

There are other ways to test for urine protein:

• One is to place the urine in a heatproof test tube and warm the upper portion of the urine in the tube over a flame for a few seconds. If protein is present, the upper portion of the urine sample will congeal or cloud up, much like the cooked white of an egg, while the lower portion of the sample will remain clear (see Figure 25).

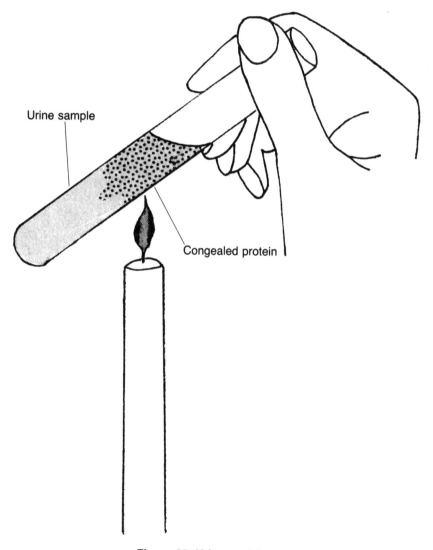

Figure 25. Urine protein test.

- Another way is to add about one teaspoon of white vinegar slowly down the side of the tube (or glass) into the urine and look for clouding.

What to Watch Out For

A false-positive test can come from:

- Residual cleaning substances in the container used to hold the urine.
- Any contamination of the urine specimen (menstruation, vaginal discharge, a prostrate infection, sexual activity).
- An alkaline urine (see Urine Tests, **Clinical Analysis: pH**).
- Recent X-rays over the abdomen.
- The use of certain drugs; check with your doctor or pharmacist.
- The test strip's being old or having been exposed to air, light or heat for a period of time.

Be sure to observe the strict time limitations stipulated in the test's directions, and only read color changes if you have normal color vision.

What the Test Results Can Mean

From 5 percent to 10 percent of the population (mostly men) will have a positive urine protein test without having an underlying disease; however, proteinuria, as protein in the urine is called, can also come from:

- Kidney disease and urinary tract conditions such as bladder infections.
- Sexually transmitted diseases.
- High blood pressure, not necessarily due to kidney involvement.
- Other forms of heart and artery disease.
- Diabetes and certain other hormone imbalances.
- Infections—no matter where they are in the body.
- Several different forms of cancer.
- Some very rare conditions such as lupus erythematosus or amyloidosis.

A positive test could also be an early warning sign of metal or chemical poisoning (arsenic, cleaning fluids, formaldehyde, fluorides, nutmeg, etc.).

A positive test should always be repeated several hours, or even a day, later; an occasional positive test can be normal. When urine shows protein, many doctors have their patients repeat the test at home for several days to save the patients time and money. The finding of protein in the urine on more than one occasion, especially when there seems to be no known or obvious nondisease cause, warrants medical consultation, even if only to rule out a defective test strip. Because persistent proteinuria may be an early warning sign of kidney or heart disease, such a test finding justifies ruling out any potential disease process as soon as possible.

Reliability

Although the test is 95 percent accurate in revealing protein when present, it can also react in the presence of drugs and show a false color change. A positive test rarely reveals the specific cause of urine protein.

CLINICAL ANALYSIS: SPECIFIC GRAVITY
(A simple screening test to assess kidney function)

The specific gravity of urine is a reflection of its density—that is, an indication of the amount of solid material dissolved in the urine specimen being tested. A somewhat newer term, more popular with the medical profession, is *osmolality*. Osmolality, although essentially meaning "specific gravity," is alleged to be a more precise measurement. Many chemicals such as sodium chloride grains (salt), urea nitrogen compounds, sugar molecules, protein particles, calcium, phosphates and sulfates that are normally dissolved in blood are filtered out of the blood by the kidneys and become virtually invisible matter in urine. The greater the amount of dissolved substances in the urine solution, the higher its specific gravity.

In a normal individual eating and drinking a typical American diet, approximately 450 gallons of blood flow through the kidneys every 24 hours. The kidneys filter out approximately 45 gallons of plasma each day and then reabsorb all but 1 quart to 1.5 quarts of fluid, which ultimately end up in the bladder. With urination, a portion of urine containing the dissolved material leaves the body and can be tested. Urine specific gravity measurements are but one of several indications as to the kidneys' ability to function properly.

Mosenthal test. The specific gravity test's principal purpose is to assist, along with several other related tests, in the evaluation of kidney function and to aid in locating that part of the kidney that might be malfunctioning. One way of doing this is to assess the kidneys' ability to concentrate urine under controlled conditions; this assessment, sometimes called the Mosenthal test, is performed as follows:

Drink no liquids (usual solid foods are permitted) for 24 hours prior to testing. Then, on awakening in the morning, test the urine for specific gravity. Return to bed and stay as relaxed as possible for another hour and then test a second urine specimen for specific gravity. Following the second test, get up and be active for one more hour (eat or drink nothing during the test) and test a third urine specimen for specific gravity. At least one of the three urine samples tested should show a specific gravity of 1.025 or higher as an indication that the kidneys can concentrate urine when liquids are withheld. If all three samples show a specific gravity of less than 1.020, medical consultation is warranted for more specific kidney evaluation. This test should not be performed when there is the slightest suspicion of kidney disease except under a doctor's supervision.

What Is Usual

Specific gravity is reported as a numerical figure based on the relative value of distilled water—1.000, since it contains no dissolved solids; therefore, the greater the amount of solid matter dissolved in solution, the higher the re-sulting number. Single urine specific gravity values usually range from 1.010 to 1.025, assuming a typical diet, typical fluid intake and moderate physical activity; throughout a 24-hour day, different measurements should show a variation of at least 0.010 in two or more samples.

A normal specific gravity measurement can also reflect many different circumstances: the time of day (after a night's sleep, without food or fluids, the specific gravity is greater and shows a higher reading than after routine daytime activities and diet); the quantity and quality of foods and fluids (the more liquids consumed, the more dilute the urine and the lower the specific gravity reading); excessive physical activity (when body fluid is lost through perspiration, there is less fluid to pass through the kidneys, resulting in a less dilute urine and a higher specific gravity reading). Thus, a single mea-surement ranging from 1.005 to 1.035 could still be normal, depending on the circumstances.

What You Need

The most common test apparatus to determine urine specific gravity is a hydrometer (frequently called a urinometer when sold primarily for urinal-ysis). It is a small, weighted glass float with a numerical scale that indicates how deeply the float sinks into the liquid being tested. The scale usually reads from 1.000 to 1.060; the greater the amount of dissolved material, the less the float sinks and the higher the specific gravity reading (see Figure 26). A hydrometer (urinometer) ranges in cost from $3.00 to $5.00, depend-ing on its size, and usually comes with a tall glass tube in which to place the hydrometer; the smaller size is quite adequate for urine testing. For re-peated measurements that is the least expensive equipment.

The newest and simplest technique for testing urine specific gravity uti-lizes a thin strip of chemically treated paper (shown in Figure 19) that is dipped into a urine sample; the color change is compared with a chart to give specific gravity values. These plastic dip-and-test strips are comprehen-sive dipsticks that not only test for specific gravity but also include other urine tests on the same strip; they cost from $0.10 to $0.30 per strip, de-pending on the quantity purchased and the number of different tests on the dipstick.

What to Watch Out For

Although routine testing of urine for specific gravity has no adverse effects, measurements that involve evaluating the concentration and dilution of urine following excessive intake and then deprivation of fluids should not be un-dertaken if there is a suspicion of kidney disease, except under a doctor's supervision. At such times it could be dangerous to deprive the kidneys of fluids.

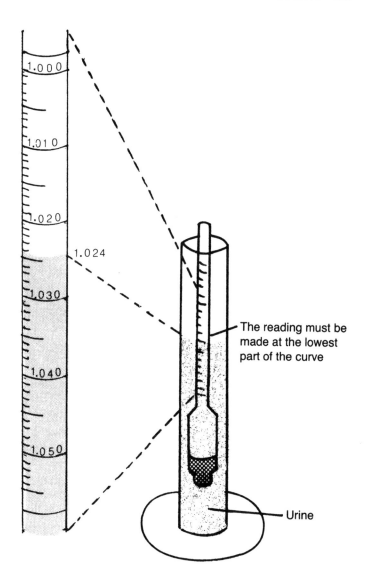

Figure 26. Urine specific gravity test, as measured by a urinometer.

As a general check on the accuracy of urine specific gravity measurements, you should be aware that a high specific gravity is usually found in urine with a deep amber or orange color, while a lower specific gravity is usually found in urine with a lighter yellow and clearer color. An inconsistency between specific gravity and color can point to disease.

When using a hydrometer, it is important to have sufficient urine in the glass cylinder to ensure that the hydrometer floats freely and that it does not touch the sides of the tube. The hydrometer must be kept scrupulously clean. The reading should come from the lowest part of the curve formed by the top of the liquid against the scale. Urinary hydrometers must be checked for accuracy regularly (by placing the hydrometer in distilled water, where it should read 1.000) since they frequently become erroneous.

If a urine specimen contains abnormal amounts of sugar, protein or other chemicals, the specific gravity readings will be abnormally high, and the effect of such substances must be taken into account to obtain a correct reading. If urine pH measures 6.0 or greater, the specific gravity readings could be falsely low; add .005 to the reading. If you have been taking diuretic drugs, the specific gravity reading will be low as a result of the excessive amount of fluid that the drugs prevent the kidneys from reabsorbing.

What the Test Results Can Mean

When urine specific gravity shows a value of from 1.015 to 1.030 in the first specimen voided that day, and assuming no intake of food or drink for the previous eight hours, it is usually a reasonable indication that the kidneys are capable of concentrating urine normally. Additional evidence of normal kidney functioning would be a specific gravity measurement of from 1.007 to 1.020 in the evening, especially after normal intake of food and drink during the day, showing the kidney's ability to dilute the urine when appropriate. An occasional deviation from what would be expected is not necessarily an abnormal result, especially when hydration, physical activity and diet are taken into account. It is the repeated observation of unexpected, abnormal values that points to a kidney malfunction or some hormone imbalance.

As an example of how the specific gravity test can hint at hormone activity (as long as all other kidney function tests are normal), when an individual is subjected to unusual stress—especially of an emotional nature—or pressure, the specific gravity may read as high as 1.040. Anxiety-producing situations can cause an antidiuretic hormone (ADH) known as vasopressin to be manufactured in greater-than-normal amounts. This hormone slows down excretion of urine from the kidneys, and the fluid that does filter through becomes very concentrated. Some doctors use this test as a means of evaluating a patient's response to emotional provocation.

Another antidiuretic hormone appraisal consists of the repeated observation of urine with a high specific gravity accompanied by an unexplained bad temper, confusion and sometimes convulsions and coma. This can, at times, come from the "syndrome of inappropriate antidiuretic hormone secretion" (SIADH), and while it may be brought on as a consequence of cancer, severe infections and many other diseases, it can also occur as a side effect of many medicines, especially diuretic drugs. The discovery of this syndrome can be a warning signal to search for some undetected disorder.

Diseases of the parathyroid gland that prevent the kidneys from excreting normal amounts of calcium in the urine can result in extremely low urine specific gravity measurements; taking too much vitamin D can also cause similar test results. And when amounts of urine voided reach from 10 quarts to 20 quarts a day, along with specific gravity measurements of 1.007 or less, it is a fairly reliable indication of diabetes insipidus, a rare disease in which the pituitary gland fails to manufacture sufficient vasopressin—the antidiuretic hormone. While the condition can be inherited, it can also occur after a head injury or subsequent to severe generalized infections.

If abnormal specific gravity measurements persist or do not correspond with usual patterns of eating, drinking and other physical activity, the test could be an early warning sign of some impending disease process. A particularly ominous observation is specific gravity measurements that stay close to the same numerical value at all times. Repeated abnormal specific gravity measurements are sufficient reason to seek medical attention.

Reliability
All tests for specific gravity are at least 95 percent accurate as to the reading. Abnormal readings that cannot be explained by diet, fluid intake, physical activity and so on are 80 percent reliable as an indication of kidney dysfunction.

CLINICAL ANALYSIS: UROBILINOGEN
(A screening test, primarily to detect liver disease but also used as an early warning sign for generalized infections)

Urobilinogen is formed in the intestine from bilirubin, a yellow pigment that is part of the liver's bile (see Urine Tests, **Clinical Analysis: Bilirubin**). Very minute amounts are filtered from blood by the kidneys and can be detected in urine. For some unknown reason, afternoon urine—collected between 1:00 p.m. and 3:00 p.m.—contains the greatest concentration of urobilinogen, and when looking for this specific substance, midafternoon is the best time for testing. As with so many other urine tests, the taking of certain drugs, such as those used to treat gout and especially antibiotics, can cause false-negative values. At times the use of aspirin products can cause a false-positive result. Unlike many other urine tests, noting an absence of any urobilinogen in the urine can be as important as finding an excess. Because urobilinogen is one of the many end products of the breakdown of red blood cells, its presence can reflect certain anemias, especially those that come from red cell destruction. Its presence in more than trace amounts can also signal liver disease. Although the urobilinogen test can be performed by itself, it is more accurate when accompanied by the urine bilirubin test as a substantiating check.

What Is Usual
It is considered normal to show no more than a trace of urobilinogen in urine, especially when the test is performed in the afternoon.

What You Need
Although there are many chemical tests for urobilinogen, the easiest is one of the dipstick methods. A single-test strip for urobilinogen called the Urobilistix is available at $9.00 for 50 strips, but it is better to use one of the dipsticks that also incorporate the test for bilirubin, usually along with several other tests; these cost from $0.10 to $0.30 per test strip.

What to Watch Out For
Keep the following points in mind when testing for urine urobilinogen:

- The urine to be tested must be freshly voided—not more than five minutes old.
- It must not be too acid, or a false-negative result can occur; if the urine is too alkaline, a false-positive result can occur. This is another reason why a multiple-test strip incorporating pH testing is more accurate (see Urine Tests, **Clinical Analysis: pH**).
- The test strips must be fresh and must not have been subjected to heat or moisture.
- Any drug use that could interfere with the test must be noted (check with your doctor or pharmacist).
- Although a very low urobilinogen level may be detected, a negative test is not sensitive enough to indicate an absolute absence of urobilinogen.
- You must have normal color vision to assess the dipstick color changes accurately.

What the Test Results Can Mean
Increased levels of urobilinogen usually mean liver or bile duct disease (any condition that prevents urobilinogen from being reabsorbed into the liver). Some other generalized infections such as mononucleosis (see Blood Tests, **Mononucleosis**) can cause an elevated urine urobilinogen level. Prolonged constipation and some forms of heart disease that slow the circulation may also cause a positive test. While a few forms of anemia can also raise urobilinogen in the urine, the test is not specific enough to warrant anything but a medical consultation if any increase is noted; when performed with a urine bilirubin test, it can help distinguish liver disease from a blood problem.

Reliability

The test's reliability is equal to that of professional laboratory testing; when interfering factors are eliminated, the test is 90 percent accurate. The Ames brand dipstick is considered the most sensitive.

CLINICAL ANALYSIS: VITAMIN C
(An aid that can enhance the accuracy of several urine tests)

Because of an ancient, genetically transmitted defect, the human is one of very few mammals that cannot manufacture their own vitamin C (ascorbic acid). And although this vitamin is not stored in large amounts in the body, it is still essential to the body's defense mechanisms (resistance to all forms of disease) and to the formation of bones and teeth. With a fairly normal diet, an individual usually ingests sufficient amounts of vitamin C to take care of the body's needs on a day-to-day basis; the addition of supplementary vitamins (commonly in pill or powder form) more than makes up for any daily deficiency—unless, of course, you are a believer in the theory that humans need far greater amounts of ascorbic acid than is presently recommended by most nutritionists. People who do take supplementary amounts of vitamin C (even as little as 300 mg a day), let alone massive or megadoses, inevitably spill any excess not utilized by the body into their urine, and large amounts of vitamin C in the urine can cause the following effects on Urine Tests:

- A false urine bilirubin test (see **Clinical Analysis: Bilirubin**).
- A false urine glucose test (see: **Clinical Analysis: Glucose**).
- A false urine blood test (see: **Clinical Analysis: Blood**).
- A false urine nitrite test (see: **Clinical Analysis: Nitrite**).
- An abnormally high acidity result on the urine pH test (see: **Clinical Analysis: pH**).

Note: This test should also be performed prior to testing feces for occult blood (see Mouth, Throat and Gastrointestinal Tests, **Occult Blood [Feces]** test); large amounts of vitamin C in the body, as reflected by the urine, can cause a false-negative feces blood test.

The test is primarily of value when used to ascertain the accuracy of other urine tests; it can, of course, also indicate an absence of vitamin C in urine, but this test alone does not necessarily mean the individual has a definite vitamin C deficiency (scurvy).

What Is Usual

Most healthy people on a balanced diet will excrete about 20 mg of ascorbic acid when measured in all urine passed over a 24-hour period. The amount may vary from a trace to 10 mg per 100 ml in a single urine specimen; and on occasion, depending on diet, a urine sample may show 40 mg per 100 ml or more at one time. When large amounts of vitamin C are taken, the test may show proportionately large amounts in the urine.

What You Need
The test can be performed using a dipstick called C-STIX, which tests only for vitamin C and which costs from $8.00 to $10.00 for a bottle of 50 sticks. There are multiple-test urine dipsticks that include a test for vitamin C; they cost from $0.10 to $0.30 per strip, depending on the quantity purchased and the number of different tests on the dipstick. The Chemstrip 9 dipstick is claimed to be free from vitamin C interference, but large amounts of vitamin C in urine may still alter test results.

What to Watch Out For
The following guidelines should be kept in mind when you test urine for the presence of vitamin C:

- The test must be performed on freshly voided urine; urine that has been left standing for more than 15 minutes may give false-negative values.
- The timing of the test is important; follow the test directions explicitly.
- If the original color on the dipstick does not match the "O" on the accompanying color chart before use, or does not match the "O" when dipped in distilled water, do not use that bottle of dipsticks.
- Certain drugs can cause false reactions; check with your doctor or pharmacist if you are using any medicine.

What the Test Results Can Mean
Large amounts of vitamin C in the urine can make urine test results for blood, glucose, nitrite and pH inaccurate.

Very little, or no, vitamin C in the urine can mean an anemia, especially in an infant who is fed nothing but milk, and can also accompany infection, alcoholism and hiatal hernia (in which a portion of the stomach extends back up through the diaphragm and can cause an indigestion type of heartburn; see Mouth, Throat and Gastrointestinal Tests, **String Test**). Some people with cancer show a very low level of vitamin C, even with a normal diet and vitamin C supplements. Repeated results showing no, or very little, vitamin C warrant medical consultation.

Reliability
A positive test result is 90 percent accurate in indicating excessive vitamin C in urine and is a sufficient basis for questioning the results of other urine (and feces) tests.

BLOOD TESTS

Analysis of the chemicals and other constituents of blood has long been used to help diagnose illness and search for early warning signs of impending disease. There are now more than 2,000 different analytical procedures that can be performed on a blood sample.

Blood carries oxygen, enzymes, hormones and essential nutrients to all parts of the body; it also carries away carbon dioxide and other waste products of metabolism to the lungs, kidneys and skin. Thus, when something goes wrong anywhere in the body, cellular and/or chemical changes can occur in the blood and may reflect a disease or disorder. When tests are performed to study the red and white blood cells or platelets, such testing is usually referred to as hematology; when testing is limited to electrolytes, enzymes, fats, gases, hormones, minerals, proteins and protein products, sugars or organ products such as from the liver, it is usually referred to as blood chemistry studies.

Although blood is composed of a great many substances, for testing purposes it is separated into four categories:

- Whole blood—which includes all the cellular material, red and white blood cells, along with platelets (thrombocytes) and fibrinogen (for clotting), and the serum, or liquid portion, with all its components as well. (Blood from a fingertip is an example of whole blood.)
- Cellular material alone.
- Serum—the clear liquid portion of the blood after it has clotted and the clot (consisting of all cellular material) has been removed.
- Plasma—the pale yellow liquid that remains after blood is collected in a receptacle containing an anticoagulant (heparin or a special chemical compound to prevent clotting); the cellular material, minus the fibrinogen, is removed through centrifugation or by allowing the blood to stand while the solid elements settle to the bottom.

Most clinical laboratories test either serum or plasma because the chemical composition of the blood cells can sometimes be inconsistent; for certain chemical tests only serum can be used. In performing home blood testing, however, only whole blood is used, and it is sufficiently stable and accurate for the tests described in this book.

OBTAINING A BLOOD SAMPLE

What You Need

In order to obtain a blood sample, you should have the following materials:

- A sterile needle or lancet. Those who prefer a needle commonly use a 25-gauge, one-inch-long hypodermic or syringe-style needle; it is best to use individually wrapped, presterilized, disposable needles, which cost from $0.05 to $0.08 each. Most people prefer disposable lancets that let you control the depth of penetration. One commercial brand, called Monolets, costs about $0.05 each. These lancets can also be used with automatic (push-button) pricking devices such as the Autolet, which costs approximately $25.00; the Autoclix, which costs approximately $20.00; or the Penlet, which looks like a small ballpoint pen and costs approximately $10.00. Such devices really do help eliminate much of the anxiety and discomfort of trying to stick oneself.
- Gauze pads or cotton plus rubbing alcohol, or readily available, individually wrapped, alcohol-soaked "swabs," "prep-pads" or Zephirin towelettes, which cost $2.00 per 100.

Where to Stick
There are four areas where a drop of blood is easily obtained. They include:

- *The fingertip*—the most common site (either the index, middle or ring finger); if you make the puncture just slightly to the side of the center of the tip, it is reportedly less painful (some people find that pressing the thumbnail hard against the fingertip about to be punctured also lessens the discomfort).
- *The soft portion of the earlobe*—said to be the least painful area of all. If the earlobe is used, it is usually possible to collect additional drops of blood for additional or repeat tests from the one puncture site without the need for resticking by simply flicking the earlobe with the fingertip.
- *The back of the heel*—supposedly the easiest site to obtain a drop of blood from young children.
- *Alongside the tip of the big toe*—also used mostly with children.

What to Do
Proceed as follows to obtain the sample:

- Wash the area well with soap and water, then dry.
- Rub the selected site with an alcohol-soaked gauze pad or "swab" and let the alcohol evaporate before making the puncture.
- Make a small puncture hole with the needle or lancet.

- Wipe away the first drop of blood that appears with a piece of sterile gauze or cotton.
- Use the next full drop of blood for the test.
- After the blood sample has been obtained, hold a piece of sterile gauze or cotton to the puncture site for a few minutes until the bleeding stops.
- Cover the puncture with a bandage such as a Band-Aid.

What to Watch Out For
Keep the following pointers in mind when obtaining a blood sample:

- Do not puncture an area that is swollen or seems infected.
- Be sure the puncture site is at body temperature; warm it, if necessary, by applying warm cloths or soaking in warm water just before washing.
- Be careful not to squeeze or milk the puncture area to try to force bleeding; this can dilute the blood sample with fluids from adjacent tissues and cause a false test result.
- Never use a needle that has been used by someone else or even one that has been sterilized by boiling; there is always the risk of transmitting disease this way.
- Avoid puncturing the same area repeatedly.
- Never use any material if there is the slightest doubt about its sterility.
- If testing someone else's blood, do not touch the blood sample; it could carry an infection.
- Some blood tests require precision measurements; do not attempt such tests if you cannot be exacting in your technique.

Note: When taking blood, make a note of your position. Blood taken while standing, as opposed to reclining (whether testing is done at home or in a doctor's office or laboratory), can show much higher values for certain tests (for example, cholesterol, hemoglobin).

Most people find that when a blood sample is to be obtained for the first time, it is best to perform the task in front of a doctor; this not only lends reassurance about the technique but also assures that the blood sample is properly obtained.

Reporting Blood Test Results
Depending upon the type of test, blood values may be expressed in many different ways. Most chemical determinations are reported in milligrams per 100 milliliters, or mg per 100 ml (milligrams per deciliter, or ml per dl—a deciliter = 100 milliliters—is now becoming more common). This is an arbitrary measurement, indicating how much of a chemical would be found if 100 ml (3.5 ounces) of blood were evaluated: obviously, only a minute amount of blood is examined, and so 100 ml was chosen for purposes of standardization. Blood glucose and hemoglobin results are reported this way, al-

though it is not unusual to report only the milligram amount as a solitary numerical figure (for instance, a blood sugar level of 110 mg per 100 ml would be reported simply as 110). Clotting time is reported in seconds of time, and many other tests performed merely to determine whether a substance is present or not—such as for sickle-cell hemoglobin—are reported as positive if present and negative if undetectable.

AIDS
(Have you been exposed to, and *possibly* infected with, the acquired immunodeficiency disease syndrome?)

First, understand the meaning of *AIDS*. *Acquired* means that the illness most likely came from contact with someone or something carrying the causative organism. *Immunodeficiency* means a partial or total inability to fight off an infection, an allergy or even a cancer; the body is incapable of producing its usual antibodies, which are the body's primary defense against any disease (these normally consist of protein globulin molecules and certain white blood cells that can destroy agents that can cause disease—such as bacteria, viruses and pollens—or combine with these agents and make them useless). *Syndrome* is a medical term that refers to a particular group of symptoms (subjective complaints) and signs (objective findings) that are fairly consistent in all patients who have the same disability. AIDS, therefore, is not a distinct disease but rather a generalized condition that weakens the body's natural defenses and allows other specific diseases, such as a particular kind of pneumonia, cancer, fungus or skin affliction to ravage the body and even kill the individual. Medical professionals may use the term *HIV*, which stands for "human immunodeficiency virus."

At this time a precise definition of AIDS is virtually impossible; the Public Health Service, which usually spells out the required indications and circumstances for any contagious disease, has literally changed or altered its criteria of signs, symptoms and laboratory evidence for AIDS at least once a year since this condition was formally recognized in 1981. Actually, information about AIDS seems to accrue and change almost daily, so that what is written today may well by out of date tomorrow. It must be assumed, however, that most people not only are aware of the illness but also know most of its unique characteristics as well as the fact that it is prevalent among homosexuals and intravenous drug abusers, called high-risk groups. While attributed to a particular virus infestation called the human immunodeficiency virus, or HIV (previously known as *HTLV-III*, for "human T-lymphocyte virus, type III," to differentiate it from the types I and II, which cause other diseases; or *LAV*, for "lymphadenopathy-associated virus"), there is still some question in the minds of a few medical experts about whether the real cause is known.

What is tentatively agreed upon is that the causative agent, be it HIV or something as yet unknown, does render useless the particular lymph white blood cells that normally help fight off diseases. As a result, the most common manifestations include swollen lymph glands, fever, extreme fatigue, cough and breathing difficulties, candidiasis (white fungus patches in the mouth, sometimes called thrush), black and blue blotches and growths on the skin, vision difficulties and signs of brain damage, to name but a few. The most recent evidence indicates that once the disease is acquired, it may not show any of its symptoms and signs for from several weeks to several years.

There are many different tests for AIDS; most reveal the presence of antibodies to the implicated HIV virus that are produced after the AIDS virus does, in fact, infect the body. The most common, routine test is called an *ELISA* (referring to the technique of using enzymes to detect antibodies). At present, anyone who has a positive ELISA-AIDS antibody test should have that test repeated. If it is positive a second time, a more specific test (called a *Western Blot*) is performed; only if all three tests are positive is the individual then considered positive. It should be mandatory, and it could prevent much grief, that no one be told that his or her AIDS test is positive unless and until all three tests are positive. A positive test, however, does not mean that the individual actually has active AIDS and will manifest its symptoms and signs; it is generally accepted, however, that someone whose test shows antibodies specifically indicating an exposure to AIDS must be assumed to be contagious and capable of passing the condition to others. There are even more precise tests for the presence of the virus and some of its component parts that are being performed by certain laboratories. Whether you go to your physician directly, to a laboratory or obtain blood from your fingertip at home, the test performed is identical. There are several laboratories that will furnish you with a kit to obtain your own blood sample and send it back for testing using your own selected anonymous number or code; you then call in and the test results are furnished, usually along with some counseling. There are also laboratories that allow you to "drop in" for AIDS blood testing without requiring identification—essentially a do-it-yourself test. Regardless of how you choose to be tested, if you do desire such testing, consider the test no more than a screening examination; before you come to any decision about how to react to your test results, you should seek a medical consultation.

What Is Usual

No test result should indicate the presence of AIDS virus or antibodies to the HIV virus, presently suspected to be the cause of the loss of immunity.

It must be noted, however, that there have been cases where a negative AIDS test occurred in people who later developed the physical and mental manifestations of AIDS; it is believed that in these cases the test was performed too early in the course of the conditions's progress, for it seems to take weeks—and even months for some individuals—after exposure before antibodies appear in the blood. Along the same lines, a negative test is no assurance that HIV is not active in the body.

What You Need

There are several companies that plan to offer home test kits for AIDS; many advertise in local newspapers. Some do limit the mailing of their kits to residents of the state where they are located. The following are some of the companies that may supply these kits:

- Discreet Medical Testing Inc. (902 N. Grand Ave., Santa Ana, Calif. 92701)
- National AIDS Testing Hotline Inc. (Fort Lauderdale, Fla. 33310)
- Scientific International Inc. (Fairhope, Ala. 36533)
- USAT Laboratories Inc. (3841 Old Canejo Rd., Newbury Park, Calif. 91320)
- MikroMed Systems Inc. (1661 N. Swan, Tucson, Ariz. 85712)

In general, the cost runs from $30.00 to $50.00, including all necessary material and a prepaid return mailing package although the test itself costs from $1.00 to $2.00. Most of these laboratories will repeat the ELISA test if the first one is positive and also perform a Western Blot test at no extra charge. In addition, many doctors will take your blood and send it to a laboratory for anonymous AIDS testing for the same fee, also essentially a do-it-yourself test.

(Note: At the time this book was written, there was a question as to whether the FDA would allow testing by mail.)

While the ELISA-type test is the most common in use at the present time, many new techniques have been and are being developed. Baxter Healthcare International (Deerfield, IL 60015) now sells a finger-tip blood 5-minute AIDS test developed by Cambridge Bioscience. The test costs $10.00 to a doctor.

What to Watch Out For

If you have any reason to believe that you have been exposed to AIDS, do not accept a negative test as absolute; repeat the test monthly for at least six months. At the same time, taking the test may well imply that you are part of a high-risk group. Most of all, be aware that taking the test and awaiting the results (it can take several days to two weeks with some laboratories albeit the actual test performance time is five minutes) can be extremely stressful; you may need professional help just to cope with that anxiety.

What the Test Results Can Mean

A negative rest result only means that you have no detectable AIDS antibodies in your blood at the time of the test—assuming the test was accurate; only you know whether you may have been exposed to and/or infected with HIV. It does not mean that you are immune to AIDS. A single positive ELISA test result does not necessarily mean that you have AIDS (or ARC, meaning AIDS-related complex—a positive test without *all* the full-blown signs and symptoms of AIDS). As noted, a true-positive result should be based on two positive ELISA tests and a positive Western Blot. At present, only about 30 percent of those with a positive test result seem to come down with the condition itself (although there are some doctors who feel that this figure is far too low). A positive test warrants a medical consultation to learn the latest information about how to stay healthy and become aware of the latest treatments. Depending on your conscience, a positive test should warrant your informing intimate relations and taking measures to protect those intimates from infection. At least, do not donate blood or other body specimens.

Reliability

The accuracy of all ELISA/AIDS antibody tests is not good—even the Western Blot, now considered the most accurate, is not perfect. In many surveys, of those who show an initial positive AIDS antibody test, more than half later turned out to be in error—false-positive. And for some as yet unexplained reason, women seem to have 10 times as many false-positive tests as do men. In general, a single positive routine test for AIDS is considered to be about 20 percent accurate; when a second test is positive along with a positive Western Blot as a third test, the tests together are considered to be 85 percent accurate. There are newer confirmatory tests that are claimed to be 95 percent accurate; at present they cost about $80.00 each. More precise tests for the actual suspected virus and/or its particles are available through professional laboratories. The new 5-minute test has not proved very accurate when performed by physicians (a great many false positives); it is, however, better than 90 percent accurate when performed by trained technicians.

Note: Also see Blood Tests, **Cholesterol** for a discussion of the association between low blood cholesterol values and AIDS.

BLEEDING AND CLOTTING TIME
(A test of how quickly blood coagulates after an incision or injury)

Although they are two essentially different tests, bleeding and clotting time are usually tested together as a crude measure of how quickly bleeding will be stopped by normal body responses—a process called hemostasis. More specifically, bleeding time reflects the condition of the blood vessels—particularly the smallest ones called capillaries—by measuring how well they constrict and close off following an injury. Bleeding time also indicates how well the blood's platelets (tiny cells that clump together to plug each broken capillary) are performing. Clotting time, on the other hand, is a generalized indication of the performance of all the other body chemicals that contribute to clotting: antihemophilic substances, enzymes, minerals (calcium), proteins (prothrombin, the specific clotting factor disabled when anticoagulant drugs are prescribed) and vitamin K.

The two tests offer screening information to help detect bleeding tendencies, whether inherited or resulting from anemia, lead poisoning, liver disease, cancer or radiation exposure; the use of drugs such as adrenalin, aspirin, some antibiotics, oral contraceptives, coumarin products (warfarin), phenylbutazone (for arthritis) and cortisone preparations; or dietary deficiencies of calcium and vitamin K. The tests are especially valuable prior to medical or dental surgery and before certain drugs are prescribed for a prolonged period of time.

Another test that can suggest a bleeding tendency but does not require sticking the finger to obtain blood is the **Capillary Fragility** test (see Heart and Circulation Tests); it primarily measures the strength of the capillary walls and whether or not sufficient platelets are present.

What Is Usual

If you stick your fingertip with a lancet or needle and, with the edge of a clean piece of blotting paper or gauze, gently remove the drops of blood as they appear, the bleeding should stop after 30 seconds and before 3 minutes; this is a measure of bleeding time. For people over 50 years of age, the bleeding time may normally be shortened; and by the age of 70 it may be shortened by as much as 1 minute. If, on the other hand, you put that drop of blood on a clean glass slide or dish and touch it with a pin every 30 seconds, you should see evidence of a clot (a thin, sticky thread stuck to the pin) sometime between 6 minutes and 16 minutes. A thin glass capillary tube may also be used; when you touch an open end of such a tube to a drop of blood, the blood is automatically drawn up into the tube by capillary action. Then, simply break a segment of the capillary tube periodically, starting at one end, until you see evidence of a clot (a thin thread of blood remaining between the two pieces of broken glass) sometime between 6 minutes and 16 minutes; the time that elapses until this thread is observed is the clotting time.

What You Need

To perform the test, you must have one or more drops of blood (see Blood Tests, **Obtaining a Blood Sample**); some blotting paper (see Blood Tests,

Hemoglobin) or gauze pads; a few plain microhematocrit capillary tubes, which cost from $1.50 to $2.00 for 100; and a watch or clock. Automated devices to measure bleeding time are now available, but these tend to leave scars and are not advised for home use.

Note: For patients taking anticoagulant drugs, there is a new home device to determine prothrombin time (a much more precise measurement of clotting time); it is called the Biotrack Protime Test System and is used under the direct supervision of a doctor.

What to Watch Out For
Be sure that the needle or lancet is sterile and that the blotting paper or gauze is clean or sterile. Keep in mind that any medicine you are taking can alter the test results; check with your doctor or pharmacist to see whether your drugs can interfere with the test (even a few aspirins a day can double your bleeding time).

What the Test Results Can Mean
A prolonged bleeding and/or clotting time can be an early warning sign of several different bleeding diseases; some are secondary to another pathology in the body—especially liver disease. Any abnormally long bleeding or clotting time warrants medical consultation. If bleeding time is prolonged but clotting time seems normal, it often indicates thrombocytopenia (a decrease in the number of platelets); with hemophilia-type diseases the bleeding time may be within normal limits while the clotting time is prolonged. These tests, or something similar, should always be performed by the doctor or hospital before any type of surgery.

Reliability
Much can depend on how deep or shallow a puncture wound is made; a forceful stick can cause a false-prolonged bleeding time and vice versa. In general, these tests are about 70 percent accurate when properly performed. A careful review of one's past and family history can be an even more accurate indication of bleeding and clotting time, and any questionable indication of a familial bleeding tendency warrants a medical consultation.

BLOOD TYPING
(Knowing your blood type can be lifesaving)

Most people are aware that individuals can have different types of blood; that is to say, one person's blood group may contain antigens that are not compatible with another's. Should the two different groups of blood be mixed through a transfusion, the red blood cells can be destroyed, leading to a fatal reaction. The most common blood type grouping is called ABO, and blood is typed, or categorized, as A, B, AB or O, depending on which antigens are present or absent. Other blood groupings include the Rh factor (expressed in terms of whether it is present or not) and the MNS system; there are nearly 100 known blood groups at present. Knowing one's blood type, especially in an emergency (injury, accident) can save your life in two ways: first, by avoiding a transfusion of incompatible blood and, second, by saving the time that would otherwise be required to make a blood type determination.

While you can usually find out your blood type, including your Rh status for free by donating blood, you can also have this service performed at most medical laboratories for from $5.00 to $25.00. You can also determine your own blood type at home, as well as someone else's, should a transfusion be needed in a foreign country.

What Is Usual
The most common blood type is O; it is found in 45 percent of whites, 49 percent of blacks, 80 percent of American Indians and 40 percent of Orientals. Type O blood can usually be transfused into any individual (there are a few exceptions); in contrast, a person with type O can safely receive only type O blood. Type A is the next most common; type AB, containing both A and B antigens, is the least common.

What You Need
ABO dipsticks should be available in 1989 from Immucor Inc. (3130 Gateway Dr., Norcross, Ga. 30091); the retail price is yet to be determined but averaged $0.05 per dipstick for research studies. You simply place a drop of fingertip blood (see Blood Tests, **Obtaining a Blood Sample**) on the tip of the dipstick, and positive or negative reactions to either A or B, neither or both are indicated in about one minute.

What to Watch Out For
Follow the directions exactly; failure to do this has been the only real cause of error. Do not attempt to interpret the test if you are color-blind.

What the Test Results Can Mean
This test is not an illness indicator; its primary purpose is to prevent illness should a transfusion ever be needed.

Reliability
With the exception of a very few people with rare blood types, the test is as accurate as professional laboratory testing—better than 95 percent.

CHOLESTEROL
(A relatively useless, albeit most commonly performed, test alleged to indicate longevity and immunity)

If there is any one medical test that epitomizes the inaccuracy inherent in most medical testing, it is the cholesterol test. There are two reasons for such consistently deceptive results: first, the test itself. At present, there is no one standard way of performing the test; there are instead a great many techniques, and no two of them will consistently produce identical values on the same blood sample. When the American College of Pathologists sent a sample with a specific amount of cholesterol to more than 5,000 laboratories (the actual value was 262.6 mg per dl, but this was not known to the labs), over half the labs came up with test results so erroneous as to be useless—some were off by more than 200 mg per dl. Had those values been accepted by doctors across the country, thousands of patients could have been put on a dangerous, but totally useless, drug regimen. Thus, any cholesterol value must at this time be considered suspect in itself.

The second problem in measuring blood cholesterol concerns the individual. Believe it or not, just as with blood pressure, the amount of measurable cholesterol in your blood can change by as much as 100 mg per dl within seconds! As but one example: Can you recall lying in bed late at night and being awakened by a noise that made you think of an intruder? You know how soon your heart started pounding—within a few seconds. That was how long it took for your brain to signal your adrenal glands to secrete adrenalin hormones (epinephrine, norepinephrine) to help you to react to fear; adrenalin causes your heart to beat more quickly and strongly—among other signs that reflect nervousness. That same adrenalin also causes your blood cholesterol to rise just as quickly. If you are apprehensive over a needle stick, if you are startled by a loud noise at the time your blood sample is taken, even if you are affected by nothing more than your fear of a "bad" test result, that alone can cause your cholesterol test to indicate that you are ostensibly about to die of a heart attack—assuming, of course, that you believe in the still scientifically unfounded relationship that today is the sole basis for performing the test at all.

By now just about everyone has been proselytized with the cholesterol dogma: Eat too much of it (or eat too much of certain fats that cause cholesterol to increase in the body), and the end is near. Incidentally, research now shows that the amount of cholesterol you eat has little or no effect on your blood cholesterol levels. Most people also now know that cholesterol is not a fat but a solid alcohol called a steroid and is absolutely essential for your body to manufacture sex hormones and for your brain and nervous system to grow and function. Few people seem to know, however, that this substance also increases in the blood when the thyroid gland is not operating properly; with hepatitis, herpes and kidney disease; and even when a host of drugs such as diuretics and asthma medications are taken. Taking female hormones and certain vitamins as well as suffering from anemia will lower blood cholesterol values. And over the years there has been a fairly consistent relationship between people's having a low blood cholesterol value and their also having cancer, certain mental problems and a loss of immunity. In studies where drugs were used to lower cholesterol, although the amount of heart attacks in the drug-taking group was in truth reduced less than 2 percent when compared to a group not taking the drugs, the amount of accidents, homicides and suicides was more than doubled in those who took the drugs. Jail studies show that the most violent prisoners have the lowest cholesterol levels. And in San Francisco, doctors who specialize in **AIDS** (discussed under Blood Tests) consider a cholesterol level lower than 135 mg per dl as a definitive sign of the immune deficiency AIDS-related complex.

Be that as it may, should you still want to measure your cholesterol, or check your laboratory results, you can now do so at home. What you will measure is *total* cholesterol. There are many different forms of cholesterol; some, called high density lipids, are even considered good for you.

What Is Usual

To be quite honest, no one really knows what a "normal" blood cholesterol level is. If the accepted laboratory standards for all other medical tests are used, in which "normal" consists of the results found in 95 percent of the population, then any value up to 280 mg per dl for people under 50 years of age is within normal limits and up to 350 mg per dl as one gets older. If, on the other hand, you accept the doctrine of the American Heart Association and the National Institutes of Health, anything over 200 mg per dl implies impending death.

What You Need

Blood cholesterol values can be measured using the Technimed test from Home Diagnostics Inc. (6 Industrial Way West, Edentown, N.J. 07724). This is a one-minute test in which a drop of blood is placed on a special paper. The cost is about $2.00 per test.

The Clinicard screening device from Chem-Elec Inc. (P.O. Box 372, North Webster, Ind. 46555) can also be used. Here the drop of blood is placed on a special card, and the result is available in three minutes. The cost is $2.50 per test.

At present, both tests will probably have to be obtained from a doctor.

What to Watch Out For

More than anything else, try to be as relaxed as possible when performing this test. Be sure to ask your doctor or pharmacist about the effect of any drugs you are taking—even those not requiring a prescription; aspirin, for example, is but one drug that can change cholesterol values. And ask your doctor whether any illness you may have will alter the test's values. Be sure your color vision is normal; several patients have reported difficulty in distinguishing between the closely related shades of blue-green that denote the different blood values.

What the Test Results Can Mean

Here is a most unique situation; in essence, the test results mean what you want them to mean. If you feel that an elevated cholesterol level is, in fact, associated with heart disease, then you should consult with your doctor as to what action to take. If you are performing the test to assess your immune status, a low cholesterol value also warrants a medical consultation. Should you observe that your cholesterol value changes with stressful situations, you might want a medical consultation to find ways of moderating your reaction to stress. The very fact that you performed this test could, in itself, be an indication of excessive apprehension.

Reliability

At present this test—even if performed by a professional—must be considered no more than 50 percent accurate; you could toss a coin. If, however, you are fully convinced about the cholesterol hypothesis, then measure your cholesterol at least 10 times, at various times of the day and on various days of the month, before averaging all those values. Even then, the accuracy of this test is still questionable. The most recent research no longer considers the *total* cholesterol test an accurate, albeit ostensible, risk factor for heart disease.

Keep in mind that if blood is taken for a cholesterol test while you are standing, the result could easily be up to 50 points higher than if sitting. If you measure your cholesterol at various times during the day, or over a period of several days, there can be differences of more than 170 points; none of these extreme variations are related to immediate food intake.

And, finger-stick blood is not equivalent to blood taken from a vein; it usually gives a much higher cholesterol value (up to 50 points more, even while sitting).

DRUG MONITORING
(Increasing drug efficiency and preventing toxic reactions)

First off, it must be pointed out that drug monitoring has nothing to do with identifying drug abuse (see Urine Tests, **Clinical Analysis: Drug Abuse Identification**). Drug monitoring is quantitative and protects you from having too little or too much of a particular drug in your body; an insufficient amount is relatively useless while more of any drug than is necessary can cause dangerous side effects, even death, and offers no benefits. Drug abuse testing, on the other hand, is primarily qualitative, to detect the use of illegal drugs, especially in individuals whose occupation may endanger the lives of others; the specific amounts of the drug are relatively unimportant.

Many prescribed drugs have a very limited therapeutic range; that is, there is only an extremely small difference between the amount needed to produce their expected effect and the amount that can be toxic. The difference between efficacy and toxicity is sometimes measured in micrograms (mcg), or millionths of a gram (it takes 28 grams to equal one ounce); phenytoin (Dilantin), an anticonvulsant drug, will usually only prevent epileptic seizures when there are more than 10 mcg per milliliter, or ml, in the blood (it takes 5 ml to equal one teaspoon); yet the drug starts causing dangerous side effects when blood levels go above 20 mcg. Theophylline, one of the primary drugs used to treat asthma and some other lung conditions, must also reach at least 10 mcg per ml in the blood to help make breathing easier; once the amount in the blood exceeds 20 mcg, the drug can cause agitation, confusion, seizures and even fatal irregularities of the heart's rhythm. When it comes to digitalislike drugs, a variation of one-billionth of a gram in the blood can make the difference between a therapeutic and a toxic effect.

Many factors can alter the amount of a drug in the blood in addition to the obvious—how much of the drug is taken. Some drugs are not well absorbed when taken with, or within an hour of, certain foods. Taking some drugs concomitantly may have an effect on either or both of those drugs when it comes to absorbtion, metabolism and excretion (here one's kidney function plays an important role).

The time that a drug was taken, in relation to the time when the amount of that drug in the body is tested for, is especially important when monitoring for toxic levels. Thus, the amount of a drug in the blood at the time of testing may not reflect the amount of the drug actually taken. And many doctors use drug monitoring as a means of determining whether a prescribed drug was used correctly or even whether it was used at all; studies have shown that two out of every three patients do not properly follow directions for a drug's use, while one out of three never even has their prescription filled.

There are several relatively simple tests for drug monitoring that can be performed at home. While most use a drop of blood from the fingertip, some doctors have found that saliva, substituted for blood, is just as effective in determining the presence and amount of a drug in the body. The primary advantage of home drug monitoring is cost and convenience; it costs a doctor about $15.00 for each test kit as compared to close to $80.00 for the same test performed in a commercial laboratory. In addition to saving on the cost of the test itself, the patient need not go to, or pay for, an office visit.

What Is Usual

Virtually every drug, even nonprescription drugs such as aspirin, has what is known as a therapeutic range—a lower blood level where effectiveness usually begins and an upper blood level where there is usually no increase in efficacy but where toxic side effects commonly occur. Not all drugs require blood-level monitoring, since, in most cases, the therapeutic range is wide enough to be safe. Depending on the drug, there are certain, different, drug levels that are usual. When a prescribed drug is taken, there should be some indication of the drug's presence in the body.

What You Need

At present, while home test kits for drug monitoring do not require a prescription, they are best obtained from your doctor; if you are in fact taking a drug that is usually monitored, you should be under a doctor's care. One such test kit, as an example, is the AccuLevel theophylline test, which comes complete with all supplies, takes about 40 minutes (including 35 minutes of waiting time) and costs the doctor about $15.00. It comes from Syntex Medical Diagnostics (Palo Alto, Calif. 94304). There are also test kits for various anticonvulsant drugs and prothrombin time (used when taking an anticoagulant drug).

What the Test Results Can Mean

In general, monitoring drug use, where applicable, allows a more efficacious, less costly and safer use of that drug. In fairness, it should be mentioned that there are physicians who are not convinced that therapeutic drug monitoring does prevent a drug's toxic side effects; they admit a relationship between higher-than-necessary drug blood levels and minor side effects such as nausea, vomiting and diarrhea but feel that elevated drug levels do not always correlate with serious drug reactions. Obviously, each individual can react differently to the same amount of drugs, but drug monitoring under the physician's direction has been known to be lifesaving. In many cases your doctor can give you an antidote to take if your blood level of a drug goes too high.

Reliability

The amount of a drug in the body, as determined by drug monitoring, is considered to be at least 90 percent accurate. As to the blood level of a drug and its effects, a great deal depends on how much time has elapsed since the drug was taken, how often the drug is taken and especially how long the drug has been used; the longer a drug is used, the greater the chances that it may build up in the body. Some drugs may be metabolized or pass out of the body within a few hours; others may show activity for days after a single dose. In most cases, a certain, known amount of a drug in the body is necessary to be effective; drug monitoring is the only way to determine whether that level has been reached while preventing an overdose.

GLUCOSE
(A reflection of carbohydrate metabolism)

Note: If you have diabetes or some other blood-sugar-related condition, this screening test is not for you.

Blood glucose measurements, sometimes called blood sugar measurements, really only measure the amount of one form of sugar, glucose, floating free in the blood at the time of the test. The results primarily show how well the body handles carbohydrate metabolism, and secondarily they show how well all organs related to that metabolism are functioning. No matter what form of sugar (sucrose, or ordinary granulated table sugar; fructose, which is found naturally in fruits; lactose, found in milk products) or other carbohydrates (grains, vegetables) we eat, the body ultimately metabolizes them to glucose (or dextrose, as it is sometimes called).

Of interest is the recent research that dispels many old ideas about which foods affect blood glucose levels. Carrots, corn flakes, potatoes, rice and whole-grain bread, as but a few examples, tend to elevate blood glucose the most; while ice cream, orange juice, pasta and peanuts seem to have the least effect. And the form of the food can also make a difference. Mashed potatoes and ground lentils raise blood glucose levels much more than baked potatoes and whole lentils.

Usually, glucose is stored in the liver until it is needed as fuel by the body for many and varied functions: movement of muscles, beating of the heart, breathing, even thinking. If not enough stored glucose is available to fuel these activities, it can then be manufactured from proteins and fat elsewhere in the body. After glucose is produced, how well it is utilized by the body depends a great deal on the hormone insulin, which is secreted by the pancreas—a gland just behind the stomach. The disease known as diabetes is essentially one in which inadequacy or unavailability of insulin prevents proper glucose utilization.

Most often, blood glucose is measured as a single test for screening purposes. It may also be used to note the effects of stress or anxiety on an individual. And blood glucose measurements are valuable in preventing certain complications that may arise during pregnancy, while dieting, while taking various drugs and subsequent to some forms of poisoning.

Glucose tolerance. Should two or more blood glucose test results suggest abnormal values, the glucose tolerance test (GTT) may be performed. For this test the individual ingests a measured amount of glucose, usually in liquid form, and the blood glucose levels along with urine glucose levels (see Urine Tests, **Clinical Analysis: Glucose**) are measured each half-hour for the first two hours and then hourly for the next three hours, although some doctors feel that measurements at one-half, one and two hours are sufficient. This is supposed to be a more precise evaluation of carbohydrate and glucose metabolism than when a single test is performed. Glucose levels in the blood can also reflect other non-insulin-related disorders, however, and are influenced by injuries, a variety of hormone-caused diseases, infections and even physical exercise.

Many drugs can also cause an elevated blood glucose level, although it is usually temporary. These drugs include:

- Atromid-S—used to lower blood cholesterol
- Birth control pills (oral contraceptives) and other estrogens
- Phenytoin (diphenylhydantoin), whose trade name is Dilantin
- Cortisone products—used to treat asthma, arthritis and many skin conditions
- Decongestants (for colds and allergies)
- Diet pills that contain decongestants
- Diuretic drugs
- Thyroid preparations
- Caffeine in large amounts
- Nicotine
- Nicotinic acid (niacin or vitamin B_3) in large doses over a prolonged period of time
- Vitamin A in large doses
- Lithium
- Tagamet—the trade name for a drug used to treat ulcers
- Tranquilizers such as Thorazine
- Acetaminophen—an aspirin substitute found in many nonprescription products such as Tylenol, Anacin-3, Pamprin, Syne-Aid and Nyquil
- Some of the newer angina and blood pressure medicines

Drugs that can lower blood sugar levels include:

- Alcohol
- Beta blockers—a generalized descriptive name for some of the new antiangina and blood pressure medicines
- Aspirin in large doses

What Is Usual

If, after an individual has gone without any food or drink for two hours or more, the blood glucose level measures anywhere between 60 mg and 120 mg per 100 ml, this is usually considered normal. Some doctors, however, now consider an occasional level of up to 140 mg per 100 ml as still being within normal limits. After 50 years of age, and as aging continues, it is not unusual for fasting blood glucose levels to be slightly higher (120 mg to 130 mg per 100 ml). After someone either eats food or drinks a prescribed amount of glucose solution, the blood sugar level should rise no higher than 180 mg per 100 ml and then return to normal limits within two hours. Here again, though, there are now doctors who feel that a sudden rise to 240 mg per 100 ml may not necessarily indicate diabetes or other related disease and may be normal for certain individuals. When a glucose tolerance test is performed, the blood sugar level should start out within the accepted normal range, rise markedly in one-half hour and start down at about one hour's time. It should be within normal limits after two hours, although some people show a drop below their starting figure three or four hours later (see Figure 27).

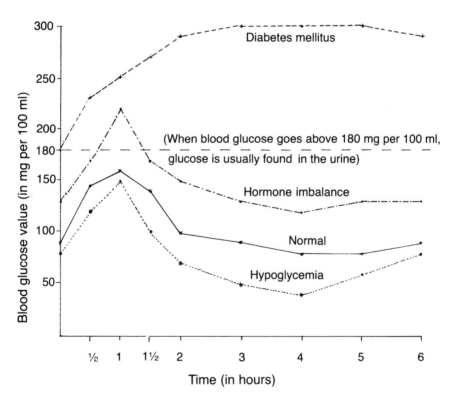

Figure 27. Glucose tolerance test.

What You Need

The test requires a drop of blood (see Blood Tests, **Obtaining a Blood Sample**). The simplest way of measuring the amount of glucose in that drop of blood is to apply it to the tip of a chemically treated plastic test strip, wait one minute, and then wipe it or wash it off and compare the color on the strip with its accompanying color chart, which is calculated to show relative glucose values. One such strip is called Chemstrip bG, and although the numerical values read 20 mg, 40 mg, 80 mg, 120 mg, 180 mg, 240 mg and 800 mg per 100 ml, it is easy to arrive at values in between those given on the color chart for a reasonably accurate test result—certainly accurate enough for any home testing. Chemstrip bG test strips cost from $10.00 to $20.00 for a package of 25, or about $0.60 per test.

Another test strip is called Dextrostix. Here the drop of blood must be washed off with water rather than wiped with cotton, and the timing must be absolutely precise. The range of values that can be observed with this test runs from 0 mg to 250 mg per 100 ml—a smaller range, but allowing a bit more accuracy in comparing the colors. Dextrostix cost from $0.70 to $0.80 per test.

A somewhat similar test strip is VISIDEX II. No water is required for washing this test strip; simply wipe or blot off the test area. A smaller amount of blood is needed, and the test result color will remain stable for up to four days, so that the doctor can also check the findings. At about $0.70 per test, it does offer greater convenience when away from home.

Test strips are quite adequate for screening at home. For those with diagnosed conditions where regular monitoring is called for, there are a great many different electronic meter devices that display a digital readout of the glucose value from the test strip. Some of these machines offer "voice" readings of values, for those with vision problems, and some have memory banks that retain the values for days or weeks so that the doctor can review them. When a meter is required, or desired, check with your doctor to find out which brand he or she has found to be easiest to use and most accurate.

Measured amounts of glucose, for glucose tolerance testing, are available in a bottled solution (under several brand names), at a cost of $1.50 per bottle. Your doctor will tell you how much to drink, depending on your weight and condition.

What to Watch Out For

Even before you begin testing, you must be sure that the test strips have been kept absolutely airtight and dry in their containers; air, especially humid air, leaking into the bottle can deteriorate the test strips and cause false and misleading results. If there is any doubt, open a sealed bottle and compare the results of a test with a strip from the old and new containers. Before testing, be certain that the strip-tip color matches the base standard on the color chart; do not use the strip if the colors do not match. Usually, a deteriorated test strip will be darker than the standard, or it may show a brownish hue. Most doctors agree that you should not use a test strip from a bottle that has been open more than four months, regardless of the expiration date.

Keep in mind that stress or even anxiety over a seemingly unrelated situation can cause false, elevated blood glucose levels. Most doctors request that their patients make a note of any physical activity, unusual emotional state and dietary intake for the two-hour period prior to testing. Do not test yourself for blood glucose, and particularly for glucose tolerance, immediately after any injury, illness or stressful situation; do not perform these tests for screening purposes while dieting or after any recent weight loss.

Before a glucose tolerance test is performed, it is important to eat a diet containing normal amounts of carbohydrates for several days to a week prior to testing. Many patients tend to cut down drastically on carbohydrates when they plan to have this test, and such dietary alterations can cause false-abnormal results. One's physical activities for three days prior to testing should also be usual.

Be sure your color vision is normal, since the difference in shades of color between normal and abnormal on some test strips is slight.

What the Test Results Can Mean

A single elevated blood glucose test result may not be significant. Repeated values greater than 140 mg per 100 ml after fasting, however, warrant medical consultation. Only after all the many extraneous factors that can cause a rise in blood glucose levels have been taken into account is a professional investigation undertaken to ascertain the reason for the abnormally high blood glucose level. These extraneous factors include:

- Emotional state.
- Food intake for the two or three days prior to testing.
- Exercise or other physical exertion for the two or three days prior to testing.
- Age—blood glucose levels seem to rise normally with age.

In addition to diabetes, many other conditions can alter the blood glucose level:

- High blood pressure
- Pregnancy
- Obesity
- Infections
- Heart disease
- Certain cancers

- Various disorders of the pituitary, thyroid, adrenal and pancreas glands
- Recent injuries, especially head trauma or wounds that cause severe bleeding
- Use of certain drugs, particularly some of the diuretics
- Smoking

A lower-than-normal blood glucose level (below 60 mg per 100 ml) can reflect different disorders of the same endocrine glands cited above; it can also reflect inadequate nutrition, prolonged exercise, vomiting for several hours, high fever for several days, liver disease and other metabolic problems, including hypoglycemia. To justify a diagnosis of hypoglycemia, however, blood glucose levels must be lower than 50 mg per 100 ml at least three different times, and symptoms such as sweating, palpitations, weakness and bizarre behavior should be evident along with the low blood glucose levels. Many doctors feel that when the glucose tolerance test for hypoglycemia is to be performed, a normal meal should be eaten two hours before drinking the glucose solution in order to avoid a false "rebound" hypoglycemia. Other doctors think that bottled glucose solutions should not be used for this test; rather, a well-balanced, mixed meal should be the stimulating food instead of the commercially prepared mixture.

Glucose levels in the urine should correspond to glucose levels in the blood (see Urine Tests, **Clinical Analysis: Glucose**).

With a glucose tolerance test, if blood glucose levels are still elevated two hours after drinking the glucose solution, the most likely cause is diabetes; as with other abnormally high levels with a single glucose test, however, the cause could be hormonal, injury, infection or emotional. Lower-than-expected glucose values, especially after two hours, can indicate hypoglycemia, pancreatic infection or other causes of excessive insulin production, inadequate production of other body hormones and even anorexia nervosa. Values that are either higher or lower than normal warrant a medical consultation.

Recently, some doctors have employed the glucose tolerance test as a means of detecting certain patients believed to be at greater risk of having heart disease, especially if the patients have inherited elevated blood lipid levels, high blood pressure and a fast pulse and are also obese.

Note: When comparing blood glucose values from fingertip blood to values obtained from a clinical laboratory where only the serum portion of blood was tested, many doctors suggest that you add another 10 percent to 15 percent of the fingertip blood result for a more comparable evaluation. For example, a fingertip blood value of 140 mg per 100 ml is equivalent to a value of about 155 mg per 100 ml from a laboratory test performed on the serum portion of blood taken from a vein.

Reliability

The test strips are considered 95 percent accurate in reflecting the blood glucose level when the test is properly performed. As a regular screening test for those who have a family history of diabetes, it is deemed to be 80 percent accurate. However, when used for general screening purposes, the accuracy is felt to be only 70 percent because of the many conditions that can cause an abnormal result.

HEMOGLOBIN
(A nonspecific test, primarily for anemia)

Anemia itself is not a disease; most often it is a sign or reflection of some illness within the body. Some symptoms of anemia include: tiredness, weakness, dizziness, feeling cold all the time and fainting; some signs include jaundice, impotence and emotional problems. More recently, a low hemoglobin level reflecting iron deficiency is considered to be a signal of impaired immunity; some doctors now feel that a lower-than-normal hemoglobin level increases susceptibility to infection.

Hemoglobin is an iron-protein substance inside red blood cells that picks up oxygen when the cells pass through the lungs; at the same time, it releases carbon dioxide (a waste product of metabolism) to be exhaled. The amount of oxygen the blood can carry to body organs and tissues is related to the amount of hemoglobin present. There can by many different types of hemoglobin in the blood; some are abnormal and indicate a disease or disability that reduces the body's oxygen supply. A few examples:

- Carboxyhemoglobin is formed when normal hemoglobin combines with carbon monoxide, most often as a consequence of smoking or exposure to auto exhaust or faulty gas heater fumes (see Environmental Tests, **Carbon Monoxide**). When carboxyhemoglobin is present, the skin may turn cherry-red.
- Methemoglobin is formed when normal hemoglobin combines with nitrites or nitrates in food, when heart disease patients use excessive amounts of nitrate drugs, from some aspirinlike drugs and certain sulfa drugs, and even when too many iron-supplement pills are taken. When methemoglobin is present in large amounts, the skin may appear bluish (cyanosis) because although methemoglobin picks up oxygen, it will not release it (see the discussion of nitrogen dioxide in Environmental Tests, **Air Pollution**).
- Hemoglobin S is associated with sickle-cell anemia (see Blood Tests, **Sickle-Cell Screening**); the red blood cells are sickle-shaped and usually carry insufficient oxygen.

• Hemoglobin A or A-2 is an inherited abnormal form associated with Cooley's anemia (sometimes called Mediterranean anemia because it was first discovered in people living adjacent to the Mediterranean Sea); it can cause stillbirth as well as other blood problems—generally later in life.

When testing for anemia, the usual screening tests, even those performed by a doctor or laboratory, measure all the various hemoglobins present without differentiating them. Since dietary iron is the primary source of hemoglobin, any inadequate intake of this mineral can reflect itself through low hemoglobin levels. A recent study revealed that women who ate red meat at least five times a week had far less anemia than women who relied primarily on fish and poultry or vegetarianism for protein. A loss of blood from an injury, during surgery, following a blood donation or with menstruation can also be reflected as an anemia at times.

What Is Usual
Men average from 14 grams to 16 grams of hemoglobin per deciliter of blood; women average from 12 grams to 15 grams; young children can average from 11 grams to 13 grams and still be considered within normal limits. Hemoglobin used to be measured as a percentage of what was considered the ideal—15.5 grams, or 100 percent. Thus, men were considered to be normal at 90 percent or better (14 grams) and women at 80 percent or better (12.5 grams). Although hemoglobin levels do not change significantly with age, they are usually lower in black people (thought to be a consequence of the frequency with which blacks inherit sickle-cell and Cooley's anemia). Posture can change hemoglobin levels; they can be much lower if measured when the patient is lying down, especially after sleeping, than when measured with the patient in a sitting position.

What You Need
The simplest way to measure blood hemoglobin is to use the Tallquist Hemoglobin Scale. After you obtain a single drop of blood (see Blood Tests, **Obtaining a Blood Sample**), usually from a fingertip, the drop is placed on a small square of special white blotting paper, and the color of the blood drop is then compared with a color scale that accompanies the booklet of blotting papers (see Figure 28). The blotting paper booklet (containing 152 test squares) and a color scale are available from Medical Charts and Specialists (75 Oser Ave., Hauppage, N.Y. 11788) for $4.12. Easy-to-follow directions accompany the booklet. More precise hemoglobinometers are available for $100.00 to $1,000.00, but for screening purposes the Tallquist scale is more than adequate.

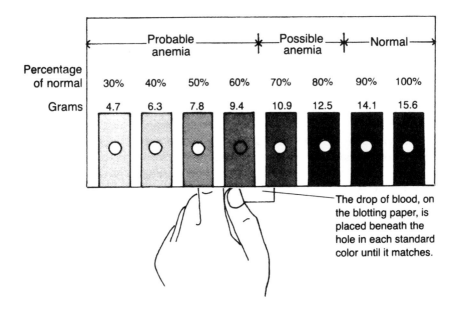

Figure 28. Blood hemoglobin test (for anemia).

What to Watch Out For

Use only one drop of free-flowing blood on the blotting paper and compare the color of the blood sample with the color chart within 30 seconds. Use natural light for color comparison; artificial light can distort the colors. Do not attempt to perform the test if you are color blind.

What the Test Results Can Mean

If the color of the blood spot on the blotting paper indicates a lower-than-normal hemoglobin level, and a repeat test shows a similar result, it warrants a medical consultation. Decreased hemoglobin levels most likely mean an anemia, but they do not even hint at the cause. Liver disease, thyroid disorders, heavy smoking, certain cancers and some inherited conditions can also lower hemoglobin levels indirectly. Naturally, any loss of blood will cause temporarily lower hemoglobin levels. Many prescription drugs can cause anemia as an adverse side effect, which, if not detected early enough, can be fatal. And there is a condition (called by various names: runner's anemia, jogger's anemia, sports anemia) in which, seemingly due to nothing more than regular physical activity, a slightly lower-than-normal hemoglobin level occurs. Most doctors feel that this comes from a resultant increase in the amount of blood plasma, which "dilutes" the red blood cells, and does not require treatment.

Should the blood spot seem to be darker than the 100 percent color when compared to the chart, it could indicate a condition called polycythemia (too many red blood cells). This may also mean that the blood is too viscous (thick) to flow easily, and some doctors consider such an abnormally elevated hemoglobin level an early warning sign of the susceptibility to a stroke; some doctors also feel that a high hemoglobin level is the cause of certain mental problems as a consequence of poor circulation to the brain. Heavy smoking can cause what seems to be an elevated hemoglobin level by increasing the number of red blood cells to supply more oxygen to the tissues. Living or working at high altitudes or being dehydrated (not having sufficient fluids) just prior to testing can also cause high hemoglobin levels. A repeated elevated hemoglobin level warrants a medical consultation.

Reliability

The Tallquist Hemoglobin Scale, while not the most precise hemoglobin measurement, is considered sufficiently accurate for screening purposes. It is used in many countries around the world because of its simplicity and is also used by the U.S. armed forces. Its results have been found to be within 15 percent of those provided by the most accurate devices. At the same time, when the most accurate device was used by professional nurses, as many as 40 percent of the test results were wrong.

MONONUCLEOSIS
(A test for the Epstein-Barr virus; a possible clue to persistent tiredness)

Infectious mononucleosis is also known as dormitory disease, glandular fever, the holiday disease, the kissing disease and student's disease. Its latest, somewhat related appellation is the "yuppie disease" or "yuppie flu," since it seems increasingly to affect young and ostensibly successful upwardly mobile businesspeople as soon as they suffer their first setback. This persistent form of the illness (lasting for more than six months) has since been officially labeled chronic fatigue syndrome. The origin of the many names becomes obvious when one realizes that the condition arises primarily in young people from 10 years to 30 years of age, with most cases occurring between 15 years and 20 years (although there have been rare cases in 1-year-olds and in people over 60), especially in those who room together or who otherwise have repeated close contact.

The causative virus can stay in the saliva for more than a year after the person has had the disease. It almost always produces enlarged, tender lymph glands (most often along the side of the neck). And its most common symptoms—fatigue, lethargy, loss of appetite and malaise—are, more often than not, first observed by the young person's parents when their son or daughter comes home from school or college. Other frequent symptoms and signs of the disease include a sore throat (the most common complaint in those in their teens), fever, headache, muscle and stomach pains, swollen eyelids and a rash that can imitate German measles or a drug reaction or that may look like tiny hemorrhages under the skin. In other words, infectious mononucleosis, in itself an uncomfortable but rarely dangerous disease, can imitate a great many other far more serious conditions and can be very difficult to diagnose. (See Mouth, Throat and Gastrointestinal Tests, **Mouth, Tongue and Throat Observations**).

The cause of infectious mononucleosis is a herpes-type organism called the Epstein-Barr Virus (EBV), but because it is difficult to isolate and identify this virus, most tests to help diagnose this disease depend on finding mononucleosis-specific antibodies in the blood. Antibodies are disease-fighting substances formed in the body whenever it is invaded by microorganisms (bacteria, viruses, etc.); they are usually specific against the infecting germ. The test simply shows whether or not antibodies to the Epstein-Barr virus are present. Antibodies generally appear in the blood of a person with infectious mononucleosis within four or five days after he or she contracts the disease (a day or so before symptoms appear), but they may not be present in a sufficient amount to be detected by testing until two weeks to three weeks later; they may then remain at detectable levels for six months or more.

Several studies have shown that young people with a negative mononucleosis test (no antibodies evident) are much more susceptible to the disease when they leave home for college living; those with a positive test seem to have a degree of immunity.

The test is not perfect. There are other diseases and viruses than can, on occasion, cause a false-positive result. And there are some people who, even though the presence of the disease can be confirmed by other means, still show a negative test; a few of these, however, will show a positive test several months after recovering from the disease.

What Is Usual

A negative test is considered normal, although there are some doctors who believe that virtually everyone has been exposed to EBV by the age of 20 and can carry some degree of infection, with one out of three ultimately showing symptoms. An individual with the symptoms and signs that usually accompany infectious mononucleosis has more than a 90 percent chance of showing a positive test reaction if, in fact, the symptoms and signs are from that particular disease. A negative test in the presence of symptoms warrants looking for a different cause for the symptoms.

What You Need

A drop of blood (see Blood Tests, **Obtaining a Blood Sample**) is placed on a glass slide; then the MONO-TEST (FTB) is performed. This test, which is marketed by Wampole Laboratories (Cranbury, N.J. 08512), is an easy two-minute procedure. It costs $30.00 to $35.00 for a 10-test kit.

The test comes with specific instructions, which must be followed explicitly to obtain accurate results.

What to Watch Out For

The following guidelines apply when testing for the presence of mononucleosis:

- If you keep the test material refrigerated, warm it to room temperature before use.
- If you are testing someone else's blood, keep in mind that it may contain live virus and avoid contact with the blood.

What the Test Results Can Mean

Usually, the symptoms and signs of infectious mononucleosis are such that they warrant medical attention. If, however, they seem mild or inconsequential, a mononucleosis test might help point to a diagnosis. If the test is positive, no matter how slight the symptoms, a medical consultation is warranted.

More recently, evidence of Epstein-Barr virus antibodies has been used to screen for certain cancers.

If the test is negative and you still have doubts about whether you might be harboring EBV, repeat the test in one week. If the symptoms become annoying or persist, medical attention is warranted no matter what the test result; infectious mononucleosis can have drastic, albeit rare, complications. A negative test without symptoms or signs of any illness usually indicates a susceptibility to the disease and could offer useful information should a mysterious illness occur at a later date. Keep in mind that several research studies have failed to show a direct link between EBV and "yuppie disease"; while some doctors attribute the "yuppie flu" to psychoneurosis, at the present time neither EBV nor psychoneurosis has been proved to be the cause. One random study of more than 500 people younger than 50 years of age showed that 20 percent complained of persistent tiredness similar to chronic fatigue syndrome—almost half of them to the point of being bedridden at times—yet they showed no statistically greater incidence of positive EBV tests.

Reliability

A positive test, while about 90 percent accurate as to the presence of EBV, is only about 60 percent accurate as an explanation of symptoms.

RHEUMATOID FACTOR (ARTHRITIS)
(A test that may help explain the cause of joint pains)

The symptoms of arthritis—pain and stiffness in the joints, usually but not always accompanied by swelling, redness and warmth of the afflicted joints—can come from many different diseases. When the joint stiffness is worse after inactivity, especially first thing in the morning, and when there are repeated bouts of fever, along with weight loss and generalized weakness, the most likely diagnosis is rheumatoid arthritis, a prolonged inflammatory-response disease that affects the entire body. It usually occurs between 20 years and 60 years of age and more than twice as often in women as in men.

Although the specific cause is still unknown (some doctors feel that it comes from a virus, while others blame genetics, diet and even emotional stress), at least three out of four people with rheumatoid arthritis produce special antibodies called rheumatoid factor, which can be detected in the blood. Antibodies are manufactured in response to, and to help combat, infections and many other disease antigens (the disease-provoking substances). Unfortunately, other nonarthritic conditions can also cause a rheumatoid factor reaction—especially liver, lung and heart problems; syphilis; and certain worm (parasite) infestations. The test is performed primarily on patients with arthritis, or on those with unexplained eye or skin conditions, to help confirm a diagnosis and select proper treatment. Rheumatoid factor usually does not appear in the blood until months after the disease begins, and it can persist for several years. A negative test does not rule out a diagnosis of rheumatoid arthritis, but it can help distinguish between rheumatoid arthritis and other rheumatoid conditions that damage joints, muscles, collagen or connective tissue and various bodily organs.

What Is Usual
There should be no evidence of rheumatoid factor in the blood (a negative test).

What You Need
A drop of blood (see Blood Tests, **Obtaining a Blood Sample**) is placed on a designated dot on a paper slide that is part of a RHEUMANOSTICAN DRI-DOT kit, which costs from $30.00 to $35.00 and contains enough material to perform 25 tests; two large test tubes, which cost from $0.50 to $1.00 each; and some calibrated capillary tubes, which cost $2.00 per 100.

What to Watch Out For
Keep the following points in mind when you perform the test:

- This test kit comes with positive and negative control samples; when using the kit for the first time, test yourself with the controls to be sure that you are performing the test properly.

- Do not use a test kit if the seal or envelope has been broken, if there is only one dot on the slide (there should be two—one peach-colored and one clear) or if the slide appears to be moist.
- Use a clock or watch that has a sweep-second hand or a digital display that shows seconds, or use a stopwatch, to time the one minute that the test takes.

What the Test Results Can Mean

This test is a prime example of the fact that any medical test result alone— be it positive or negative, within normal numerical limits or higher or lower than what is usually found in ostensibly normal, healthy people—is not con- clusive proof of the presence or absence of a suspected disease or condition. A positive rheumatoid factor test, even if accompanied by the usual symp- toms and signs of rheumatoid arthritis, is but one peg on which to hang a proper diagnosis. It must be kept in mind, however, that the test is not definitive and that a positive reaction can also occur with:

- Other forms of arthritis-mimicking conditions such as gout, ankylosing spondylitis (stiffening of the spine, primarily), psoriasis, colitis, gonor- rhea and other joint infections.
- Diseases of collagen (which is the connective tissue under the skin, around organs, bones, muscles and other structures that helps hold everything together), such as systemic lupus erythematosus and scleroderma.
- Generalized infections, such as tuberculosis, leprosy, syphilis and endo- carditis (infection of the lining of the heart).

And a positive reaction has been known to occur in evidently healthy peo- ple with no signs of arthritic involvement. A positive test warrants medical consultation.

A negative test simply means that rheumatoid factor antibodies are not present or are present in such minute amounts as to be undetectable. It would seem that the symptoms alone that provided sufficient provocation to perform this test would warrant medical consultation, even if the test result were negative.

Reliability

If rheumatoid factor antibodies are present, the test is 97 percent accurate in detecting them. However, the test will be positive in only 70 percent to 85 percent of patients who have rheumatoid arthritis; it can also be positive in 40 percent of patients with systemic lupus erythematosus; and it can be positive in up to 90 percent of patients with Sjogren's syndrome (a condition believed to be related to rheumatoid arthritis in which there is dryness of the eyes, nose, mouth and vagina along with generalized body pains). A positive test alone is not sufficient to make a diagnosis of rheumatoid ar- thritis, but it can be of help.

SEDIMENTATION RATE
(A very nonspecific test that can, at times, be helpful in monitoring certain illnesses)

The erythrocyte sedimentation rate, so called because it measures how fast and how far red blood cells (erythrocytes) settle as a sediment toward the bottom of a specially marked tube in an hour's time, is one of the most common tests performed by physicians. Most often called a "sed rate," it is a poor screening device, being "positive" in response to literally hundreds of different diseases and conditions. It is primarily used by doctors to follow the progress of certain illnesses such as arthritis and some infections. The faster the red blood cells fall in the tube, the more indicative it is of the possibility of some body disorder. Recently, a simple method of performing this test at home has been marketed, and some doctors give their patients the equipment to test themselves on a regular basis, where indicated; it can reduce the cost of this test from an average $20.00 (in addition to the cost of an office visit) to less than $1.00.

What Is Usual
A doctor's office laboratory may use one of several different types of tubes to measure the fall of the red blood cells; therefore, depending on the tube, usual values may vary slightly. In general, a "normal" man's cells fall at a rate of from 1mm to 12mm in an hour; cells of women and the elderly may fall at a rate of up to 20mm per hour, and the rate would still be considered normal.

What You Need
The test requires a drop or two of fingertip blood (see Blood Tests, **Obtaining a Blood Sample**) and a MicroSed tube. At present, you may also need a special reservoir cup to collect the blood and some normal saline solution for diluting the blood; your doctor will give you all the necessary supplies when he or she shows you how to perform the test (no experience or special training is necessary). The material is also available from Ulster Scientific Inc. (P.O. Box 902, Highland, N.Y. 12528) and costs the doctor about $60.00 for 100 tests.

What to Watch Out For
Although the test requires careful measurement, it takes only a minute or two to collect the blood and place it in the tube; it then takes one hour before the measurement is made. The tube must be kept upright for the hour's time, and some doctors give their patients a special rack for that purpose.

What the Test Results Can Mean

Since the test is primarily used to follow the course of an illness—as a measure of the success of a drug, for example—the slower the sed rate becomes, the greater the indication that the therapy is working. If the sed rate remains high, it could indicate that the wrong drug is being used. When the test is used as a screening device, as it sometimes is, it must be kept in mind that it never indicates any specific illness and cannot be used as a definitive diagnostic measurement, albeit many doctors still use the sed rate as a means of ostensibly uncovering some occult disease. Since this test is usually performed under your doctor's direction, your reports of the results to him or her will determine whether or not an office visit is necessary.

Reliability

The home test has proved as accurate as similar tests performed professionally in laboratories, and sometimes even more accurate. In general, all tests of this type are at least 90 percent accurate in measuring the sedimentation rate; as a means of predicting the prognosis of an illness, the test is considered about 75 percent accurate. One use of the sed rate, however, is to eliminate the possibility of some hidden disease; a normal sed rate is about 90 percent accurate in ruling out suspected illnesses.

SICKLE-CELL SCREENING
(A test that can help identify an inherited sickle-cell trait or the disease itself)

Sickle cells are red blood cells that carry a misshapen molecule of hemoglobin called hemoglobin S (see Blood Tests, **Hemoglobin**), which, in turn, causes these cells to assume a "sickle" shape (somewhat like the curved blade of the farm implement) instead of the usual doughnut shape of normal red blood cells. Because of their elongated shape, sickle cells usually cannot pass through tiny arteries and capillaries and can cause small clots (thromboses), which prevent adequate blood from reaching distant tissues. Sickle cells are also much more fragile than normal red blood cells and tend to break easily, causing anemia. These changes occur more frequently in situations where lower-than-normal amounts of oxygen are present—such as when flying, especially if the plane depressurizes, after injuries, during surgery and with physical exertion—and can precipitate a critical, sometimes fatal, condition.

   Sickle-cell problems have two distinct aspects: sickle-cell anemia, in which the individual inherits two sickle-cell-causing genes, one from each parent, and actually contracts the disease, and sickle-cell trait (sickling trait), in which only one sickle-cell-causing gene is inherited and the individual does not have the disease. If, by chance, two people with sickle-cell trait mate, they can pass the disease on to their offspring.

The disease shows itself through severe episodes of pain, especially in the abdomen and bones when these organs are deprived of blood; weakness and jaundice from the anemia; as well as nerve and muscle disorders when the brain is afflicted. Those with only the trait rarely show any symptoms unless exposed to extremes of diminished oxygen or subjected to extreme physical exertion. However, both those with the disease and those with only the trait may at times show physical signs (blood in the urine, swelling of the hands and feet, and pain imitating appendicitis or gallstones) that can confuse doctors and cause them to suspect some disease other than sickle-cell anemia unless the sickle cells are known to be present; thus, the importance of screening for sickle-cell hemoglobin.

Although the disease and the trait are found primarily in blacks (1 out of every 400 inherits the disease; 1 out of every 10 inherits the trait), they are also found in Caucasians of Mediterranean or Middle Eastern origin, Southeast Asians, East Indians, Caribbeans, and Central and South Americans.

Many states have already passed laws or regulations for screening newborn children to help detect a variety of inherited and metabolic diseases (for example, see Urine Tests, **Clinical Analysis: Phenylketonuria Screening**); some are mandatory, and some are voluntary. Several, but not all, states include the search for sickle-cell trait and disease as part of the program. In some instances, primarily because most people wrongly fail to distinguish between the trait and the disease, discrimination has resulted. A few airlines would not let black employees fly because of a fear that any decrease in oxygen could cause a crisis situation; insurance companies either refused to insure blacks or, if they did, raised their premiums; and even the military considered rejecting blacks with the sickle-cell trait, not just the disease. Then, if it became public knowledge that someone had the trait alone, the chances for employment could be reduced and a social stigma might be attached to the individual. Thus, the opportunity for confidentiality in screening for sickle-cell trait and anemia can be of particular personal value.

The latest recommendation of the National Institutes of Health is that all newborns be screened for sickle-cell anemia regardless of ethnic background, especially since there are now proven treatments to lessen the adverse effects of the disease.

What Is Usual
No evidence of hemoglobin S should be detected in the blood.

What You Need
To perform the test, you should get a Sickledex Tube Test kit, which costs from $30.00 to $35.00 for a package of 12 tests. A drop or two of blood (see Blood Tests, **Obtaining a Blood Sample**) is placed in the tube. This test only detects the presence of hemoglobin S and does not differentiate between the trait and anemia.

You can also use a SICKLEQUIK test tube, which costs $39.50 for a package of 25 tubes. You simply put two drops of fingertip blood in the tube, wait about 10 minutes and, by comparing the colors of a floating sediment layer with the solution that forms under it, you can detect both the sickle-cell trait and sickle-cell anemia itself.

What to Watch Out For
Do not test infants younger than 6 months of age; they may have been tested at birth. If hemoglobin S is present but in low levels in infants, the test could show a false-negative result; it should be repeated professionally a few months later. There are 10 states that now automatically provide for, but do not mandate, the test; other states authorize such screening, some when children reach school age, but parents may refuse on religious or other grounds.

What the Test Results Can Mean
Any positive result warrants medical attention to determine the true extent and status of the condition. If there are signs and symptoms similar to sickle-cell disease, especially if generalized anemia exists (see Blood Tests, **Hemoglobin**), a medical consultation is warranted, even if the test is negative. Of great importance, the patient requires proper counseling in order to understand all aspects and ramifications of either being a carrier or having the disease.

Reliability
The test itself is considered 95 percent accurate. There have been reports of misdiagnosis, however, especially when routine screening of newborns is performed.

UREA NITROGEN (Blood Urea Nitrogen, BUN)
(A measure of protein metabolism and kidney function)

Urea is produced in the liver and is the main nitrogen-containing end product of protein metabolism. Normally, there is very little urea in the blood, and what is present is usually eliminated into the urine by the kidneys. A diet high in protein can cause a temporary increase in blood urea nitrogen (BUN), as can excessive exercise with profuse perspiration and other activities that cause dehydration or starvation, such as vomiting and/or diarrhea. A low-protein diet can decrease BUN values. And the use of a great many drugs can alter BUN levels:

- Antibiotics, such as Chloromycetin and streptomycin
- Diuretic drugs

- Blood pressure medications, such as methyldopa
- Salicylates, such as aspirin and related products
- Sedatives, such as chloral hydrate
- Steroid hormones, such as cortisone products

Although the BUN level is primarily an indicator of kidney function, it can be altered by so many other non-kidney-related conditions that it should be considered only as a rough screening test for kidney disease and as an early warning signal for other latent body pathology.

What Is Usual
Most people show a BUN value of from 10 mg to 20 mg per 100 ml of blood. Some doctors accept up to 25 mg per 100 ml as usual with aging. Repeated values within this range are reasonably indicative of normal kidney function. It is possible to have a value lower than 10 mg per 100 ml following a low-protein diet and during a normal pregnancy.

What You Need
The test is performed with a drop of blood (see Blood Tests, **Obtaining a Blood Sample**) and an AZOSTIX (a plastic strip with a chemically treated tip, similar to those used in blood glucose and urine testing), which costs from $14.00 to $18.00 for a package of 25. (Incidentally, the prefix *azo* refers to nitrogen, and *azotemia* means too much urea nitrogen in the blood.)

What to Watch Out For
Here are some cautions for BUN testing:

- Do not use an AZOSTIX if the chemically treated tip has a yellowish color.
- Do not use an AZOSTIX more than 60 days after the bottle has been opened, no matter what expiration date is given.
- Do not use a small drop of blood; a large drop is required.
- Use a clock or watch with a sweep-second hand or a digital display that shows seconds, or use a stopwatch, for this test; exact timing of one minute is extremely important.
- Color distinction is critical; be sure you have normal color vision.
- Be sure to take into consideration any drugs you are using; consult your doctor or pharmacist to see whether your medicines will interfere with this test.

What the Test Results Can Mean
Any test result that is between 15 mg and 25 mg per 100 ml should be repeated the next day. If still greater than 20 mg per 100 ml, a medical consultation is warranted. A test value greater than 25 mg per 100 ml should

be considered abnormal, and even if the cause can be explained by diet, physical activity or drug use, it warrants medical attention. There are other tests that a doctor can perform to ascertain whether the high BUN level is from a disease.

Most often, an increase in BUN is an indication of kidney trouble; it may be from an acute infection, from repeated damage due to chronic infection or from a tumor. Any other condition that causes less blood to flow through the kidneys—such as heart failure, bleeding (especially in the intestines), shock and even extreme stress—can cause an elevated BUN value. Other factors that can increase the BUN include: heavy-metal poisoning;; thyroid disease; diabetes; gout; many different hormone disorders; infections elsewhere in the body, such as pneumonia and pancreatitis or simply a high fever; and any blockage of the urinary tract, such as from a kidney stone, bladder infection or enlarged prostate (see Urine Tests, **Clinical Analysis: Nitrite**). A BUN level greater than 30 mg per 100 ml warrants immediate medical attention.

On occasion the BUN value can be lowered by liver disease, certain drugs (especially antibiotics), a condition called amyloidosis (an accumulation of a starchlike material throughout the body) and nephrosis (a degenerative disease of the kidneys that causes water retention, or edema). A persistent decreased BUN level warrants medical consultation.

Reliability
When compared with complex laboratory techniques, the plastic-stick method proved to be quite satisfactory as a screening test. Normal readings are considered 90 percent accurate. When BUN values between 20 mg and 40 mg are observed, about half of those turn out to be falsely high. Values greater than 40 mg per 100 ml are again 90 percent accurate.

HEART AND
CIRCULATION TESTS

BLOOD PRESSURE
(One of the simplest, yet best, preventive general health tests available)

The term *blood pressure* generally refers to the pressure in the arteries as opposed to the veins. To take one's blood pressure is to measure the pressure (tension) of the blood within the artery walls. (Pressures in the capillaries and veins are quite different.) The end result is affected by a number of factors: the force of each heartbeat, the elasticity or resilience of the walls of the artery, the amount of blood flowing through the arteries at any one time, the viscosity (thickness) of the blood, the number of molecules of various substances (such as protein and sodium) in the blood, the amount of certain hormones and enzymes (such as adrenalin from the adrenal gland and renin from the kidneys) circulating in the blood and the functioning of the autonomic or sympathetic nervous system (over which a person has no direct control) in response to changes in posture, stressful situations and other stimuli. (See Heart and Circulation Tests, **Cold Pressor and Finger Wrinkle.**)

Every day, on the average, the heart pumps 2,000 gallons of blood through 70,000 miles of blood vessels. The blood pressure is altered during every heartbeat, reaching its highest point when the heart muscle is most contracted (forcing blood into the arteries) and its lowest point when the heart muscle relaxes after each heartbeat. The heart muscle contraction is called systole, and the medical term for the highest point of one's blood pressure is *systolic*. The momentary resting phase of the heart is called diastole, and the low point of one's blood pressure is known as *diastolic*. The difference between these two pressures is called the pulse pressure.

The measurement of blood pressure is really the measurement of how much pressure must be applied around an artery to close off its circulation. This is most commonly done by applying a cuff or sleeve around the upper arm and then inflating that cuff with air to put sufficient pressure on the brachial artery (the largest artery that runs down the arm) and its surrounding skin and muscles to close it off. The amount of pressure is determined by reading an air pressure dial or a digital display or by noting how high a column of mercury is pushed up a calibrated glass tube. The latter is considered the standard against which all other measurements are compared, and blood pressure readings are usually reported in millimeters of mercury (mm Hg), no matter what technique is used. When closure, or collapse, of the brachial artery occurs, the pulse can no longer be felt at the wrist or heard through a stethoscope or other electronic sound detector placed on the inside of the arm in front of the elbow. As the pressure is gradually reduced by allowing air to escape from the cuff, the point at which the pulse is once again detected is recorded as the systolic blood pressure. The pulse will continue to be detected as long as sufficient pressure is applied from the outside to cause the blood's pulsations to rebound off the artery wall. When the outside pressure becomes low enough so that there is no measurable resistance against the artery wall, the pulse's sound will no longer be detected (it can still be felt at the wrist); this point is recorded as the diastolic blood pressure.

Home blood pressure testing is usually limited to measurement of an upper arm, but it can be a good idea, initially, to measure the pressure in both arms and even in the upper legs, as most doctors do. Also, when first starting out to test your blood pressure, you should measure it while standing, sitting and lying down; wait at least five minutes after assuming a new position before you take your blood pressure (see Heart and Circulation Tests, **Orthostatic Blood Pressure**). Blood pressure tests should also be performed at various times of the day—with a note as to your activities, emotions and environment. Blood pressure can rise if you are afraid or angry. If you outwardly express your anger, your blood pressure should return to its usual level in a short time; if you hold your anger inside, or feel guilty after expressing it, your blood pressure can remain elevated for a much longer time.

One way of measuring your reaction to stressful situations is to take your blood pressure before, during, immediately after and then 30 minutes to 60 minutes after playing a competitive video game to win. Studies have shown that people who react strongly to such a challenge with a rise in blood pressure of more than 20 mm systolic and/or 15 mm diastolic, or whose blood pressure goes above 160/95, are much more prone to develop hypertension (high blood pressure) and heart disease in later life.

A great many drugs can cause high blood pressure. Some of the most common include medicines to treat asthma, birth control pills or estrogens alone, certain antidepressant medications and tranquilizers, a few of the new nonaspirin products used for arthritis and even penicillin.

At the present time it is believed that large amounts of sodium (salt) in the diet can contribute to high blood pressure (see Body Observations, **Salt Measurements**). But because all the facts are not as yet scientifically proved, you should not severely restrict your salt intake without first consulting your physician. Some people challenge their sensitivity to salt by measuring blood pressure before and after eating very salty foods. And there are some people who react with elevated blood pressure when they eat a great deal of licorice, while others show a rise in blood pressure after drinking liqueur made of anise; it is postulated that licorice causes sodium to increase in the blood, and the sodium holds excess water in body tissues. There have also been reports that ginseng, tobacco and some antacid preparations can contribute to high blood pressure.

High blood pressure also seems to run in families; children of parents with hypertension are much more prone to develop the condition. People who are overweight have a greater incidence of high blood pressure than do those who are thin. Blacks seem much more predisposed to hypertension than do whites. Where there is a family history of hypertension, many doctors recommend that children of the family start regular blood pressure screening at the age of 6. Small increases are considered predictive of potential problems in later years, and the earlier the risk is discovered, the easier the hypertension is to control.

And it is probably not surprising that blood pressure is usually lower than usual while you are asleep and a bit higher than usual when you are working at your job. It is almost always lower when measured at home and almost always higher when tested in a doctor's office. When blood pressure measurements are regularly, but falsely, elevated whenever the test is performed by a doctor, this rise is called "white-coat disease" or "cuff reacting."

What Is Usual

The most generalized figure used as normal for arterial blood pressure is 120/80, signifying that the systolic pressure is 120 mm Hg and the diastolic pressure is 80 mm Hg when the person is sitting down at rest and relaxed. It is not unusual, however, for a person's blood pressure to vary on occasion; it can be 120/80 at one time and be 160/100 a few hours later. This should not occur more than once or twice every few months. Although blood pressure does tend to rise with age, it should stay below 140/85; higher figures point to hypertension. It should be fairly consistent (within 5 mm Hg) in both arms and legs and after standing for a period of five minutes after one has been in a sitting position.

Note: In general, read blood pressure to the nearest 5mm; more precise figures are considered unnecessary.

What You Need

The test is performed with a sphygmomanometer—a small, portable device that has a cuff that fits around the arm, allows pressure to be inflated in the cuff and includes some sort of instrument to show how much pressure is being applied. There are many kinds of sphygmomanometers, the primary difference being how they show the pressure values:

- Those using mercury that rises and falls inside a glass tube with mm measurements engraved along the side of the tube; they cost from $60.00 to $100.00 plus from $4.00 to $10.00 for a stethoscope to listen for the sounds.
- The aneroid type, which converts mm Hg into figures on a gauge or circular dial face similar to a thermometer. These come in several varieties: Some require the use of a stethoscope to listen for the sounds and, including the stethoscope, cost from $12.00 to $80.00 (much depends on the length of the guarantee); others incorporate a blinking light and/ or a distinct sound ("beep"), replacing the stethoscope with a built-in microphone synchronized to the sounds that would have been heard through the stethoscope, at a cost of $20.00 to $100.00.
- The digital type, which displays the systolic and diastolic pressures—and sometimes the pulse rate—directly; these cost from $25.00 to $200.00.
- Some new sphygmomanometers now automatically inflate the cuff to the proper level and then release the air at the proper time. Some provide printed results showing the date and time as well as blood pressure and pulse readings; these can be valuable to bring to your doctor with appropriate notes showing any environmental influences or emotional situations at or near the time the blood pressure was measured.
- There is a new device called a Minimonitor that measures blood pressure with a "cuff" that is wrapped around a finger; its accuracy has yet to be established. The cost is approximately $70.00.

The mercury type, while the most accurate, is also the most difficult to use at home; some come with a lifetime guarantee on the accuracy of the measuring portion (not including the rubber or cloth parts). The aneroid types that require a stethoscope are the least expensive but can also be the least accurate; the guarantee on the gauge's accuracy can range from three months to 10 years. The ones that do not require a stethoscope use batteries and are much better for home testing. (In general, automatic devices that do not require a stethoscope are much easier to use.) The digital type can be battery-operated and, while the most expensive, is the best for home use; most include built-in safeguards to prevent any error in technique and are usually guaranteed for only one year, because they, too, tend to need recalibration. The cuffs may be closed around the arm by cloth ties, metal hooks or Velcro; some include easy one-hand cuff application. Some have automatic self-deflating cuffs; others require the turn of a valve screw or the push of a button. Only a personal trial of the various types will show you which is easiest to use in relation to cost. The digital-display type has the advantage of not requiring you to watch the measurements when testing blood pressure, something that can cause anxiety and provoke a false reading.

Before purchasing any syphygmomanometer, be sure to try it out at the pharmacy or store to make certain you can use the device easily and properly. Some do allow proper cuff placement with less effort than others. Then try two or three of the same model as well as one or two from different companies to see whether the readings are almost identical. Some inexpensive digital types have not been too accurate; the blood pressure device you do choose should show close to the same reading as those on several other machines—within three to five points. After you decide, it is wise to take your syphygmomanometer to your doctor's office and compare your reading with his or hers. Even though your blood pressure reading is apt to be higher in the doctor's office than when taken at home, the two readings taken in the doctor's office should be similar.

What to Watch Out For

The accuracy of your sphygmomanometer—no matter what type—is a vital consideration. Keep in mind that even when doctors' non-mercury-column sphygmomanometers were tested at random, one out of every two to three gave erroneous readings. You should check your own device against a mercury-column type at least once a year, and even more often if you are under treatment for hypertension. Your doctor simply connects your device to his or her mercury-column meter with a Y-shaped tube; the readings from both machines should be within 5 mm of each other.

Be sure to place the cuff properly; if it has a built-in microphone, be precise about positioning it according to the directions. Be sure your cuff is big enough; it should be at least five inches wide (cover that much of your arm) and encircle the arm without strain. If a large enough cuff is not used on an obese person, a false-elevated reading can result. Do not roll up a sleeve or cover it with the cuff; the arm must not be constricted by clothing. If your devise does not automatically deflate, do not let the air out too fast; the measurements should decrease at a rate of about 2 mm a second. Do not measure blood pressure in the arm whose hand is used to squeeze the air pressure bulb. The position of the arm wearing the cuff can influence the result, although its effect is greatest on systolic measurements. The best position is for the forearm to rest on a table, with the cuff at heart level; if the arm is flat (from shoulder to hand), the readings can be falsely low, while if the arm hangs by the side, the readings can be falsely high.

If you use a stethoscope, be sure there are no extraneous noises to distract you. If you use a built-in microphone, those same extraneous noises, if loud enough, could be picked up by the microphone and give a false reading. Use a bell-shaped stethoscope head rather than a flat-shaped head; it will pick up the pulse sounds better. Learn how to use the stethoscope itself; the ear tips should face forward. Be sure you know what the pulse should sound like.

Do not accept a single blood pressure measurement as being definitive. There should be at least three different tests, on three different days, that offer a similar result; otherwise, something is wrong with your equipment or your technique.

Be sure the rubber tubing, pressure bulb for squeezing air into the cuff, air valves and other parts of your sphygmomanometer that are subject to deterioration are in good condition; pinholes in the rubber, dirty valves and a worn-out cuff can cause erroneous readings.

Do not talk while taking your own blood pressure or while having it taken; conversation tends to raise blood pressure. It is also known that exposure to loud noise for only a few minutes will cause one's blood pressure to rise rapidly and for a prolonged period of time (see Ear Observations and Hearing Tests, **Hearing Function**).

What the Test Results Can Mean

Assuming you are not already under a physician's care, any consistent reading (three different times, on three different days and under different circumstances) of a systolic pressure higher than 150 mm Hg and/or a diastolic pressure higher than 90 mm Hg warrants medical attention. Persistent measurements higher than 140/85 warrant medical consultation, for they can be early warning signs of the development of high blood pressure and should be followed closely.

High blood pressure is more of a cause than a result of heart problems. At the same time an elevated blood pressure can also signify kidney disease, connective tissue disease, nervous system problems, lung disease and hormonal problems. If blood pressure measurements differ by more than 5 mm Hg in either arm or in the legs, medical attention is warranted.

Although arm-cuff blood pressure measurements performed while exercising are not too accurate, the blood pressure usually goes up 20 mm with moderate physical activity and may increase by up to 50 mm during strenuous exercise. If either the systolic or diastolic readings during moderate exercise rise by more than 20 mm, a medical consultation is warranted.

Low blood pressure measurements (hypotension), below 100 mm Hg for systolic and below 65 mm Hg for diastolic, warrant medical consultation; they could come from medicines (diuretics and other drugs such as tranquilizers), but they can also come from Parkinson-type diseases, nervous system disorders and internal bleeding.

The pulse pressure (the difference between the systolic and diastolic pressure readings) should be between 30 and 50; if higher, especially without high blood pressure, it could come from other forms of heart disease, thyroid disease or anxiety and warrants a medical consultation. If the pulse pressure is lower than 30, it warrants medical attention, for it could be a sign of a heart valve problem or an inability of the heart to contract and expand properly.

If, after you have taken your blood pressure with the standard arm-cuff-type apparatus at different times, on different days and under different circumstances, there is still some doubt about your blood pressure measurements, your doctor can arrange for you to wear a special blood pressure cuff for a 24-hour period; this can help determine true values in all situations.

Reliability

Studies have shown that blood pressure measurements, when properly performed at home, are more precise than when performed in a doctor's office or hospital. In general, they are 95 percent accurate. When taken in a commercial setting—such as in a drug store, supermarket or county fair—blood pressure measurements are considered to be only 75 percent accurate because of the environmental disruptions and common failure to properly maintain the test devices. Of interest, since home blood pressure measurement has become common (it has been estimated that 1 out of every 10 people in the United States now measures blood pressure at home), the overall average blood pressure levels have dropped nearly 10 percent when compared to office measurements. Several studies have shown that doctors may prescribe antihypertensive drugs on the basis of just one blood pressure test; it is now estimated that 1 out of every 3 patients on such drugs need not be taking them.

Unfortunately, not all makes of blood pressure measuring devices are reliable. The relative accuracy of 36 different sphygmomanometers is reported in the May 1987 issue of *Consumer Reports,* available at most libraries.

ORTHOSTATIC BLOOD PRESSURE
(A screening test for one cause of dizziness)

There are some people who experience a slight feeling of dizziness, and may even have momentarily blurred vision, every time they get up from a reclining or sitting position; usually, the dizziness seems greater the faster or more suddenly they arise. It has been estimated that at least 20 percent of the population over 50 years of age has this problem. This sometimes comes from orthostatic hypotension or idiopathic orthostatic hypotension (in medical terminology *idiopathic* usually means "of unknown origin"). Where the physical movement alone causes a greater-than-normal drop in blood pressure because of the sudden gravitational shifting of blood to the lower part of the body, the consequent reduction of the blood supply to the brain is believed to be the cause of dizziness. However, the same symptoms can also be produced by a few other disease conditions, most of which can be easily and successfully treated if detected early enough. Measurements of the blood pressure and pulse (see Heart and Circulation Tests, **Pulse Measurements**) while you are relaxed and sitting, or even while lying down, and again after you suddenly stand can help discern whether a medical problem exists, although it can only hint at the specific cause—usually, but not always, related to the sympathetic nervous system (see Heart and Circulation Tests, **Cold Pressor and Finger Wrinkle**) or to the use of certain medications.

What Is Usual
If you measure blood pressure after lying quietly for five minutes, just prior to standing and then again right after standing, the systolic pressure usually drops by from 5 mm Hg to 15 mm Hg. At the same time, the pulse rate usually increases by from 10 beats to 20 beats per minute. After five minutes of standing, the blood pressure usually returns to close to what it was while you were sitting or lying down, and the pulse rate returns to within 10 beats per minute of its sitting rate.

What You Need
You should obtain a blood pressure measuring device (see Heart and Circulation Tests, **Blood Pressure**) and a watch or timer (a pulse-measuring device is optional).

What to Watch Out For
If you know that you experience dizziness when you rise suddenly, be sure you have someone with you to prevent you from falling. In fact, this is one of those tests that is best performed with another person taking and recording the measurements. Do not attempt the test if you are taking any medicine to lower your blood pressure.

What the Test Results Can Mean
Should your systolic or diastolic blood pressure fall more than 15 points after you stand, this observation warrants a medical consultation, if only to establish the diagnosis of orthostatic hypotension. If the pulse rate increases by more than 25 beats a minute, accompanying the unusual fall in blood pressure, it could signify an anemia, diabetes or some other hormone dis-

order, internal bleeding or a very rare adrenal tumor called a pheochromocytoma. If, when the blood pressure falls, your pulse rate increases only very slightly or decreases, it could signify a nerve, heart or circulation problem, or it could also be the consequence of any one of many different drugs, especially tranquilizers, sleeping medicines, alcohol or narcotics. Any pulse alteration of more than 20 beats per minute warrants medical consultation. When there is a variation from what is usual in both blood pressure and pulse rate, it warrants medical attention.

Reliability
The test is considered to be 80 percent accurate in detecting orthostatic hypotension.

CAPILLARY FRAGILITY
(Tourniquet; Rumpel-Leede)
(A possible clue to why you are black and blue)

If you seem to bruise easily when you bump into something, it may well be that your capillaries (the tiniest of all blood vessels and the ones that connect the arteries to the veins) are unusually fragile; that is, they break more easily than they should and release blood into the tissues. Bleeding, especially under the skin, is usually described by three terms: *petechiae*, or tiny dotlike hemhorrages that resemble scarlet fever; *purpura,* or red-brown or blue-brown patches, larger than petechiae but usually smaller than a 10-cent piece; and *ecchymosis*, or large black-and-blue bruises.

One way to test for capillary fragility is to perform a modification of the blood pressure test. Place the blood pressure cuff around an upper arm and measure the systolic and diastolic readings. Once these readings are determined, set the pressure on the cuff halfway between those two readings and leave it that way, on the arm, for five minutes. The pressure is then released entirely, and two minutes later the inside of the forearm of the arm that had the pressure applied is examined for petechiae. It is usual to draw a one-inch diameter circle (the size of a quarter) on an unblemished part of the forearm prior to applying the pressure and only count the petechiae that appear within that circle. This is one of a series of tests to measure hemostasis, or how well the body responds to stop bleeding following trauma (see Blood Tests, **Bleeding and Clotting Time**). Since a tourniquet similar to the ones used by laboratory technicians when they draw blood from the arm is often used, the test is sometimes called a tourniquet test; it is also known as the Rumpel-Leede test, after the two German doctors who first reported the observation.

For some unknown reason, women with red hair and women over 50 years of age may show petechiae (a positive reaction) without any disease condition.

What Is Usual
Two minutes after the blood pressure cuff has been removed, there should be no petechiae inside the circle on the forearm. However, some doctors feel that up to 5 tiny spots in a man and up to 10 in a woman are still within normal limits.

What You Need
The test requires a blood pressure measuring device, a watch and a 25-cent piece to make the circle.

What to Watch Out For
The following precautions should be observed when testing for capillary fragility:

- Do not put excessive pressure on the blood pressure cuff; be precise about using the midway pressure between systolic and diastolic.
- Do not use a blood pressure cuff with an automatic deflating device; it will not hold sustained pressure.
- If petechiae appear, do not count them until two minutes after the cuff is removed.
- Do not circle an area on the forearm that contains spots, bruises or other marks that could be mistaken for petechiae.

What the Test Results Can Mean
Although the test essentially measures capillary fragility, the most common cause for 10 or more petechiae to appear is thrombocytopenia (an abnormally low number of platelets); this, as well as weakened blood vessel walls, can reflect:

- An inherited condition.
- A secondary result of many diseases (such as cancer, kidney disease, leukemia and liver disease) and infections (such as flu or tuberculosis).
- The use of drugs, especially aspirin, but also certain antibiotics, barbiturates, diuretics and medicines used to treat arthritis, cancer and epilepsy and taking large amounts of fish oil capsules.
- Excessive exposure to X-rays or radiation.
- High blood pressure and diabetes; a positive test in a patient with diabetes could be a warning sign of diabetic eye disease (retinopathy), and some diabetics will show a decrease in the number of petechiae as their diabetes becomes better controlled.

- Scurvy (a deficiency of vitamin C that can occur in alcoholics and food faddists who have poor nutritional habits).
- Simple aging; elderly people can develop purpuric spots—especially on the forearms and backs of the hands—for no explainable reason.

A positive reaction (more than 10 petechiae within the one-inch circle) warrants a medical consultation.

Reliability
The test is considered 80 percent accurate as an indicator of a bleeding tendency.

COLD PRESSOR AND FINGER WRINKLE
(A screening evaluation of one's heart, circulation and nervous system)

The cold pressor and finger wrinkle tests, in which the hand is placed in cold and/or warm water (along with the **Orthostatic Blood Pressure** test; see Heart and Circulation Tests), help evaluate the sympathetic nervous system component of the overall autonomic nervous system. The word *pressor* refers to stimulation of the nerves that control the walls of the arteries. The autonomic nerves operate automatically—that is, without any conscious or willful control. They are comprised of two opposing systems: the sympathetic, with more of an excitatory action, and the parasympathetic, with its antagonistic action (see the discussion of the cold face reflex test under Brain and Nervous System Tests, **Reflex Testing**). Together the two systems help control the heart rate (pulse); blood pressure; rate of breathing; constriction and relaxation of the bronchial tubes; size of the pupils; digestion in, and evacuation of, the gastrointestinal tract; urination; sweating; salivation; tears of crying; stuffiness in the nose; some physical reactions to sexual stimulation; wrinkling of the skin; and even such prosaic activities as yawning.

These nerves act primarily without the purposeful control that is employed in deliberate movement. Emotions also indirectly influence the autonomic nervous system; fear, for example, can provoke the sympathetic nerves to quicken the pulse or dilate the pupils. As with blood pressure and blood cholesterol levels, if you are lying in bed and hear, or even think you hear, a strange noise—as if someone were trying to break in—usually, you can immediately feel your heart beat much faster, and you may even begin to perspire profusely. That is but one instance of how the sympathetic nervous system works. The brain's perception also causes the adrenal glands to secrete a great deal of adrenalin (epinephrine), which acts on many different body organs. And numerous drugs can cause autonomic system reactions: Many medicines used to treat asthma (especially those that act like adrenalin) can also cause a marked increase in the heart rate and a sharp rise in blood pressure. Conversely, many drugs used to treat high blood pressure can cause a type of impotence of the sympathetic nervous system. When the sympathetic nervous system does not seem to reflect normal activity, it can indicate heart and/or artery disease, certain anemias, some nerve disorders or infections, a few hormone imbalances such as diabetes, and even the ill effects of alcohol and other forms of drug abuse.

What Is Usual

First, you should establish your usual blood pressure and pulse rate. Then, when you place your hand in a container of ice-cold water for no more than one minute, the impulses felt by the skin and blood vessels near the skin's surface are carried through the nerves to the autonomic system, which lies adjacent to the spinal cord. The sympathetic part of the system then sends out impulses to the heart and arteries, causing the heart to beat about 10 beats per minute faster than usual and the arteries to constrict, which raises the systolic blood pressure some 10 mm Hg to 20 mm Hg.

Normally, the inner wall, or lining, of the artery is composed of only one thin layer of cells. When the nerve impulses provoked by the ice-cold water travel up the arm to the sympathetic nervous system, they are then transmitted from the sympathetic nervous system to all the various body organs under its control. In particular, when the impulses reach an artery, they cause the artery's muscle layer to contract, narrowing the opening of the artery through which blood is carried. The subsequent increased pressure on the blood flow is reflected by a rise in blood pressure (see Figure 29).

If an artery's inner wall is partially obstructed due to an abnormal increase of cells—such as happens with atherosclerosis—the artery opening, or blood passageway, is already so small that any contraction of the artery muscle layer causes only a slight change in the artery opening, and this is reflected by little, if any, change in the blood pressure (see Figure 30). After the hand is removed from the ice-cold water, the pulse and blood pressure should return to normal within 5 minutes to 10 minutes.

When you place your hand in warm water for at least half an hour, a different part of the sympathetic nervous system, not directly connected to the heart, reacts and should cause the skin of the fingers to wrinkle or shrivel. In addition, most people perspire within the 30-minute period.

What You Need

For the cold pressor test you need a basin of ice-cold water, preferably from 33 F to 37 F (about 2 C), a blood pressure measuring device (see Heart and Circulation Tests, **Blood Pressure**) and a watch (a pulse-measuring device— see Heart and Circulation Tests, **Pulse Measurements**—may also be em-

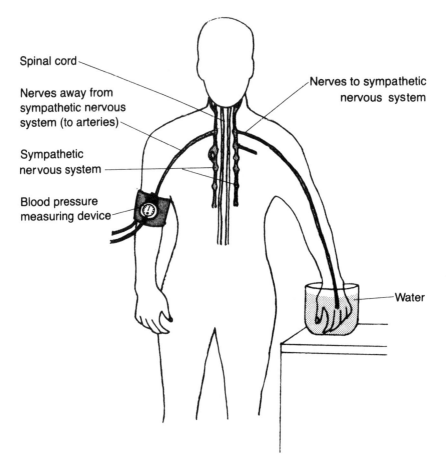

Spinal cord

Nerves away from
sympathetic nervous
system (to arteries)

Sympathetic
nervous system

Blood pressure
measuring device

Nerves to sympathetic
nervous system

Water

Figure 29. Cold pressor test.

ployed). For the finger wrinkle test, all you need is a basin of warm water, preferably at about 100 F (38 C).

What to Watch Out For
If you have ever had any form of chest pain, you should consult your doctor before performing the cold pressor test; some physicians feel that this test is quite similar to, if not better than, the exercise stress electrocardiogram test, in that it can put an extra burden on the heart and help indicate the presence of hidden or early heart disease. If you are over 40 years of age, you should also discuss the test with your doctor before performing it. Do not leave your hand in the ice-cold water for more than 1 minute, nor in the warm water for more than 30 minutes. Measure blood pressure and pulse in the arm opposite to the one in the water.

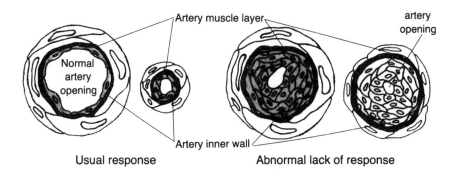

Normal artery opening
Artery muscle layer
artery opening
Artery inner wall
Usual response
Abnormal lack of response

Figure 30. Artery response to the cold pressor test.

What the Test Results Can Mean

If, within 3 minutes to 5 minutes after the hand is removed from the ice-cold water, the systolic blood pressure rises more than 30 points, it could be an early warning sign of susceptibility to high blood pressure, and you should seek a medical consultation. If, after 30 minutes, the systolic blood pressure does not rise more than 5 points or has not returned to normal (or to within 5 points of what it usually is), it could indicate atherosclerosis or some other disease of the arteries such as Raynaud's phenomenon, a condition in which cold or stress can cause blood vessels—especially in the fingers, toes, ears and tip of the nose—to contract and seriously impair one's circulation. Should the cold pressor test bring on chest discomfort or pain, it could signify a heart problem. Any one of these observations warrants medical attention.

While some people with very early disease may show a usual response, any unusual response is strong evidence of something's being wrong within the nerve–circulation system pathways.

Should the fingers show no sign of wrinkling after being in warm water for 30 minutes, it can mean that some disease process such as Guillian-Barre syndrome—a nerve infection—might exist. Severe diabetes can also prevent wrinkling. Failure of the skin to wrinkle, or failure to perspire, warrants a medical consultation. Of course, patients who have had a sympathectomy—in which the sympathetic nerve chain has been surgically removed (a procedure once performed to control high blood pressure or persistent leg cramps)—will never show the usual responses to either test.

Reliability

The test is considered to be 80 percent accurate in revealing latent heart or artery disease and about 60 percent accurate in screening for nerve-functioning problems.

PULSE MEASUREMENTS
(A possible early warning sign of circulatory or lung disease and a measure of fitness)

The pulse is a manifestation of the expansion of the arteries that takes place every time the heart contracts and forces blood into the circulatory system; each heartbeat is a pulse (stroke). The pulse is also a very sensitive reflection of the body's condition, somewhat similar to body temperature. Pulse measurements usually consist of rate, rhythm and character and can be obtained almost anywhere an artery lies near the skin surface. The most frequently used location is the wrist—with the palm up and two or three fingers of the examining hand resting on the artery just inside the outer wrist bone of the arm whose pulse is being examined (see Figure 31). The pulse can just as easily be counted by applying the fingers alongside the temples, along the side of the neck, on either leg just below the groin area and just above or adjacent to the protruding ankle bone on the inside of the foot (see Figure 32); much depends on one's weight and excess fatty tissues, of course. The pulse rate can also be noted when measuring blood pressure; each sound is a pulse beat.

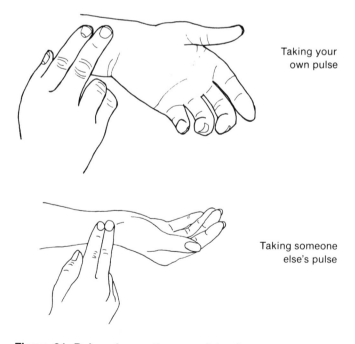

Taking your
own pulse

Taking someone
else's pulse

Figure 31. Pulse observations—wrist pulse.

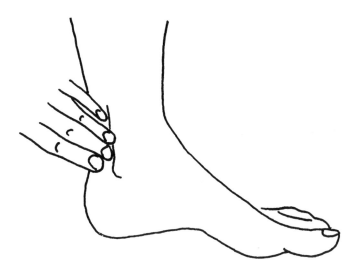

Figure 32. Pulse observations—ankle pulse.

Rhythm and character. Pulse rhythm should be observed at the same time as the rate is counted; the rhythm should be regular, with no erratic interruptions or pauses (skipped beats or extra beats) after two or three rhythmic beats. As for pulse character, each beat should feel the same—with none stronger or weaker than the others.

Except when applying pulse measurements to exercise, you should sit quietly and rest for 10 minutes before testing.

When first attempting pulse measurements, it is best to count all the beats for one full minute and then observe the rhythm and character for a second full minute. With experience, you will become able to shorten the counting time to 15 seconds and then multiply by 4.

Two-step (fitness) test. One valuable pulse test is called the two-step test. You step up and down one or two steps (at least 12 inches high), at a rate of one step per second, at least 50 and preferably 100 times (see Figure 33) and note the change in your pulse rate, particularly how long it takes after you stop stepping for your pulse rate to return to what it was before you started stepping (see Figure 34). This test, which is similar to climbing several flights of stairs, makes the heart beat faster because the heart's muscle requires much more oxygen. It is usually performed along with the **Cold Pressor and Finger Wrinkle** tests (see Heart and Circulation Tests) and can not only offer an early warning sign of heart or artery disease but can also help indicate the state of one's physical fitness.

Note: **If you have ever had chest pains, know that you have heart trouble or know that you normally cannot climb a flight of stairs without difficulty, check with your doctor before trying this test; if you notice discomfort in your chest or arms while stepping up and down, stop the test and seek medical attention.**

Many people, after first obtaining clearance from their doctors to perform strenuous activity, use the pulse rate in combination with metabolic equivalents* (METS) as a means of keeping fit. One MET is considered as resting; as activities become more strenuous, the level of effort is measured in METS, depending on how much oxygen the body needs and how many calories are being burned. Your doctor can tell you your limit in METS: driving a car or writing—under 3 METS; 3 METS—walking slowly, weeding or using power tools; 4 METS—bicycling, golf or horseback riding; 5 METS—walking briskly or playing doubles tennis; 7 METS—playing singles tennis, skiing, climbing stairs; 9 METS—running fast or handball; from 10 METS to 15 METS— very fast running (greater than marathon speed), competitive sports or shoveling snow. Your resting pulse rate, how much faster it becomes during exercise and how quickly it returns to normal can help determine any limitations on physical activity.

Training effect. Once you are cleared for physical activity, pulse measurements may be used as a means of achieving maximum fitness through exercise. Your theoretical maximum pulse rate is computed by subtracting your age from 220. Optimal exercise is said to be accomplished if you expend sufficient energy to raise your pulse rate to at least 70 percent of its maximum, and sustain that rate for 20 minutes, three times a week. You should not let your pulse rate go higher than 80 percent of its maximum. An example: A 50-year-old man would have a maximum pulse rate of 170 $(220 - 50 = 170)$; 70 percent of 170 is 119, and 80 percent is 136. His exercise should therefore be sufficiently strenuous to keep his pulse above 119 (but without exceeding 136) for 20 minutes.

Walking test. Another measure of fitness is how far you can vigorously walk in six minutes (also see Breath and Lung Tests, **Pulmonary Function Measurements**); you should be able to walk two-fifths of a mile (about 2,200

---

*Technically, a MET is related to the amount of oxygen consumed while performing various activities. It is based on the concept that the amount of exercise an individual can perform is limited by that person's breathing ability and pulse rate; it also takes the person's weight into account: 1 MET = 3.5 ml (milliliters) of oxygen use per minute for each kilogram (2.2 pounds) of body weight. Up to 3 METS is considered to be very light activity; 5 METS to 7 METS is considered moderate activity; 7 METS to 9 METS is considered heavy activity; and greater than 9 METS is considered very heavy activity.

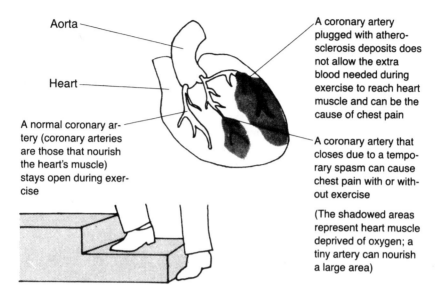

Aorta

Heart

A normal coronary artery (coronary arteries are those that nourish the heart's muscle) stays open during exercise

A coronary artery plugged with athero-sclerosis deposits does not allow the extra blood needed during exercise to reach heart muscle and can be the cause of chest pain

A coronary artery that closes due to a tempo-rary spasm can cause chest pain with or without exercise

(The shadowed areas represent heart muscle deprived of oxygen; a tiny artery can nourish a large area)

Figure 33. The two-step exercise test.

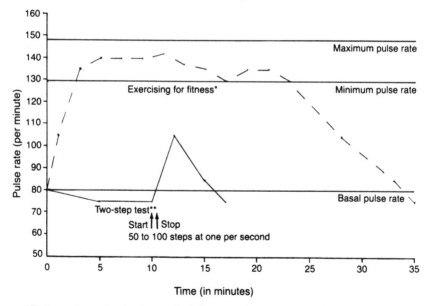

Pulse rate (per minute)

Maximum pulse rate

Minimum pulse rate

Exercising for fitness*

Basal pulse rate

Two-step test**

Start ↑↑ Stop

50 to 100 steps at one per second

Time (in minutes)

*To be performed only after medical clearance from your physician.

**Not to be performed if you have chest pains, if you cannot climb stairs without difficulty or if heart trouble exists

Figure 34. Typical pulse patterns for a 35-year-old individual with a basal (usual) pulse rate of 80 per minute.

feet) in that length of time. While this test can be performed outdoors, it can also be done in a long hallway once the distance is measured off.

Many ecological and environmental conditions can affect the pulse rate. Warmer temperatures automatically increase the rate—all other conditions being the same. Smoking, caffeine, anxiety, smog and alcohol can cause an increased pulse rate. Some of these factors can also cause occasional rhythm and character changes, such as skipped beats or palpitations. The use of drugs for other conditions (medicines for asthma, antidepressants, hormones and certain heart preparations) can all increase the pulse rate as a side effect of their intended actions. Other drugs—such as digitalis products, sedatives and some narcotics—slow the pulse rate. And someone who works at physical fitness or performs regular athletic training will usually have a much slower resting pulse rate.

What Is Usual

There is no absolute standard for pulse rate; it can vary between 60 beats and 90 beats per minute and still be quite normal. It is usually higher in women. Children may have a resting pulse rate of up to 120 per minute, as may some people after the age of 60. Many doctors take age into account, accepting a decrease in physical abilities with advancing years. This is not constant, however, and there really are no true normals related solely to age. The pulse should be regular in rhythm, although a slight increase when breathing in and a decrease when exhaling is also considered normal. After moderate exercise for one minute or two minutes, the pulse rate usually increases by 20 beats per minute and then, within five minutes, returns to what it was prior to exercise. Each pulse beat should feel as if it has the same force against the fingers as those before and after it.

What You Need

Really all that's needed is a watch or clock that has a sweep-second hand or a digital display that shows the time in seconds. However, there are many varieties of pulse monitors that count your pulse electronically and show it constantly on a digital display. Most clip around a finger or are worn like a wristwatch and do not interfere with physical activity. These cost from $49.95 to $150.00, depending on their portability and whether they also include warning devices to inform you of inadequate or excessive activity. While these gadgets are not absolutely necessary, they are convenient for anyone who plans regular pulse monitoring.

What to Watch Out For

If you have any doubt about your physical condition, check with your doctor before performing any pulse-exercise tests. Do not be surprised if your pulse rate varies 10 beats per minute up or down when measuring; that can be perfectly normal, especially if you move about at all. Check with your doctor or pharmacist to see whether any medications you are using (including those not requiring a prescription) will alter your pulse. Diuretic drugs have been known to alter the pulse's rhythm.

What the Test Results Can Mean

If your resting pulse is regularly faster than 90 beats or slower than 60 beats per minute, it warrants a medical consultation, primarily for evaluation. Thyroid disease can show its first signs by altering the pulse rate: Hyperthyroidism increases the rate, while hypothyroidism slows it. Internal bleeding and/or anemia also increases the pulse rate. An increased pulse rate almost always accompanies a fever (see Body Observations, **Body Temperature**), with the exception of typhoid fever, psittacosis (parrot or bird fever) and Legionnaires' disease. A slower-than-normal pulse rate can be an early warning sign of out-of-control diabetes, brain pathology (especially a tumor) or kidney disease. It should be possible to feel the pulse equally on both sides of the body and in all extremities. The inability to detect a pulse at both wrists and ankles warrants medical attention, since it could indicate a circulation problem.

If you notice that your pulse seems to disappear when you take in a deep breath, it could mean a chest problem (emphysema) or a heart problem and warrants medical attention. The pulse should increase slightly on inspiration (breathing in), but if the pulse diminishes, the condition is called *pulsus paradoxus*. This could be an early warning sign of a heart problem, and it can also be a warning sign of a severe asthmatic attack or other acute chest problem; it warrants medical attention.

When performing the two-step test, if you notice any chest discomfort, medical attention is warranted. If, after this test, your pulse rate does not return within five minutes to what it was prior to the test, it could be an early warning sign of heart or artery disease and also warrants medical attention. If you find that you cannot complete the test, albeit you have no chest discomfort and your pulse rate rises and falls as expected, it still warrants medical consultation as to the reason for your physical weakness.

Should the pulse rate not increase when you exercise, or not accelerate when you rise from a sitting to a standing position, this warrants medical attention; it can reflect serious heart-nerve disease.

If you find that you cannot walk more than 2,000 feet in six minutes, it also warrants a medical consultation.

If your heart rhythm is not regular (you notice extra-long pauses between one or two beats now and then), it warrants a medical consultation. While many doctors do not feel that this syndrome (called premature ventricular beats, because the heart contracts an extra time before it is filled with blood) is necessarily due to disease, there are heart problems that can also cause the same "skipped beats" or "flip-flops." Anxiety, heavy smoking and many drugs can also cause an irregular rhythm. If the character of your pulse does not seem consistent, this warrants medical attention, for it can be the first sign of serious heart disease.

Reliability

As a fitness indicator, pulse measurements are 80 percent accurate; a persistent pulse abnormality is considered 90 percent accurate as a sign of disease.

Some pulse meters have been found to be quite inaccurate when used to measure the heartbeat when you are walking or running—with errors of up to 50 beats per minute; be sure that your heart rate monitor is accurate when you are exercising. A report on 13 pulse rate monitors in the May 1988 issue of *The Physician and Sportsmedicine* indicates that chest-attached monitors are the most accurate; some others that measure the pulse in the finger or wrist or that use photocells were found to be unreliable, especially during very strenuous physical activity. Be sure to test a pulse monitor before purchasing it.

TOURNIQUET TESTS FOR VARICOSE VEINS
(Trendelenburg; Perthes)
(Tests intended primarily to see whether treatment will be successful)

Varicose or dilated veins are usually quite obvious, especially in the legs. They can result from several seemingly unrelated factors, the most common being pregnancy, injury, infection and tumors within the abdomen. Normally, they cause such symptoms as leg aches, cramps, pains, itching, dermatitis, pigmentation, ulcers and edema (see Body Observations, **Edema**).

What must always be considered, no matter what the cause or the nature of the complaints, is whether the deep veins (surrounded by the leg muscles) and/or the superficial veins (just under the skin) are involved, and whether or not the tiny veins that connect the superficial veins to the deep veins and the valves inside the veins that control the direction of blood flow are adequate. Without this information, treatment—especially surgery or sclerosing (injection treatments)—can be a painful waste of time and money. For if the deep veins cannot properly return blood to the heart when a person is standing or sitting, specific treatment of the superficial veins will usually fail.

The Trendelenburg test is performed by lying down, raising the leg to be tested up in the air so that all the blood in the veins is emptied out of the leg, applying a tourniquet around the upper portion of the thigh (to prevent immediate refilling of the veins from above) and then standing up. The Perthes test is performed by applying the tourniquet around the leg while standing, with the veins full, and then walking around with the tourniquet on for several minutes. The tourniquet, most commonly a wide piece of Velcro or rubber tubing that can easily be wrapped or tied around the leg, can be applied at various levels of the leg to help determine whether all or only some of the veins are incompetent.

What Is Usual

Obviously, varicose veins in themselves are not normal. With the Trendelenburg test, if, after applying the tourniquet to the thigh and then standing up with the tourniquet still in place, the superficial varicose veins reappear by filling slowly from the bottom up (in about 30 seconds), this usually means that the deep and connecting veins are probably adequate and treatment has a reasonable chance of success. When no obvious varicose veins exist, the filling takes place in less than 10 seconds. After 50 seconds to 60 seconds, the tourniquet is released, and if there is no additional sudden rush of blood to fill the leg, this helps confirm the findings. If the veins seem to fill rapidly (within 4 seconds to 7 seconds), from top to bottom, the deep veins are probably not competent, and removal or obliteration of the superficial veins will usually not relieve symptoms.

The results of the Perthes test are considered to indicate probable effectiveness of treatment if, after you walk around for four minutes to five minutes with the tourniquet in place, the superficial veins seem smaller or less full; this usually means that the connecting veins, the deep veins and their valves are adequate. If the veins seem to increase in size after walking, it usually means that the deep veins are incompetent.

What You Need

A tourniquet is required. A strong, one-inch-wide piece of elastic will do, as long as it can fit around the leg. Professional rubber tubing tourniquets cost from $0.50 to $1.00. Easily applied and removed Velcro tourniquets are available at a cost of from $5.00 to $7.00. An "automatic" tourniquet called the Seraket, which can be applied and removed with one hand and whose pressure can easily be adjusted, costs about $10.00.

What to Watch Out For

When performing the Trendelenburg test, do not leave the tourniquet on longer than 60 seconds. With the Perthes test, remove the tourniquet as soon as the veins seem to increase in size, no matter how little time has elapsed, and do not leave it on more than five minutes. Do not attempt either test if there is any leg infection or leg pain.

What the Test Results Can Mean

For home use the tests are performed primarily to ascertain whether surgery or sclerosing will be likely to succeed; they are more of a confirmatory procedure. In many instances the use of elastic support stockings or panty-hose may be the only possible treatment to relieve symptoms. It is believed that if elastic supports are used early enough, the condition can be pre-vented from progressing, and subsequent therapy, if utilized, will be more successful. Varicose veins, once they appear, warrant medical attention to find the specific cause; many times, removal of the cause also eliminates the varicose veins.

Reliability

The test is considered to be 90 percent accurate when used to help diagnose the cause of varicose veins and determine whether or not surgery will be successful.

BREATH AND LUNG TESTS

PULMONARY FUNCTION MEASUREMENTS
(Screening for lung problems)

Measurement of dynamic lung functions—how much air the lungs can hold, whether the lungs easily transfer oxygen to the blood and how well inhaled air can be expelled—can provide valuable clues to incipient heart and breathing problems. When performed on a regular basis, these tests can also offer early warning signals of latent lung disease. In addition, lung-air tests are helpful in evaluating treatments as well as in following the progress of therapy. Dynamic lung measurements are only a small part of overall pulmonary function testing, which usually includes additional laboratory-controlled breathing tests as well as gas diffusion tests, which quantitatively show the effectiveness of the transfer of oxygen from the lungs to the blood and the transfer of carbon dioxide from the blood back to the lungs.

There are two basic categories of lung pathology: the obstructive type and the restrictive type (see Figure 35). The obstructive type, characterized by an abnormal resistance to air flow both into and especially out of the lungs, is the most common cause of shortness of breath (dyspnea). It can come from:

- Asthma, brought on either by an allergy or by repeated lung infections, cold air, exercise and even certain odors, such as from colognes.
- Bronchiectasis, a condition in which the bronchi lose their ability to contract and thus can no longer help expel mucous; this usually follows prolonged severe lung infections.
- Chronic bronchitis as an active, usually long-standing, infection.
- Cystic fibrosis, in which excessive mucous production blocks air movement within the bronchi (sec Breath and Lung Tests, **Skin Saltiness**).
- Emphysema, in which the lungs' elasticity is insufficient to permit them to expel air easily.
- Drugs, particularly those used to treat heart disease, glaucoma and joint pains.

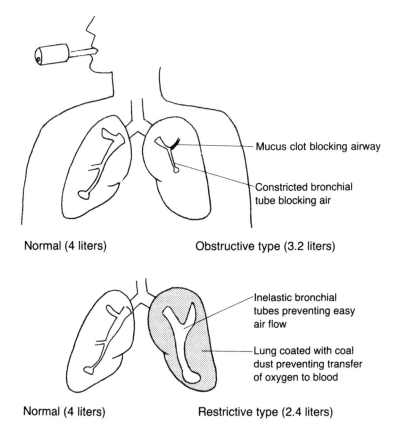

Figure 35. Obstructive and restrictive lung pathologies.

With the restrictive type of lung disease, the lungs are usually unable to fill with adequate amounts of air, or if air does enter the lungs, the normal free and easy passage of oxygen to the blood is impaired. Restrictive lung problems can come from:

- An injury to, or deformity of, the ribs or the chest wall; any condition that causes severe pain when you try to take a deep breath can also result in a similar problem.
- Pulmonary fibrosis, in which normal lung tissue is replaced by scarlike tissue; this can come from an old infection or from inhaling irritating particles such as asbestos, coal dust, cotton dust, fungi and a host of industrial chemicals.
- Certain nerve or muscle diseases that affect the diaphragm or rib cage, such as myasthenia gravis or muscular dystrophy.

• Any loss of lung tissue, either as a result of its being replaced by a growing tumor or as a consequence of surgery.
• Pulmonary edema, in which fluids fill the air spaces within or surrounding the lungs, such as happens with pleurisy or heart failure.
• Pregnancy, if the enlarged uterus presses up on the diaphragm; this, of course, is only temporary.

For home testing, the simple "match test," the forced vital capacity test, two or three breathing tests using a spirometer (an instrument that records the exact amount of air passing through it and, at times, the rate of air passage during a specific period of time), or a test using a peak flow meter can offer information concerning the possible presence of lung problems.

Match test. The match test is performed by holding a lighted paper match six inches from the open mouth, taking in as deep a breath as possible and then exhaling the air as forcibly as possible in order to blow out the match (you must not pucker your lips to increase the force of the airflow but instead keep the mouth wide open). The ability to perform this test successfully usually means that the chances of there being a lung problem are remote.

The forced expiratory time (FET) test. Another "open-mouth" test requires a watch or clock that has a sweep-second hand or a digital display that shows seconds (a stopwatch is more accurate but is not required). In the match test the goal was to determine the force of exhaled air; in the forced expiratory time test, the goal is to measure the time it takes to exhale all the air that the lungs can hold. With a watch in front of you, breath in as deeply as you possibly can. With your mouth wide open, exhale as forcibly and as fast as you can and count the seconds from the instant you start to exhale until the very last bit of air is expelled. You should repeat this test several times and record your best (shortest) time. Most people without any lung impairment can exhale all their lung air in from two seconds to four seconds. If it takes you more than five seconds to exhale all your lung air, it could be a warning signal of either an obstructive or a restrictive type of lung problem. It warrants spirometry testing and/or a medical consultation.

Forced vital capacity (FVC) test. The forced vital capacity test measures just how much air the lungs can forcibly exhale after taking in as large a breath as possible (see Figure 36). This is really the simplest recordable standardized indication of the lungs' condition.

While a spirometer is the usual instrument to measure forced vital capacity, a very inexpensive device called the VITOMETER can also be used. It does not measure the forced expiratory volume in one second (FEV_1), but

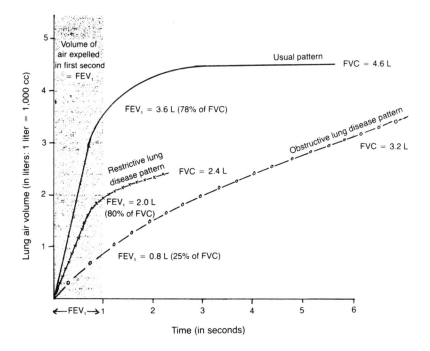

Figure 36. Typical patterns for forced vital capacity (FVC) and forced expiratory volume in one second (FEV₁) tests.

it is quite effective in determining the most fundamental indicator of lung function. With this test the maximum amount of air that can be expelled at one time is determined by blowing into a special, calibrated, transparent collection bag. This meter comes with charts that take into account one's age, height and sex to determine normal values. It is available from pharmacies and medical supply stores or from HealthScan Inc., which can be reached at (800) 962-1266. The cost is from $3.00 to $5.00

Forced expiratory volume in one second (FEV₁) test. This spirometer test is usually performed at the same time as the forced vital capacity test; it measures the exact amount of air being blown out during the first second of the FVC test (see Figure 36). The FVC and FEV_1 tests together can sometimes discriminate between an obstructive and a restrictive type of lung condition.

Maximal voluntary ventilation (MVV) test. This spirometer test offers a record of the greatest amount of air that a person can forcibly breathe in and out in one minute's time (the test is usually conducted for 12 seconds to 15 seconds and the amount multiplied by either 5 or 4). Formerly called maximum breathing capacity, this test is a relative indication of the lungs' physical fitness, since it also takes into account the muscles that help you breathe and how well you coordinate all breathing-related activities. A Propper-type spirometer is required for this test.

Peak expiratory flow rate (PEFR) test. This test measures the maximal expiratory flow rate during a forcible exhalation after you have taken in as much air as your lungs can hold; it is not necessary to exhale every bit of air. This test requires a peak flow meter. This particular device is being recommended more and more by doctors because of its low cost, simplicity of use and minimal maintenance. The PEFR test is a reasonable reflection of the amount of air exhaled in approximately the first second when compared to the FEV_1 test; another difference is that the exhalation of air is translated into a rate-time result—some meters report it in liters per minute (L/min.), others in liters per second (L/sec.). The PEFR test (sometimes called the peak flow rate) is commonly used by asthmatic patients at home to assist the doctor in monitoring their condition, evaluating drug effectiveness and identifying early warning signs to prevent impending severe attacks. For nonasthmatics it can offer an indication of obstructive lung disease. For patients prone to heart failure, regular measurements of the peak flow rate can help avoid emergency hospitalizations.

Walking test. Many doctors measure the time and distance that a person can walk before breathlessness appears as a test of lung function. It being assumed that an individual without lung problems can walk briskly just about one mile in 12 minutes, the onset of breathlessness before that time is said to correlate well with the forced vital capacity test (there are doctors who feel that walking one-half mile in 6 minutes is just as good a test). If, for example, you find yourself out of breath after walking only half a mile, it is reasonable to assume that there could be a pulmonary function problem, and it warrants a medical consultation.

Another version of the same test compares an individual's walking ability to that of others. If you can walk up hills or stairs as well as ostensibly normal people your own age and walk alongside them as fast as they walk without getting out of breath, the chances that you have a lung or breathing problem are remote. If you cannot climb stairs or hills without breathlessness, or have to stop for breath while walking along level ground, it warrants a medical consultation. If you cannot find a measured one-mile track, drive your automobile around the block, noting on the odometer how long a mile is, and use that for your test distance.

What Is Usual

Dynamic lung functions are evaluated by measuring the quantity of air exhaled in liters (L) or cubic centimeters (cc). (One liter is equivalent to 1,000 cubic centimeters and is slightly more than a quart.)

The forced vital capacity test values depend on one's age, height and sex. The larger (usually taller) a person is, the larger the lung capacity is expected to be. The younger a person is, the more elastic the lung tissues and chest muscles, and this should result in an ability to exhale air from the lungs much more forcibly. And since men usually have larger chest wall dimensions, along with stronger chest muscles, they are expected to have a greater forced vital capacity than women. Even ethnic or racial groups may have slight differences in what is considered normal. In general, the normal values for some pulmonary functions tests may be up to 15 percent lower in blacks than in whites.

All FVC test devices come with a chart or table that shows expected test values for different ages and heights as well as by sex. Two examples: A man 5 1/2 feet tall, from 25 years to 55 years of age, should have an FVC of at least 4 liters (4,000 cc); a woman 5 feet tall, from 15 years to 55 years of age, should have an FVC of at least 3 liters (3,000 cc). But such figures are not absolute; a deviation of 20 percent either way from the values shown on the chart or table supplied with the device is still considered within normal limits, and many doctors do not consider a 25 percent deviation abnormal. Thus, if the expected value is supposed to be 4 liters, any result from 3 liters to 5 liters can also be normal.

The forced expiratory volume in one second test is really a refinement of the forced vital capacity test. Usually, a person without a lung problem will forcibly breathe out from 75 percent to 80 percent of the total forced vital capacity within the first second of exhalation. If, for example, the forced vital capacity was four liters, then at least three liters should have been expelled within the first second of exhalation (see Figure 36).

The maximal voluntary ventilation test, which measures the amount of air going into and out of the lungs during a 12-second or 15-second period of time (as opposed to a single forced exhalation) while a person breathes as hard and as fast as possible, is most often expressed as liters per minute (L/min.). After 12 seconds or 15 seconds, the total recorded air volume is multiplied by 5 or 4, and the result should be at least 15 times to 20 times the forced vital capacity volume. Someone with a forced vital capacity of 4 liters should have a maximal voluntary ventilation rate of at least 60 L/min. and closer to 80 L/min. A well-trained athlete can have an MVV of more than 30 times the FVC.

The peak expiratory flow rate test also takes an individual's age, height and sex into consideration (as does FEV). Each test instrument, no matter of what design, is accompanied by "predicted normal values" expressed in L/

min. or L/sec. Many doctors consider a test result within 75 percent to 80 percent of the usual flow rate, as shown on the tables, to be within normal limits. Patients with asthma or other lung conditions usually establish their own baseline in consultation with their doctor so as to be aware of significant changes. In general, a man 5 1/2 feet tall, from 25 years to 55 years of age, will show a PEFR of from 500 L/min. to 600 L/min. (6 L/sec. to 9 L/sec.). A woman 5 feet tall, from 15 years to 55 years of age, will average from 400 L/min. to 500 L/min. (5 L/sec. to 8 L/sec.).

What You Need

A spirometer is considered the basic lung function measuring device. These instruments come in many shapes and sizes—the VITOMETER is one such device—all easily hand-held. The simplest spirometers will only measure forced vital capacity. The Propper-style compact spirometer uses a dial showing divisions in tenths of a liter and costs from $100.00 to $140.00; it will also measure maximal voluntary ventilation.

Many peak flow meters are available, but keep in mind that these instruments measure PEFR only. To name a few:

- The Healthscan Assess Peak Flow Meter, which costs $20.00.
- The Vitalograph Pulmonary Monitor, which costs $18.00.
- The AirMed mini-WRIGHT peak flow meter, which costs $29.95.

Check with your doctor; his or her patient experiences may have led to a preference for a particular model.

What to Watch Out For

Be sure that your lung function device is working properly. Although all hand-held Propper-type spirometers can be sufficiently accurate for home testing, they do tend to become inaccurate after a period of time. One way to verify the accuracy of your device is to check it out with the machine in your doctor's office. Another way is to have someone whose FVC is known to be normal help calibrate your device.

Avoid even the slightest breathing through the nose while testing. If this seems difficult, apply a nose clip or pinch the tip of your nose. Be sure that your lips are sealed tightly around the mouthpiece while exhaling.

Do not spit into a test device; this can cause a low value, which would falsely indicate disease.

It really does not matter whether you sit or stand when performing spirometry, but you should assume a position that will allow you to take in the largest possible breath and blow it out as forcibly and continuously as you can until every bit of air is exhaled. Testing while lying down, however, can cause much lower values.

Do not accept only one test result, or even the first few; rest and repeat the tests until two or more results are almost identical and then record the highest value.

What the Test Results Can Mean

The most common indication of a possible chest problem is a reduced forced vital capacity test. If your test result is 70 percent or less of what would be expected for your age, height and sex, it could mean either an obstructive or a restrictive lung condition. If less than normally expected FVC values are observed on three or more occasions, a medical consultation is warranted.

If the forced expiratory volume in one second is less than 75 percent of your FVC, a lung problem is more apt to be of the obstructive type. A reduced maximal voluntary ventilation is also an indication of an obstructive type of lung condition, and a medical consultation is warranted.

If the forced vital capacity is reduced, but the forced expiratory volume in one second and the maximal voluntary ventilation tests are near-normal, it may be a sign of a restrictive type of lung problem, and a medical consultation is warranted.

Bronchodilator inhalation challenge test. A supplementary procedure that tends to point to an obstructive-type problem, and one that also helps indicate how treatable that problem might be, is the bronchodilator inhalation challenge test. After establishing your baseline values for FVC and FEV_1, you inhale once from a bronchodilator dispenser containing epinephrine (adrenalin); Bronkaid Mist and Primatine Mist are two such products. With lung problems due to allergy, the epinephrine will usually increase the FVC within 15 minutes. Although these drugs are sold without a prescription, do not use one of these inhalers until you first discuss it with your doctor; they can cause a rapid heartbeat, elevate blood pressure and produce nervousness. Many doctors advise their patients who have asthma to obtain a spirometer or peak flow meter and keep a record of their breathing difficulties—such as when they occur and what seems to provoke them—and the measurable amount of relief obtained with the use of various medicines.

Another observation that can indicate lung problems is a large difference between FVC and FEV_1 measurements from day to day. People with obstructive types of lung disease tend to show such variations, which warrant a medical consultation.

And recent research indicates that a reduced forced vital capacity, or changes in the peak flow rate, over a 24-hour period, even in the absence of any lung problems, seems to be a warning sign of impending heart failure.

A decreased peak expiratory flow rate of less than 80 percent of the predicted values accompanying the peak flow meter warrants a medical consultation. While this drop in the PEFR most often indicates an airway obstruction due to asthma, it is also a reasonable single, simple evaluation of lung function. It can be very valuable in uncovering asthma before the onset of wheezing and breathing difficulties due to exercise or exertion. For someone with known asthma, regular testing with a peak flow meter can offer an early warning signal of an impending asthmatic attack and can thereby enable the individual to take action to ward off that attack.

Peak flow meters have proved of value to those trying to stop smoking. The obvious objective improvement in lung function in an ex-smoker along with the evident loss of lung power should the person begin smoking again offer a real incentive to abstain from smoking.

The most recent medical research has associated impotence with the obstructive type of lung disease; it seems that sexual dysfunction increases in direct proportion to the degree that lung function test values are reduced (see Genitourinary System Tests, **Nocturnal Penile Tumescence Monitoring**). Evidence of impotence accompanied by any decrease in lung function certainly warrants a medical consultation.

If any dynamic lung function test shows repeated deviation from what is expected, a medical consultation is warranted.

Reliability

All home-performed pulmonary function tests are considered to be at least 90 percent accurate, and repeated abnormal test results justify a medical consultation.

APNEA MONITORING
(Snoring can be hazardous to an adult's health; breathing problems in an infant can be fatal.)

Apnea means the sudden, involuntary stopping of breathing; it can last for a few seconds or for several minutes, and it can be fatal. At this time there is no mutually agreed-upon reason for the condition, but the blame has been variously ascribed to:

- An obstruction somewhere in the bronchi, windpipe (trachea) or back of the throat; blockage of the breathing passage can come from enlarged tonsils, the tongue's folding back on itself or a loss of tone in the throat muscles.
- Hypersomnolence, or excessive sleeping; when accompanied by obesity, it may be called the Pickwickian syndrome (from the Charles Dickens character).
- An upper respiratory infection (cold or flu), even a very slight one.
- Drugs such as narcotics, sedatives, tranquilizers and alcohol.
- Heart rhythm irregularities.

- Pathology in the part of the brain that controls respiration (resembling epilepsy, only without convulsions).
- Hypoglycemia (see Blood Tests, **Glucose**).
- Gastroesophageal reflux (see Mouth, Throat and Gastrointestinal Tests, **String Test**).
- Hormone-caused metabolic disorders.
- Severe allergic reactions to almost everything, with dust and milk leading the list (see Allergy Tests, **Patch Testing**).
- Prematurity or low birth weight, especially if accompanied by anemia.
- In an infant, smoking on the mother's part during pregnancy.

One form of the condition is called obstructive sleep apnea and is reportedly the most common cause of breathing failure during sleep. It consists of a periodic lack of breathing and interrupted sleeping and is believed to afflict more than 21 million Americans, 9 out of 10 of whom are men, most of them overweight, middle-aged and usually with high blood pressure (see Heart and Circulation Tests, **Blood Pressure**), although a few young children with enlarged tonsils have had the problem.

The most common warning sign of sleep apnea in an adult is snoring—usually quite loud and sudden in its onset following quiet sleep; the snoring reflects the difficulty in breathing. While on occasion a bed partner's description of the snoring pattern can be an early warning sign of sleep apnea, some doctors advise patients suspected of having the condition to place a long-playing, or voice-activated tape recorder next to the bed and record the snoring sounds during the night; the doctor can then listen to the tapes of those snoring episodes and at times make the diagnosis. More often than not, however, adult apnea is diagnosed in a hospital-based sleep-disorder center, where breathing, brain waves, hormone changes and heart rate are recorded during snoring episodes.

A second form of sleep apnea occurs in infants, and from 1 to 2 out of every 1,000 babies—most commonly between 2 months and 4 months of age—seem to suffer from this as yet indistinct condition. Some doctors consider sleep apnea to be the cause of sudden infant death syndrome (SIDS), in which an infant who seemed in perfect health at night is found dead in bed the next morning (called cot death in England), but there is no professional pediatric consensus on this theory either. All that is agreed upon at this time is that any apnea in an infant lasting more than 20 seconds (or even less if there is any change in the infant's color from pink to paleness or blue, or if the heartbeat slows down) warrants immediate medical attention.

One phase of testing for infant sleep apnea, after initial medical studies indicate its possibility, is monitoring the infant's breathing and/or heart rate in the home 24 hours a day—especially while the infant is sleeping. Cost-wise, it is virtually prohibitive to perform the same task for several months in a hospital, where even specially trained nurses on 8-hour shifts in an intensive care setting, using direct observation in place of monitors, miss nearly 40 percent of apnea episodes. Battery-operated electronic detectors in pads are placed under the baby (in essence, they become the crib's mattress, although some do go beneath the mattress) or around the baby's chest as a nightshirt that constantly monitors every breath and/or heartbeat, no matter how slight. They do not require the attachment of wires or electrodes and do not actually touch the baby's skin. Respiration and heart rate are displayed on a connecting instrument by means of flashing lights, digital displays or dial gauges. Your doctor can advise you as to which type would be best for your particular circumstances. The monitors detect any cessation of breathing or change in the heart rate and give off a loud alarm along with very bright flashing lights should breathing stop or the heart slow for 10 seconds (some monitors can be set to show apnea for anywhere from 5 seconds to 20 seconds, depending on the doctor's recommendations; some have remote receivers that can be carried everywhere).

These monitors require special training, usually by the pediatrician or nurses in a hospital. It is necessary for parents to learn how to use the monitor and what to do should the alarm go off, as well as to receive counseling on the monitor's psychological impact on the whole family.

What Is Usual
Obviously, it is normal not to have any breathing difficulties. Where apnea exists in children, however, the usual warning is a parent's seeing the child suddenly lose his or her usual skin color, at times even turn blue, and become limp and unresponsive.

What You Need
With the advice and cooperation of your physician, you can purchase or rent an infant sleep-apnea monitor. There are many different kinds; some keep track of breathing only, while others also disclose the slightest change in the heartbeat. In general, the machines sell for $700.00 to $2,500.00; they rent for $85.00 to $200.00 a month (in most instances they are not needed for more than two to three months). They are usually sold or rented through medical supply stores, although some hospitals also offer this service. Battery-powered machines are not affected by power failures.

For detecting adult apnea the simplest device is a voice-activated tape recorder placed alongside the bed to detect the amount and type of snoring. There are tape recorders that will operate for up to six hours without the tape's having to be changed (contact AMC Sales [Box 928, Downey, Calif. 90241]). A doctor with special training in sleep problems can usually determine whether the snores are potentially dangerous. More precise "snore detectors" are also available (one is called the Vitalog Sleep Monitor), and home-use apnea monitors can be obtained through your doctor (one is called Night Watch; another is called Portable Sensing System, or PSS, from Dr. Richard Millman of Brown University [Providence, R.I. 02912]; a third is called the Sleep Oximeter, from CNS [Eden Prairie, Minn. 55344]). While such devices can cost from $200.00 to $700.00 for one night's use, they can save several thousand dollars now charged by sleep-in sleep-disorder laboratories.

What to Watch Out For

You will have to learn to deal with the potential tension that can come from having an infant sleep-apnea monitoring machine in your home. Even though such stressful feelings cannot compare with the anxiety about the baby's condition, the machine's possible interference with family and social life can be emotionally traumatic. Be sure you know that you will have adequate support from all family members at home; be equally sure that all family members understand everything that home monitoring entails.

Accept the fact that there will be false alarms; no machine is perfect. Do not become so dependent on the machine that you refuse to give it up when your doctor says it is no longer needed.

What the Test Results Can Mean

Ten years ago there were approximately 10,000 unexpected, sudden infant deaths believed to be related to sleep apnea each year. Where sleep-apnea monitoring devices were properly used at home on children suspected of having the condition, the survival rate is claimed to be almost 100 percent.

Any suspicion of sleep apnea in a child or adult (episodes of loud snoring are considered an early warning sign) warrants medical attention; obstructive sleep apnea is a dangerous condition. Recent research shows that frequent snoring may be a risk factor for heart disease and stroke.

Apnea monitoring at home must always be decided on an individual basis. If used solely to prevent SIDS, there is at this time no absolute guarantee of effectiveness in spite of the reported successes. For those particularly interested in this subject, write the National Institutes of Health (Bldg. 1, Rm. 216, Bethesda, Md. 20892) for a copy of its *Consensus Development Conference Statement* (vol. 6, no. 6) *on Infantile Apnea and Home Monitoring.*

Reliability

While snoring by itself may not be dangerous, much depends upon whether the snoring is habitual and frequent or only occasional; habitual snoring has proved to be about 80 percent accurate as a warning sign of apnea. Although there have been no truly scientific studies to prove the efficacy of infant apnea monitoring, when SIDS is excluded, there are claims that monitoring saves lives in close to 100 percent of the cases in which it is used.

BREATH ALCOHOL
(A test that could save your life—and the lives of others)

While testing for the body's alcohol content—whether through breath, blood or urine—is most often related to the legal question of drunken driving, breath alcohol levels can be of even greater value if measured prior to driving after drinking. There are many people who actually test themselves, at home, with known amounts of beer, liquors and wine to learn just how much they can consume before reaching the legal level of "being under the influence." Others test their guests at the end of a party (some states make a host responsible for any damages by a drunken guest). People vary tremendously in how much alcohol it takes to impair their mental and physical abilities; and different states have widely varying limits on what blood alcohol level constitutes a violation of the law. Knowing how much alcohol it takes for you to reach impairment (some people cannot drive a car safely after only one or two drinks) can prevent many alcohol-caused diseases and could save lives.

Scientific studies have shown that proper testing of breath alcohol is as accurate as, and equivalent to, direct blood measurements. Breath alcohol tests measure the body's content of ethyl alcohol, or ethanol, the kind of alcohol used for consumption. This type of alcohol should be distinguished from isopropyl alcohol, or propanol, commmonly used as rubbing alcohol, antifreeze or a solvent; and methyl alcohol, also known as methanol or wood alcohol, which is used in plastics manufacturing and for cleaning purposes. Small amounts of the latter two alcohols can be fatal.

An ounce of average 86 proof liquor (*proof* is twice the percentage of alcohol in the beverage) contains about the same amount of alcohol (10 grams, 10,000 mg or ⅓ of an ounce) as do eight ounces of beer or four ounces of wine. After alcohol is consumed, it reaches its peak blood level in about half an hour. Three ounces of an average liquor will usually produce some symptoms of intoxication and can cause a blood alcohol level measurement of over 0.05 percent (in a few states sufficient for a person to be considered legally drunk). Ten ounces of the same proof alcohol will usually produce stupor or coma; blood alcohol measurements reflect this state with a level of 0.4 percent. Twelve ounces of ethyl alcohol at one time have caused death. It takes from two hours to three hours to eliminate each ounce of alcohol from the body.

Most states consider a 0.10 percent body alcohol measurement, whether by blood or by breath, as evidence of intoxication (in England 0.08 percent is the legal limit); some states, however, insist on a measurement of 0.15 percent before issuing a citation. A level of 0.10 percent means that there are 100 mg of pure alcohol in every 3⅓ ounces of blood; as a comparison, it takes only one-thousandth as much (0.1 mg) Dilantin (a drug used to treat epilepsy) in the blood to be effective enough to prevent convulsions.

What Is Usual
Obviously, no measurable amount of alcohol in the body would be normal. Legally, a breath alcohol level of less than 0.05 percent is rarely considered intoxication.

What You Need
The test is performed with a portable, battery-operated breath alcohol meter, which can cost anywhere from $39.95 to $500.00. After you breath into the device, it may signal alcohol content by colored lights: Green means less than 0.05 percent; yellow means from 0.05 percent to 0.10 percent; red means more than 0.10 percent. Other alcohol breath test meters show the exact alcohol content on a dial gauge or in digital-display numbers. These instruments may be used repeatedly. One-time disposable tests include BE SURE or Breath Scan; they cost from $1.00 to $2.00 per test.

What to Watch Out For
Do not attempt to measure breath alcohol for at least 15 minutes after your last drink; during that time there is enough alcohol in your mouth and saliva to cause a false result. Do not attempt to test yourself if you just brushed your teeth or rinsed your mouth with mouthwash; many toothpastes and mouthwashes contain alcohol and will cause false results for up to 10 minutes. If you are diabetic, you can have a falsely elevated breath (blood) alcohol test if you are also forming ketones in your body (see Urine Tests, **Clinical Analysis: Ketones**). Do not smoke just prior to taking the test; tobacco smoke can at times distort some color tests. Many inhaled medications, such as those used for asthma, contain alcohol and can give a false-positive result for up to 15 minutes after use.

Be sure that the device is operating properly. In 1982 more than 1,000 Breathalyzer machines (used primarily by police departments) were found to be defective, causing erroneous breath alcohol readings.

What the Test Results Can Mean
Testing could, of course, help save hundreds of dollars, prevent the loss of your driver's license, keep you out of jail and avoid humiliation—not to mention the lives that might be saved. Keep in mind, however, that the breath alcohol test does not indicate how much alcohol was imbibed or whether alcoholism exists, nor does it necessarily indicate your degree of impairment; it simply reflects the blood alcohol level at the time the test was performed. It cannot tell whether alcohol was used within 30 minutes prior to the test, which could cause a higher blood level a short while after the test is taken. Most of all, the test can help to keep social drinking within reasonably safe limits and could be a means of preventing alcoholism (see Mental Ability and Personality Tests, **Alcoholism**).

Reliability

When operating properly, most devices—even the least expensive ones—are rarely more than 10 percent off in their results. Thus, these devices are considered at least 90 percent accurate. Newer analyzers, such as those used by the police since 1987, are said to be 99.9 percent accurate. While the single-use tubes are not as accurate as the meters, they are accurate enough for preventive use.

One way to check the accuracy of a breath tester is to compare the value it indicates with the chart shown in Figure 37, which gives the estimated percentage of alcohol in the blood after drinking. It is measured according to body weight and the number of drinks consumed. While this chart is not precise, it offers a reasonable basis for verification. Any test device should show a warning when the breath alcohol level reaches 0.05 percent and indicate drunkenness at 0.10 percent.

Figure 37. Estimated blood alcohol levels after drinking.

Drinks:	1	2	3	4	5	6	7	8	9	10	11	12
100 lbs.	.038	.075	.113	.150	.188	.225	.263	.300	.338	.375	.413	.450
120 lbs.	.031	.063	.094	.125	.156	.188	.219	.250	.281	.313	.344	.375
140 lbs.	.027	.054	.080	.107	.134	.161	.188	.214	.241	.268	.295	.321
160 lbs.	.023	.047	.070	.094	.117	.141	.164	.188	.211	.234	.258	.281
180 lbs.	.021	.042	.063	.083	.104	.125	.146	.167	.188	.208	.229	.250
200 lbs.	.019	.038	.056	.075	.094	.113	.131	.150	.169	.188	.206	.225
220 lbs.	.017	.034	.051	.068	.085	.102	.119	.136	.153	.170	.188	.205
240 lbs.	.016	.031	.047	.063	.078	.094	.109	.125	.141	.156	.172	.188

SOURCE: Government of the District of Columbia.

BREATH ODOR AND SPUTUM
(Early warning clues to heart and lung disorders)

Sputum is the mucus secretion from the lower respiratory system (lungs, bronchi, trachea and larynx), sometimes called phlegm; it is the primary source of breath odor. Secretions from the nose, throat and sinuses are from the upper respiratory system and are not considered part of the sputum. Sputum is usually obtained by coughing, and while it is most often cultured and examined under a microscope for bacteria, fungi or cancer cells, the amount, consistency, tenacity, color and odor of sputum can also offer clues to heretofore hidden pathology. The sputum produced right after awakening can be revealing, but the total amount collected over a 24-hour period is more helpful.

The odor of one's breath can offer many clues to internal disease. To be sure, a mouth reflecting poor oral hygiene (see Dental Tests) can give off an unpleasant smell (see Brain and Nervous System Tests, **Smell Function**), but proper brushing and cleaning will usually eliminate this source of an offensive odor almost immediately. Disease-reflecting odors, on the other hand, can exist with good mouth care and usually will not disappear after brushing, albeit they may be masked momentarily by a strong mouthwash or by food or drink that has an overpowering odor. Certain drugs such as lithium, antifungal medicines and DMSO (dimethyl sulfoxide) can cause unpleasant breath; check with your doctor or pharmacist. Recognition of certain breath odors (not always an easy task on yourself), along with careful observation of your sputum, can help you detect early warning signs of allergies; diabetes; heart, liver, lung or kidney disease; sinusitis; and even stomach lesions.

What Is Usual
Breath should have no distinctive odor (other than odors derived from prior intake of foods, beverages, cleansing agents, tobaccos or even chewing gum).

The production of sputum is not common; normally, the lungs excrete about three ounces a day, and this is usually swallowed unconsciously and is not evident. But even a healthy person sometimes coughs up a teaspoonful a day. This could be a normal response to environmental irritants such as smog or inhaled chlorine fumes; in such instances there is usually only a small amount of sputum, and it is clear (unless slightly contaminated with soot), watery, colorless and without odor.

What You Need
You should get a clean, dry paper-cup-like container, large enough to hold all your sputum for a 24-hour period; some doctors advise two paper cups: one for sputum produced upon awakening and for the first hour thereafter and the second for sputum produced during the rest of the day. Do not use facial tissues to collect sputum, for they can mask sputum characteristics.

What to Watch Out For
If you are not sure whether your breath is odoriferous, do not hesitate to have a relative or friend test you. Do not attempt to hide any breath odor with mouthwash or other artificial disguises.

Do not fail to keep a record of how much sputum you produce at various times during the day, along with any possible provocative incidents associated with its production (bad air quality, dust, physical activities, body position). Do not confuse expectoration (spit), saliva or nasal secretions with sputum; do not let these substances mix with sputum.

What the Test Results Can Mean

A foul breath odor—while often the result of poor mouth care, a zinc deficiency (see Brain and Nervous System Tests, **Zinc Deficiency Taste Test**), dental problems or sinusitis—can also be the first indication of a lung infection or a stomach tumor (blocking the easy passage of food), especially if it follows several days of constipation; it may also indicate cancer, leukemia or liver disease. A particularly foul odor, especially when associated with belching, could indicate infestation by an intestinal parasite (see Mouth, Throat and Gastrointestinal Tests, **Feces Observations**). Unusually bad breath odor warrants a medical consultation to determine its cause. Acetone may be noticed on the breath before it appears in the urine and can be an important warning sign for people with diabetes; it warrants medical attention. An acetone odor could, of course, also indicate that you are on a reducing diet involving the intake of a very few or no carbohydrates or that you have been fasting for several days. An ammonia odor could be the first sign of kidney or liver disease, and it, too, warrants medical attention.

The repeated production of large amounts of sputum (more than one or two tablespoonfuls in the morning or more than three tablespoonfuls a day) is not normal; it alone warrants a medical consultation. If sputum production is markedly increased the first thing each morning, it usually means drainage of infected or allergic lung areas by gravity; the shift from lying down to standing allows different portions of the lung to drain any overabundance of secretions.

If sputum is thick, stringy and tenuous but clear, it is likely an allergic response, such as with asthma; if you are not already under medical care, it warrants a consultation. If thick but colored, it most often signals a lung infection; green, yellow, pink or rust-colored sputum often accompanies various forms of pneumonia and lung irritation by substances used in industrial processes; foul-smelling sputum could mean a lung abscess; red or red-streaked sputum most often means blood. All such warning signs are sufficient to warrant immediate medical attention, especially if you are taking anticoagulant drugs.

A frothy-type sputum, often pink-colored, usually comes from heart failure and the lung edema (excess fluid in the lungs) that results from the heart's inadequate performance. Usually, breathing difficulties will already have necessitated medical attention, but if not, bubbly, watery-pink or red-tinged sputum certainly warrants it. Should you ever notice little calciumlike particles in your sputum (somewhat like tiny shaved bits of chalk), it could be the first indication of a fungus infection of the lung or the consequences of exposure to certain minerals such as coal or silicone; it warrants a medical consultation.

Patients who use a Bronkometer (a measured-dose aerosol device for inhaling an asthma medication) at times have pink-tinged sputum. It is believed to be due to the antioxidant preservative in the medicine and is not considered harmful, albeit asthmatics must learn to differentiate the cause of pink sputum. It is also possible that inhalation of other preservative chemicals may cause the condition. Any pink-colored sputum still warrants a medical consultation.

Reliability

As an early warning sign of heart and/or lung disease, observations of breath odor and sputum (once the mouth is ruled out as the cause) are considered to be 80 percent accurate. For other conditions, such as allergies and gastrointestinal diseases, these observations are right about 70 percent of the time.

Sputum cytology. Sputum cytology is the microscopic study of the many various individual cells produced by the lungs and the respiratory passages. When these cells are examined from a deep sputum sample, they can reveal both normal as well as abnormal physiological processes—including the possible early detection of cancer. In the past a primary difficulty had been obtaining both sufficient and proper sputum samples; in many instances hospitalization was necessary. A home sputum-collection kit is now available from your doctor; it is called Novacyte (Xsirius Medical Inc., 27520 Hawthorne Blvd., Rolling Hills Estates, Calif. 90247) and costs $90.00. Sputum is collected—the best way is by spontaneous deep coughs—on first arising; if necessary, the collection can be made over several days to ensure its adequacy. It is then sent to the proper laboratory (in a preaddressed container) for study, and the results are reported back to your doctor.

The test can be particularly valuable for smokers and industrial workers, since it allows the detection of very early, possibly precancerous, cell changes, enabling preventive measures to be taken at the earliest opportunity. In general, the test is considered to be 85 percent accurate in detecting lung disease; it is considered better than 95 percent accurate in ruling out lung cancer when the test results are negative.

SKIN SALTINESS
(A possible early warning sign of cystic fibrosis)

Cystic fibrosis is an inherited condition that, 30 years ago, rarely allowed children to live past 5 years of age. It is believed that more than 1 out of every 2,000 white children are born with the disease; it is rare in blacks and Orientals. Today, if the condition is diagnosed early enough, a nearly normal life span is possible. Although cystic fibrosis is primarily a disease of the pancreas (whose fluids help the body digest and metabolize foods) and other glands and tissues that secrete fluids, its most severe effect is on the mucus of the lungs, and it is now considered more of a lung disease.

While there are several early signs of the condition, most of these are often attributed to something else: Foul-smelling bowel movements are attributed to feeding problems, suspected food allergies and the introduction of new foods to the baby's diet; a potbelly is attributed to a good appetite and increased food consumption; stomach cramps, are attributed to occasional constipation; and a chronic cough is attributed to a supposed family tendency toward allergies or catching colds easily. As a child gets older, the disease seems to concentrate on the lungs, where extremely thick, sticky mucus (sputum) plugs up the airways and causes all sorts of respiratory troubles. Wheezing and almost continuous coughing are the primary symptoms. But most of all, there is an unusual amount of sweating, and the sweat of an individual with cystic fibrosis contains much more salt than usual—so much more, in fact, that it has been known to corrode metal and ruin any leather goods with which it comes in contact.

While a diagnosis of cystic fibrosis is usually made by precise laboratory evaluations of the sodium and chloride in the sweat, one of the earliest and simplest techniques to help detect this condition is the skin saltiness test. All that is required is to regularly kiss the cheeks or forehead of an infant—daily, and at different times of the day, for the first few years of growth—to check for saltiness.

What Is Usual
Normal skin, especially in a cool room and not following any physical activity, should have no salty taste at all.

What You Need
You need both a willingness to express affection for your child in a physical manner and a reasonably normal sense of taste (see Brain and Nervous System Tests, **Taste Function**).

What to Watch Out For
Any unusual bowel and/or lung problems in an infant, even without skin saltiness, that cannot be easily explained warrant medical attention.

What the Test Results Can Mean
If at any time the skin "tastes" unusually salty, it warrants medical attention. Performing the test can result in the early detection of cystic fibrosis. One

out of 10 people with the disease may show no outward symptoms until adulthood. It has been suggested that if every infant were tested for skin saltiness, cystic fibrosis might be totally eradicated.

Reliability
The test is considered to be 80 percent accurate.

EYE AND VISION TESTS

VISUAL ACUITY
(Detecting vision problems before they become serious)

Tests of visual acuity (vision) measure the ability of each eye to perceive the size and shape of an object at standard distances. They also measure the ability of both eyes, working together, to discern the distances and depths of objects and their relationship to one another (which object is nearer or farther away); this is called stereopsis, fusion or depth perception.

The most common vision test uses the Snellen chart, in which the individual is asked to read rows of distinct boldface letters of various sizes at a distance of 20 feet (see Figure 38). For those who cannot read, there are charts that show the letter *E* in various positions (ⴹꟼⴴꟺ) or use figures such as a house, an animal, an apple or an umbrella; the positioned *E*s and the figures range from ³⁄₁₆ inch to 3½ inches in height, with it being considered normal to see a ⅜-inch letter clearly at 20 feet. This is recorded as 20/20. The first number indicates the distance in feet between the chart and the person being tested; the second number indicates how far away from the chart a person with normal vision could be and still read the smallest figures that can be read by the person being tested. Thus, 20/20 indicates the ability to read the "20" line at a distance of 20 feet; 20/40 means that at 20 feet the individual being tested could only read a line that someone with normal vision could read at 40 feet; and 20/200 means that at 20 feet the person could only distinguish the large letter that normally could be read at 200 feet. For close-up vision an individual should be able to read typical newspaper print at a distance of 14 inches.

Astigmatism is an inability to see and discern letters in one plane. For example, when you look at a clock, visual acuity could be normal (20/20) for all numbers except those that would form a straight line from the 11 to the 5, which might seem blurred or darker than the rest (see Figure 39).

Tests of visual acuity should be performed at home at least four times a year. An infant's vision can be checked by holding up a rubber ring to see whether it is grasped; first test both eyes, then cover each one and test the uncovered eyes separately. Some form of the Snellen chart can be utilized from the age of 3½ on. Pupillary reflex tests (see Eye and Vision Tests,

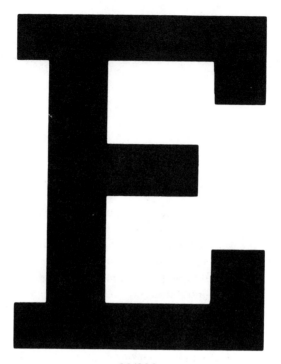

20/200

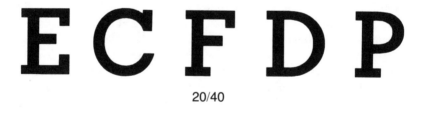

20/40

20/20

Figure 38. Visual acuity testing chart.

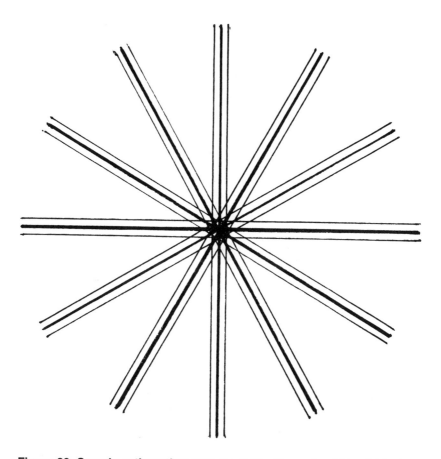

Figure 39. Sample astigmatism test chart (the lines should be 12 inches long and ⅛ inch thick).

Pupil and Pupillary Reflex) can also offer clues about an infant's vision. Observation of the pupils to see that they both seem to focus on the same point, rather than one's looking in a different direction from the other, will help detect strabismus, which causes a loss of depth perception (see Eye and Vision Tests, **Strabismus**). After the age of 40, it is good preventive medicine to check your vertical line perception once a week. With one eye closed or covered, look at a telephone pole, flagpole or lamp pole with the other eye; the pole should appear to be perfectly straight vertically and completely intact.

Pinhole test: If there is some question as to whether letters on a Snellen chart or distant objects are clear and/or distinct, the pinhole test may help resolve the matter. Simply punch a pinhole in an opaque piece of cardboard and look through that hole at the same letters or objects again. The tiny

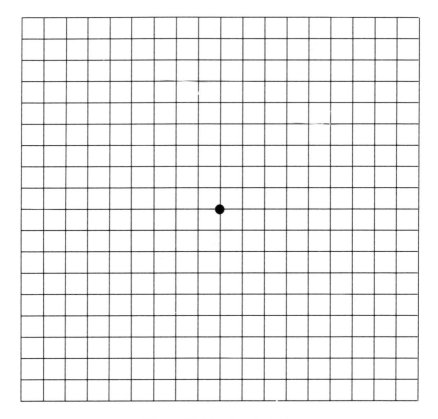

Figure 40. The Amsler Grid.

hole acts somewhat like a camera lens that has been closed down to allow the greatest depth of field (focusing on near and far objects at the same time). In many instances viewing through a pinhole improves visual acuity.

Another eye test to help detect the first signs of visual impairment is the Amsler Grid (see Figure 40). Although primarily used to uncover a condition called macular degeneration (the macula, located in the center of the retina in the back of the eye, is what allows sharp, clear, detailed vision at the focal point when you look at an object, such as when reading or sewing), the Amsler Grid can also offer an early warning sign of vision problems that can be treated to prevent subsequent blindness. Simply hold the Amsler Grid about a foot away from you and, with both eyes open, stare at the dot in the center of the grid. Then close one eye and see whether any of the squares around the dot disappear, do not seem straight or change in any other way. Again, look with both eyes, close the other eye and repeat your observations with the open eye. This test is a refinement of the test for vertical line perception (looking at a telephone pole, flagpole or light pole). Any change in the grid lines warrants medical attention. Many physicians feel that this test should be performed regularly—at least once a week—to detect the first signs of any visual impairment. The sooner treatment for macular degeneration begins, the less chance there is of permanent disability. The most common form of macular degeneration is called "age-related," since it is typically found in individuals past the age of 65 (more than 150,000 cases a year). For some as yet unknown reason, it is seen most often in people with blue eyes, cigarette smokers and those with inadequate nourishment; however, many doctors feel that the condition is inherited.

The legal definition of blindness is 20/200 or worse with the use of the most efficient corrective lenses.

What Is Usual

Although 20/20 vision is considered normal, up to 20/40 vision without the aid of glasses is also considered within normal limits, and most states will issue a driver's license to someone with 20/40 vision without requiring corrective lenses. You should be able to read fine print $\frac{1}{16}$ inch high (for example, the print in this book) at a distance of from 12 inches to 14 inches. It is considered usual, however, to lose some close-up vision after one reaches 40 years of age, since the muscles in the iris lose some of their strength and cannot perform accommodation (see Eye and Vision Tests, **Pupil and Pupillary Reflex**). You should also be able to look at two objects, one in front of the other, the farther about 10 feet away and the nearer 5 feet to 7 feet away, and know which one is in front and approximately how far in front it lies. When you look at an astigmatism test card 20 feet away, the lines should seem uniformly dark (that is, none of the lines should appear lighter or darker).

What You Need

The Snellen charts cost from $2.00 to $4.00 and are the most convenient testing device. You can also use Figure 38 at a distance of 20 feet. Printed cards to reveal astigmatism cost about $3.00 but can easily be made by drawing a one-foot-diameter circle and then drawing three parallel lines $\frac{1}{16}$ inch to $\frac{1}{8}$ inch thick as if you were connecting the numbers on the opposite sides of the face of a clock (from 12 to 6, from 3 to 9, etc.); you can use Figure 39 if you hold it two feet away, but it is not as accurate as the full-size card. A piece of firm cardboard with a pinhole in the center is also needed.

An excellent eye test kit is available for $1.00 from the Minnesota Society for the Prevention of Blindness (1208 Pioneer Bldg., St. Paul, Minn. 55101). It includes a modified Snellen chart with a pinhole apparatus, an Amsler Grid and a glaucoma survey with easy-to-follow directions. It is well worth the time, postage and $1.00 to order this kit.

The Minnesota Society for the Prevention of Blindness also offers a unique booklet for testing vision in children from ages 7 to 11 called *The Bright Eyes Kids Eye Book*. In addition to providing a special Snellen-type chart, the booklet explains vision, a visit to an eye doctor, how eyeglasses work and eye safety. If the booklet is not available through your own eye doctor, the Minnesota Society for the Prevention of Blindness will provide it at a cost of $2.00 to cover printing and mailing.

The newest form of vision-testing device is called the contrast-sensitivity chart. It consists of circles or letters of various shades or degrees of gray along with shaded dark lines of varying widths separated by diminishing spaces. Testing vision with this type of chart helps detect the ability to see clearly in various light conditions (bright sunlight, dusk, at night). One such chart is called the Arden gratings, and it, along with other similar contrast-sensitivity charts, is available from most eye doctors.

Another way of testing infants is to hold two large cards—one showing a bold pattern in a circle and the other showing a plain circle—in front of the baby, who usually will stare at the one with the pattern; failure to do so warrants a medical consultation.

What to Watch Out For

Have sufficient light on the eye chart but without any glare. Keep in mind that these eye tests are only for screening purposes; some doctors feel that the Snellen chart tests are too sensitive, especially for children, and may indicate visual defects where none really exists.

What the Test Results Can Mean

The inability to read fine print when held 12 inches from the eyes or to see Snellen chart letters labeled 20/40 without the aid of lenses usually indicates a visual defect. If you look at the same letters through a card with a pinhole in it and they seem clearer, this usually means that a prescription lens will improve vision. Although there is still some debate on the matter, many doctors believe that the sooner visual defects are discovered and treated, the less chance they have of progressing; it has also been claimed that wearing hard contact lenses will stop the progression of myopia, or nearsightedness. Thus, any variation from normal visual acuity warrants a medical consultation. If there is obvious deviation of one eye (it may only be intermittent), crossed eyes or squinting of one eye, these are signs of strabismus, and medical attention is warranted.

If, when you look at a vertical pole, it seems bent, curved or not intact (some segments missing), it could be an early warning sign of glaucoma, cataract or retinal problems and warrants medical attention.

Reliability

Visual acuity screening tests are considered 90 percent accurate. Recently, however, there have been some cases of eye disease (less than 5 percent) in which tests still show normal visual acuity; the newer contrast-sensitivity tests seem to eliminate this small amount of false-negatives such as can occur with multiple sclerosis and early glaucoma.

VISUAL FIELD
(A vision screening test that can also indicate diseases not involving the eyes)

Visual acuity is the ability to see an object directly in front of you (see Eye and Vision Tests, **Visual Acuity**). Visual field measures the eye's ability to see other objects within the periphery of one's line of vision—being aware of something or someone off to the side, above or below while staring straight ahead. While both tests help evaluate the eye and the nerves that serve it, visual acuity testing tells more about how the lens of the eye works, while visual field testing helps assess the performance of the structures within the eye and aids in determining just where eye, eye-nerve or brain problems may be located. It is quite possible to have a markedly diminished visual field and still have normal visual acuity. Home visual field testing is only a rough form of screening, but it can be very valuable in identifying early warning signs of disease.

What Is Usual
If you stare at a point about three feet in front of you with one eye (the other eye being covered), you should still be able to see an object that comes within the circumference of an area formed by your eyebrow, the bridge of your nose, your foot and to your side about as far back as your ear. The easiest way to check these peripheral fields is to sit opposite someone, with your noses about three feet apart, close your right eye while the person opposite closes the left one, and while staring at each other's nose (a finger pointing toward the examiner's nose helps concentrate the examinee's attention), both should see a moving fingertip or bright object at the same location in the periphery on the same side as the open eyes (see Figure 41). The test is then repeated with the opposite eyes.

What You Need
Nothing is required, other than patience and the willingness to keep staring at one point (your partner's nose) while performing the test.

What to Watch Out For
You may have a tendency to shift your eye toward the moving fingertip or object rather than stare straight ahead. There is a small area, just off center and to the side, where the fingertip will not be seen; this corresponds to the eye's "blind spot," or the place where the optic nerve goes from the back of the eye into the brain and contains no vision receptors. It is a normal phenomenon.

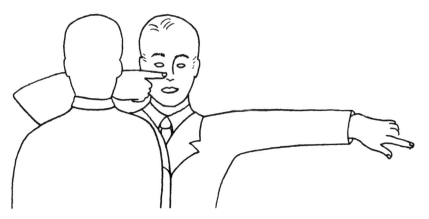

Figure 41. Visual field observations.

What the Test Results Can Mean

If you find places where the person opposite you can see the fingertip but you cannot, you should then repeat the test with someone else. If the same visual field defects remain, medical attention is warranted (and of course, a much more precise visual field examination). Visual field defects can come from glaucoma (which produces tunnel vision, in which only objects straight ahead can be seen), brain pathology (most often a tumor), nerve involvement, infections, inherited eye diseases, hemorrhages and drug poisoning—by arsenic, methyl alcohol, quinine or excessive smoking (nicotine poisoning).

Reliability

When properly performed, a visual field screening test is considered 90 percent accurate in detecting disease.

COLOR BLINDNESS
(An important observation to help one get along in the world)

About 1 in every 25 men (and 1 in every 250 women) cannot perceive the difference between red and green; however, about one-third of such people can distinguish such color sufficiently for commercial driving and flying. This condition is almost always inherited. And there are a few people who cannot tell the difference between blue and yellow. People in many occupations require absolutely precise color discrimination—for example, airline pilots, truck drivers, electricians, police officers, firefighters and military personnel.

While there are professional color charts to test for color vision, it is almost as easy to perform this screening test by using skeins of colored yarn, braiding together rose, red and green strands and yellow, blue and violet strands and asking the individual to separate the red or green strand (or the yellow or blue one) from the braid. Another form of the test is to request that three different-colored strands of yarn from one braid be matched to the same colors in a different braid.

What Is Usual

No matter how mixed up several colors are, an individual with normal color vision can discriminate not only between colors but between shades or hues of the same color.

What You Need

The test can be performed with colored objects such as yarn skeins; colored blocks or colored paper circles will do as well, but they should have similar shapes. You should have two or three shades of red, green, and pink or rose for the one test and various hues of blue, yellow and purple for the other.

If color vision testing is critical, Ishihara or Hardy-Rand-Rittler color plates, in a book, are available; they cost from $5.00 to $50.00, depending on how many different plates are needed. These plates show various shades of the primary colors in various dots to make up a numeral or shape, such as a triangle or circle, with the numeral or shape being superimposed on a background of similar dots of both contrasting and similar, but not identical, colors (see Figure 42). Someone with normal color vision can easily detect the number or figure within the many colors; someone with color blindness will see nothing definite. Recently, several advertisements (for Panasonic and Columbian Coffee) have used illustrations similar to professional color blindness test plates; they are excellent testing devices.

What to Watch Out For

Some people memorize the color plates in order to avoid having their color blindness detected. Do not confuse color ignorance, in which subtle shades of one color can be distinguished but are difficult to name, with color blindness. Color ignorance can be corrected through education.

The yarn skeins or test plates should be held 2½ feet from the eyes. Do not use sunlight or regular light bulbs as a direct source of illumination, for they can confuse shadings; a room lit by daylight is best. If more than three seconds are required to distinguish colors, or if color identification is impossible, it warrants a medical consultation.

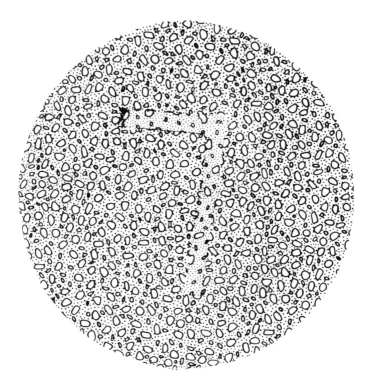

Figure 42. Color blindness observations. Although the actual color chart is made up of many different-colored dots, you should be able to distinguish a number (in this case a 7) buried among the contrasting colors.

What the Test Results Can Mean

Being aware that you are color blind can be sufficient to enable you to learn how to get along in the world (with traffic lights red is usually on top, for example), and with practice it is sometimes possible to learn to distinguish shadings to help identify colors. If you do happen to have a blue-yellow defect, it warrants a medical consultation to ascertain that the problem is not a result of alcoholism, along with the other consequences of this disease.

Reliability

Even when yarn skeins are used, this test is 95 percent accurate in detecting faulty color vision.

GLAUCOMA SCREENING AND MONITORING
(Detecting elevated eyeball pressure to prevent blindness)

Glaucoma is a condition in which the pressure of the fluid inside the eye is too high. This is somewhat analagous to high blood pressure within the circulatory system, but in this case the consequences are disturbed vision. Just as with measuring **blood pressure,** though (see Heart and Circulation Tests), when eyeball pressure is measured in a doctor's office, the results can be falsely elevated through anxiety; when measured at home, however, what at first appeared to be elevated pressure may in fact turn out to be normal. In addition, as with blood pressure, eye pressure may change from hour to hour and from day to day. And just as with anxiety's causing a false-high pressure, so can increased eye fluid pressure—especially when it occurs outside of office hours—seem to be normal at the doctor's office, indicating a well-controlled pressure when in fact the pressure may really be too elevated and ultimately cause a loss of vision.

Most often, the first signs of one type of glaucoma are blurring of vision along with pain in the eye. The eye may be red, as if infected, and the pupil (see Eye and Vision Tests, **Pupil and Pupillary Reflex**) usually is dilated and does not react to light. Another form of glaucoma starts with the loss of peripheral vision (see Eye and Vision Tests, **Visual Field**). Early detection of glaucoma can allow medical rather than surgical treatment in many cases.

Measuring the pressure inside the eye is called tonometry, and it may be performed in the doctor's office by using a tonometer. One type just touches the surface of the eye after the eye surface has been anesthetized; another measures pressure inside the eyeball by applying a brief puff of air to the eye surface, and no anesthesia is needed.

A home-use tonometer is available that allows an individual to make several measurements throughout the day, for several days, in order to ascertain the correct eye pressure. The device will also allow patients who have glaucoma to monitor their condition in order to achieve the best possible treatment results.

What Is Usual
Normally the pressure inside the eye runs between 10 mm and 20 mm of mercury (in contrast, systolic blood pressure normally runs between 120 mm and 140 mm of mercury [see Heart and Circulation tests, **Blood Pressure**]).

What You Need
At the present time, the home glaucoma testing device is rented from an eye doctor, on a week-to-week basis, and the observed measurements are related to that doctor for interpretation. Your doctor can obtain detailed

information by contacting Dr. Ran Zeimer, Dept. of Ophthalmology, University of Illinois College of Medicine, 1905 West Taylor St., Chicago, Ill. 60612.

What to Watch Out For

Although the device is simple to use, it does require a brief training period. You must learn how to instill a drop of anesthetic into the eye, how to activate the probe that contacts the eye for one second and how to use the eyepiece of the device (similar to a microscope).

What the Test Results Can Mean

A pressure measurement greater than 20 mm of mercury, normally expressed as 20 mm. Hg, is a reasonable indication of glaucoma and warrants medical attention. In most instances, the home glaucoma test will be used to follow the progress of glaucoma treatment and decreasing pressure measurements should indicate successful treatment.

Reliability

The test has been shown to be 90 percent accurate when used by someone after 30 minutes' training.

PUPIL AND PUPILLARY REFLEX
(The pupils can offer early clues to many internal diseases.)

The pupil is the opening in the very center of the eye surrounded by the colored (pigmented) circle called the iris. Within the iris are muscles that can tighten or relax, thereby causing the pupil to dilate (enlarge, or widen) or to constrict (contract, or shrink down). The two functions originate in two different areas: Dilation comes from the sympathetic nervous system (see Heart and Circulation Tests, **Cold Pressor and Finger Wrinkle**), while constriction comes from the brain. Abnormal reflexes can reflect several illnesses as well as the presence of several drugs. The pupillary reflex can be tested by observation, by light stimulation and by altering the distance of an object that the eyes are watching.

What Is Usual

On observation both pupils should appear to be the same: round, regular in shape and equal in size (see Figure 43). In a normally lighted room they should not appear unusually large or tiny. When a bright light (a flashlight beam) is directed toward the eyes or when the person goes into bright sunlight, the pupils should contract (called miosis) and appear very small. In contrast, when the amount of light diminishes or light is removed from the

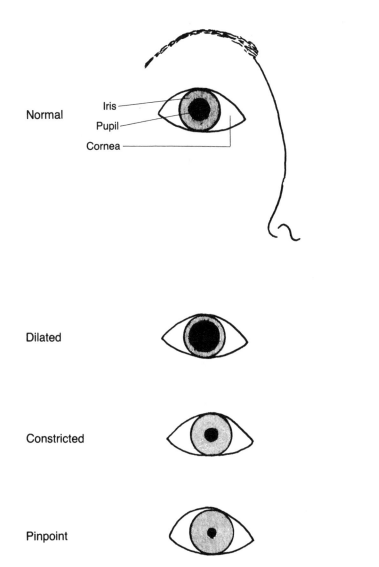

Figure 43. Pupil size.

eyes, the pupils should dilate, or widen (called mydriasis). If light is directed toward only one eye, with the other eye completely protected from the light source, that other covered eye's pupil should also contract (called consensual reaction). There should be no pain or discomfort in either eye when a bright light is directed at one eye while testing consensual reaction.

When an individual looks at an object close up, within four inches to six inches, especially after looking at a distant object, the pupils should contract (called accommodation). Pupillary reflex reactions should be prompt, but with aging the reaction time may seem slow and still be normal.

If you are taking certain drugs such as those used to relax the bowel (antispasmodics); antidepressant drugs; drugs used to treat Parkinsonism; drugs used to treat asthma, allergies or sinus conditions such as adrenalin or phenylephrine; or stimulants such as amphetamines or cocaine, the pupils may stay enlarged for a long period of time. If you are taking neostigmine-type preparations to treat myasthenia gravis, to help stimulate the bladder and sometimes to alter heart rhythm; sedatives such as alcohol, barbiturates or chloral hydrate; or narcotics such as morphine, the pupils may stay constricted for a period of time. Barbiturates and alcohol may, however, also cause dilation at times.

When an object (such as the eraser end of a pencil) is held in front of the eyes, both pupils should move together in following the object as it moves left, right, up and down.

What You Need
The test just requires a good flashlight with a bright beam (a penlight seems best).

What to Watch Out For
Primarily, you should take into consideration the use of drugs (including nonprescription products) that could interfere with the pupillary reflex; if you are taking medicine, check with your doctor or pharmacist to see whether it affects the pupils' reactions.

What the Test Results Can Mean
While unequal pupils (one larger than the other) may be normal in some people, when this condition is noticed for the first time, it is still significant enough to warrant medical attention in order to rule out any disease. It could signify brain disease, nerve disease, artery disease, glaucoma or an infection—not just an infection of the eye whose pupil is enlarged but a generalized infection as well. Unequal pupils can also be a grave sign following an injury.

An irregularly shaped pupil, in which the iris edge is not perfectly round, usually comes from an old eye infection. If one or both pupils do not react (constrict) when light is shined on them or when shifting focus from a far to a near object, it could mean a generalized infection or brain pathology, or it could even hint at lead poisoning; this, too, warrants medical attention. One particular pupillary reflex condition is called the Argyll-Robertson pupil, in which the pupils do not react to light but do react to accommodation; it is considered a classic sign of syphilis. Argyll-Robertson pupils warrant a medical consultation. If, when light is blocked from one eye while being directed toward the uncovered eye (see Figure 44), both pupils do not react equally, a medical consultation is warranted. If a person experiences eye discomfort when looking at something six inches away after looking at an object three feet away or when a light is shined into the eyes, and if the person experiences pain in the eye that is covered when light is directed toward the other, uncovered, eye, it can indicate an infection of the iris of the covered eye and warrants immediate medical attention.

Constantly dilated pupils can come from brain pathology (as a consequence of an injury, stroke or tumor), glaucoma, a lack of oxygen associated with heart or lung problems, mushroom or **carbon monoxide** poisoning (see Environmental Tests), intense fright, fear or manic-depressive behavior. Prolonged dilation can also come from using drugs that help calm the stomach (atropine and its derivatives), drugs that help breathing (adrenalin and related derivatives, including some nonprescription cold-relief preparations), barbiturates, and of course, alcohol abuse and drug abuse with narcotics such as cocaine. Constantly constricted pupils can occur in people who have a brain infection (abscess, encephalitis, syphilis), brain hemorrhage, nerve disorders or diabetes; in those who have eaten too much nutmeg; and especially in those using narcotics. In any case, medical attention is warranted. Fixed pinpoint pupils usually mean a severe drug overdose and indicate the need for immediate medical attention.

If, when an eraser tip is moved from side to side or up and down, one pupil does not seem to follow in unison with the other, medical attention is warranted.

Reliability
Abnormal pupillary reflex reactions, not explainable by an old injury or illness, are considered 90 percent accurate as warning signs of disease.

STRABISMUS (Cover-Uncover; Red Dot)
(Detecting "cross-eyes" as soon as possible)

Strabismus is a condition in which the two eyes do not see the identical image (see Eye and Vision Tests, **Visual Acuity**). But unlike the usual causes of an inability to see clearly (namely, a defect in the shape of the eyeball, which may have been inherited, or a defect in the shape of the lens of the eye), this condition is most often due to weakness in one or more of the six muscles that control the movements of each eye. It is the most common cause of diplopia (double vision). Children with strabismus usually show crossed eyes (in which one or both eyes looks inward) or wall-eyes (in which one eye looks outward). The problem may be overlooked in that as the con-

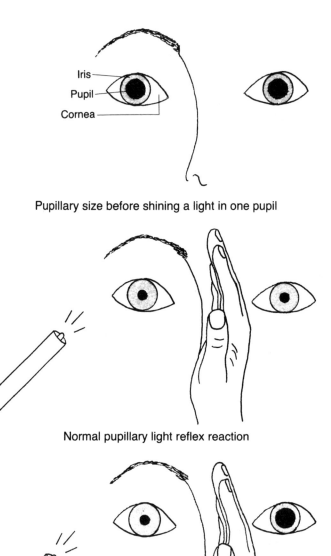

Pupillary size before shining a light in one pupil

Normal pupillary light reflex reaction

Abnormal pupillary light reflex reaction

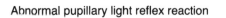

Figure 44. Consensual pupillary reflex observation.

dition begins and progresses, one of the child's eyes may not *always* be looking in different directions. A child with this condition will tend to use only one eye to see, and that eye may have normal visual acuity. If strabismus is not detected early enough, the other eye can then become "lazy" and fail to develop proper vision functions; in essence, it becomes blind. Early detection of strabismus can allow treatment by eye exercises (orthoptics) and/or eyeglasses instead of surgery. Double vision can also occur in the elderly, but this is more often due to a nerve involvement.

What Is Usual

If you stare at an object 20 feet away, both eyes should be directed at the same point. When one eye is covered and then uncovered while staring, the covered eye should not appear to an observer to shift its position. If you place a red-colored glass in front of one eye and then look at a flashlight about two feet away with both eyes, you should still see only one light.

What You Need

A flashlight and a piece of red-colored glass are used to test for strabismus. It is also possible to use a favorite toy in the case of a child, at arm's length when covering and uncovering an eye, but a 20-foot distance is more revealing.

What to Watch Out For

When testing children, it is sometimes difficult to hold their attention; try to make the procedure more of a game than a test.

What the Test Results Can Mean

If, when the eye is covered and uncovered while staring at a distant point, the covered eye moves in any direction, this provides reasonable grounds for assuming that there is an eye muscle problem; medical attention is warranted. If, when a flashlight is viewed with both eyes, one of which is covered with a red glass, two distinct lights are seen—one red and one white—it is evidence of diplopia and also warrants medical attention.

Reliability

When the covered eye moves after being covered and then uncovered, there is a 90 percent chance that a muscle imbalance exists.

EAR OBSERVATIONS
AND HEARING TESTS

EAR CANAL AND EARDRUM OBSERVATIONS (Otoscope)
(An easy way to detect certain hearing problems)

Before any **Hearing Function** test (see Ear Observations and Hearing Tests) can be performed, it is necessary to know that the ear canal is not obstructed and that the eardrum is intact and not inflamed. Many so-called hearing problems have been miraculously cured by the simple removal of wax from the ear canal. In other instances foreign bodies such as beads, parts of toys and even insects have been found blocking hearing—especially in young children. And many ear and hearing problems arise from bacteria or especially fungus infections of the ear canal as a consequence of swimming, bathing or subsequent to scratching or picking at the ear canal. Such troubles are usually called external otitis when limited to the outer ear (from the opening to the eardrum), as opposed to otitis media, or middle ear disease, which involves the eardrum and the tiny space behind the eardrum that is connected to the back of the throat; the latter usually accompanies a sore throat. The third anatomical part of the ear, the inner ear, includes the nerves that transmit sound to the brain as well as the mechanisms that help keep one's balance (see Brain and Nervous System Tests, **Dizziness and Ataxia**).

Home testing of the ear by examination is limited to the outer ear and the outer surface of the eardrum. This is easily performed with an otoscope, a battery-operated flashlight device that projects light into the ear canal while leaving an opening for viewing (see Figure 45). This instrument has replaced the once-familiar mirror with the hole in the middle that doctors used to wear on the forehead to reflect light into the ear through a speculum (a funnellike adapter to concentrate one's vision).

What Is Usual
Once you get used to handling an otoscope, it will be relatively easy to peer inside someone else's ear canal. As long as there is nothing obstructing the passage of the small end of the funnel tip of the otoscope, insert it carefully, always making sure that nothing is in its way; if you see the slightest obstruc-

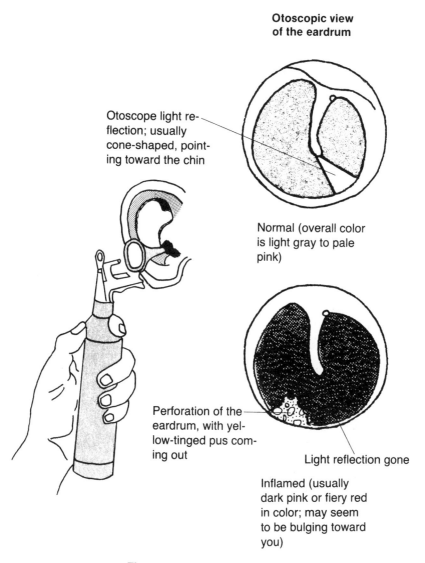

**Otoscopic view
of the eardrum**

Otoscope light re-
flection; usually
cone-shaped, point-
ing toward the chin

Normal (overall color
is light gray to pale
pink)

Perforation of the
eardrum, with yel-
low-tinged pus com-
ing out

Light reflection gone

Inflamed (usually
dark pink or fiery red
in color; may seem
to be bulging toward
you)

Figure 45. Using the otoscope.

tion, you should evaluate it before continuing the examination. Without
anything blocking the way, you should be able to see the pale, pink-colored
tunnel of the external ear canal all the way to the eardrum. The drum should
also be pink, but possibly with a gray tinge; most important, it should reflect
your light back in the form of a triangle, with the point at the center of the
eardrum and the widest part toward the chin of the person being examined
(see Figure 45).

It is also usual to see tiny flecks of brown material along the ear canal; these most often are particles of ear wax. If they do not obstruct vision or cause discomfort when touched, they should not interfere with your view of the eardrum. If the material does not seem to be ear wax, you should not perform this examination until the foreign matter is verified professionally.

What You Need

You should obtain an otoscope, which ranges from $16.00 for a Sears, Roe-buck model (which is small enough for nose examinations and also includes a lighted tongue depressor for throat examinations) up to $50.00 for an otoscope with removable speculae (funnel tips) in various sizes. Professional otoscopes cost from $70.00 up but offer no greater benefits for home use. For removing ear wax you may want to get the Murine ear wax removal system, which comes complete with a dropper bottle of cleaning solution and a soft rubber syringe for rinsing; Debrox is a similar preparation without the rinsing syringe. Both cost from $4.00 to $5.00 (a generic ear wax remover that costs $1.00 is sometimes available).

What to Watch Out For

Keep the following points in mind when examining the ears and removing ear wax:

- Do not attempt or continue an ear examination if you see anything that blocks your view of the eardrum, if there is any discomfort when the speculum touches the ear canal or if there is any discharge coming out of the ear.
- Do not attempt to remove any foreign body from the ear canal (other than wax, using an appropriate cleaning solution).
- Do not mistake the walls of the external ear canal for the eardrum; a normal eardrum has a distinctive light reflex.
- Do not be discouraged if it takes several days for all the wax to be washed out; follow the instructions that accompany the cleaning solution.
- Your doctor can give you a product for home use that can remove ear wax in 30 minutes.

What the Test Results Can Mean

If the ear canal and the eardrum seem as they should, go ahead with hearing function tests. If the walls of the ear canal look white or red, if they appear granular or if they seem to be covered with mucous, a medical consultation is warranted. If the eardrum looks bulging, blue or fiery red or if it is producing a discharge, medical attention is warranted. If, in fact, the only abnormality is that the typical light reflex is missing or cannot be seen, that, too, warrants medical attention (see Figure 45).

Incidentally, if an insect does happen to fly into an ear, a procedure that can help remove the bug is to go into a dark room or closet and shine a light into the ear; this usually attracts the insect out of the ear canal.

Reliability

It has been shown that the average person, with a few days of practice, can easily learn to use an otoscope. Other studies indicate that ear wax and/or eardrum abnormalities are correctly observed more than 90 percent of the time.

HEARING FUNCTION
(Some simple tests to help detect and prevent deafness)

Sound is heard and measured in two ways: by its intensity, more often called volume or loudness, and by its tone, sometimes called pitch, which depends upon how fast or slowly the sound waves vibrate. The intensity of sound is recorded in decibels (db). Loudness is also influenced by distance: A given noise at 20 feet will sound 10 percent louder when it is only 5 feet away. A bel is 10 db, and a sone is a subjective measurement to indicate 40 db more than one's sound threshold. Normally, it takes 10 db to 20 db of sound to be perceived (leaves blowing in a tree just above you would be an example of sound of this intensity). Some other examples of sound intensity include:

- 20 db to 30 db—a whispered voice nearby.
- 50 db to 60 db—the normal spoken voice.
- 70 db to 80 db—music at its proper volume; typical television sound; a dishwasher, washing machine or garbage disposal; a restaurant environment; freeway traffic.
- 80 db to 90 db—shouting, food processors, coffee grinders, low-flying airplanes.
- 90 db to 100 db—inside most subway trains, within 25 feet of most trucks.
- 100 db to 120 db—thunder overhead, an 11-month-old baby screaming six inches from his or her mother's ear.
- 120 db to 140 db—rock music at its typical volume, even at a distance and, naturally, much worse in closed room or car.
- 140 db or more—a jet engine within 100 feet; near the muzzle of a gun, especially a shotgun, being fired.

Each 10 db increase in sound reflects 10 *times* the amount of intensity; 80 db is 10 times as loud as 70 db, and 90 db is 100 times as loud as 70 db. The length of time that sound is heard is also an important factor when it comes to causing hearing loss. A constant factory noise (80 db) heard for more than eight hours is considered dangerous. At 90 db, such as the sound made by most power tools, ear damage can result in from two hours to eight hours. When sound reaches 100 db (a chain saw or a power mower), it can cause deafness within an hour. Rock music has caused ear damage within no more than a few seconds to a few minutes, depending, of course, on how near one is to the loudspeaker. The loudest sound recorded is that adjacent to a rocket launch (160 db), which, without protection, causes immediate, irreversible deafness and possible brain damage. Sound at 130 db can actually cause pain.

The tone of a sound is recorded in cycles per second (cps), or frequency; the lowest tones give off the smallest number of cps. The ear can normally hear sound with frequencies from 16 cps to 16,000 cps, but the typical speaking range of sound is between 500 cps and 1,500 cps. Frequency is also measured in Hertz (Hz), which stands for the number of pressure variations or cycles that occur per second; while Hz is the same as cps, it is more often said that the ear can usually hear from 16 Hz to 16,000 Hz.

Sound is perceived and conducted to the brain in two ways: air conduction (sound enters through the ear canal and is detected by the eardrum) and bone conduction (sound is detected by the bones around and behind the ear). It has been estimated that 1 out of every 10 people has some form of hearing impairment; deafness is considered one of the most prevalent chronic health problems in the United States. In many cases the impairment could have been corrected or overcome had it been detected early enough in life.

Some babies, however, are born deaf as a consequence of the mothers' having contracted certain infections during pregnancy (for example, rubella, or German measles) or having an Rh factor problem; other infants suffer deafness as an inherited congenital defect or from injuries sustained during childbirth. While it is difficult to ascertain whether an infant up to the age of 6 months can hear properly, many doctors advocate repeated home testing of a newborn's hearing starting a week after birth until evidence of hearing is observed. One such test is to sound a bell near a sleeping infant to see whether he or she awakens at the sound. By the time an infant is 6 months old, it should have become obvious to the parents that their child does or does not respond to sounds. Another sign of deafness, albeit not definitive, is failure of the child to make sounds and attempt to imitate words. It is important to be aware of any hearing defects before a child starts school; in far too many cases children have been labeled as having learning problems simply because they could not clearly hear and comprehend words and directions.

Once a person is past 50 years of age, hearing may become impaired through aging alone, or impairment may be brought about by a hard, bony growth over the hearing bones called otosclerosis. Many elderly people lose hearing so gradually that they fail to recognize the impairment and, at times, are thought to be rude rather than deaf. Between infancy and aging there are many things that can reduce or eliminate normal hearing: ear infections, sinusitis and tonsillitis (although normal hearing usually returns when the infection is cured), head injuries, brain and nerve diseases, exposure to excessive noise on the job (without using adequate protective devices) and even sociocusis—a loss of hearing due to nonoccupational exposure to recreational noises (entertainment, motor boats, motorcycles, shooting, flying) or home activities (power lawn mowers, living alongside a freeway or near an airport). More and more deafness is being observed in teen-agers and young adults as a consequence of listening to rock-type music through earphones or in closed cars or rooms.

A more recent cause of deafness comes as a side effect of drugs. Many antibiotic medications (ganamycin, kanamycin, neomycin, streptomycin), some diuretics (Edecrin, Lasix), antimalarials, a few hormones, and even large amounts of aspirin or aspirinlike preparations are considered ototoxic; that is, they damage the ear nerves if used for prolonged periods of time. Damaged ear nerves can also cause **dizziness and ataxia** (see Brain and Nervous System Tests).

There are several tests that may be performed to assess hearing function; some measure sound intensity, while others evaluate tone perception, or the frequency of sound heard. The ultimate test of hearing ability is performed with an audiometer—a device that can control the volume as well as the pitch (tone) of sound. While home-use screening audiometers can be purchased for $250.00 to $300.00, and there are even combination audiometer-otoscopes, it is best to apply the simple tests at home and, if problems are detected, seek out a skilled audiometer operator, who can usually define the type of deafness along with the potential benefits of treatment.

Sound measurements. One of the simplest and most effective ways of preventing hearing disabilities is to measure and monitor the loudness of sound around you. While this can be particularly valuable in the work environment, it can be equally valuable at home if loud noises occur persistently, albeit sporadically—for instance, loudspeakers emitting music, airplanes flying overhead, adjacent vehicle traffic, power tools, and even some air-conditioners and other mechanical appliances. Not only can loud sound damage the inner ear, it has also been reported to cause brain cell changes that, in turn, can produce behavioral abnormalities such as confusion and hostility; some feel that it is the brain's reaction to damaging noises that causes ringing in the ears.

By testing the loudness of sounds around you, and then avoiding dangerous levels of sound either through insulation or by wearing protective ear devices when exposure cannot be avoided, you can do a great deal to protect your hearing function. Keep in mind that while repeated exposure to sound louder than 85 db is known to cause some hearing loss, some people will experience a partial loss of their hearing function at even lower decibels of sound, depending on its duration.

What Is Usual

The voice and whisper tests are the simplest. You should be able to hear and repeat numbers spoken in a normal voice intensity from 20 feet away. Then you should be able to hear loud whispers from the same distance, and as the whispers become softer, they should still be heard at a 2-foot distance. Whispers represent a higher pitch (tone) than the spoken voice.

Many doctors use the ticking watch test as a screening technique. Doctors know just how far away their watch or clock must be before they can no longer hear it (assuming, of course, that the doctors know that they have normal hearing); they then measure the distance at which their patients are able to hear the ticking. You can perform the same three tests described, but be sure you know that your hearing is normal before you test someone whose hearing is in doubt.

A tuning fork (which should have a frequency of 512 cps) can enable you to perform a more refined type of test. After the tuning fork is set in motion (by tapping its sides against the palm or by squeezing the tips together and releasing them suddenly), the sound should be heard by each ear at a distance of 20 feet (hold the opposite ear closed with the palm of the hand pressed tightly over the ear against the side of the head). When the examiner compares his or her, presumably normal, hearing to that of the examinee, both should hear the sound. This is called the Schwabach test.

There are other tuning fork tests that help determine both whether air conduction or bone conduction is impaired as well as which ear is impaired. For the Rinne test (shown in Figure 46), the vibrating tuning fork is placed an inch or two away from each ear opening (as a test of air conduction); while the tuning fork is still vibrating, its base is then placed against the mastoid bone behind the ear (as a test of bone conduction). The tone should be heard for twice as long when the tuning fork is held alongside the ear. For the Weber test (shown in Figure 46), the base of the vibrating tuning fork is placed on the top of the head (or in the center of the forehead at the hairline), and the way each ear hears the sound is observed. It should be heard equally in both ears at the same time.

One particular tuning fork test used by doctors, but which can easily be performed at home, is the stethoscope–tuning fork test. The person to be tested places the earpieces of a stethoscope in his or her ears; a clamp can be placed over one of the two tubes that go from the stethoscope to the ears to test each ear separately. A 1,024 cps tuning fork is sounded and placed close to the stethoscope opening or diaphragm and also alongside the ear of the person doing the testing. The person wearing the stethoscope should hear the tuning fork's sound a minimum of 15 seconds longer than the person holding the tuning fork next to his or her ear. The test is usually performed before a patient receives any drug that can cause deafness and is designed to establish a baseline of hearing ability. Repeated testing during

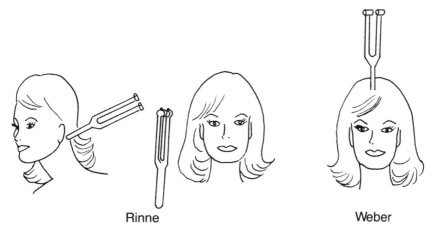

Rinne   Weber

Figure 46. Hearing tests.

administration of the medicine and for a few months after it has been stopped can help detect deafness caused by the drug; if hearing time when the person is wearing the stethoscope is reduced by more than 3 seconds, additional audiometer tests are indicated.

A fifth tuning fork test is called the Teal test; it requires two tuning forks. When a person claims that the tuning fork is not heard when placed alongside the ear, the individual is blindfolded, and the base of a nonvibrating tuning fork is placed against the bone behind the ear, while another, vibrating tuning fork is placed alongside the head about three feet away. Someone simulating deafness will claim that he or she detects the sound through bone conduction; a deaf person will hear nothing.

A hearing test is also available by telephone. Call toll-free (800) 222-3277 and you will be given a local number that when called, plays a series of tones; failure to hear all the tones warrants a medical consultation. If the number does not answer, call (800) 555-1212 and ask for the latest information on "Dial-a-Hearing Screening Test," or write Occupational Hearing Services (16 S. Orange St., Media, Pa. 19063).

What You Need
The following equipment is required to test hearing:

- An otoscope is used to be sure that the ear canal is not obstructed and the eardrum not inflamed prior to testing (see Ear Observations and Hearing Tests, **Ear Canal and Eardrum Observations**).
- A ticking watch or clock is used, or a ticking kitchen timer, at a cost of $3.00 to $4.00, might also serve the purpose.

- A tuning fork (preferably having a frequency of 512 cps), which costs from $8.00 to $10.00, should also be obtained.
- A stethoscope (see Heart and Circulation Tests, **Blood Pressure**) is optional.
- You might want a portable sound level meter, which detects sound and measures it in terms of decibels; such a meter can cost from $30.00 to $400.00 and can offer an early warning against potentially damaging sounds. The least expensive model (available at Radio Shack stores) is quite adequate for home testing.

What to Watch Out For

Be sure that you check your own hearing against that of someone whose hearing is known to be normal before you perform the tests on anyone else. Do not perform the tests if there is wax in the ear canal or if there is any suspicion of an ear infection. Check with your doctor or pharmacist to see whether any of your medicine is ototoxic. Some doctors believe that mumps vaccine can also cause deafness.

What the Test Results Can Mean

If you ever experience sudden deafness, especially if it is preceded by a brief noise in the ear, it warrants immediate medical attention.

Any persistent divergence from what most people can hear warrants a medical consultation. Any sign of diminished hearing, especially in a child, warrants audiometry and a professional ear examination. Any abnormal tuning fork test warrants medical attention. Two particular examples: If, when the Rinne test is performed, the sound is not heard when the tuning fork is removed from the mastoid bone and held adjacent to the outer-ear opening, it usually indicates an outer- or middle-ear problem—especially when accompanied by an abnormal Weber test. If, when the Weber test is performed, the sound seems louder in one ear, it usually means that the problem is in the ear that perceives the sound as being louder (as an example, perform the Weber test with your finger in one ear to block out sound). If the Rinne test is normal and the Weber test reveals hearing in only one ear, it usually indicates an inner-ear problem in the ear that hears the sound.

If, when you test the intensity of sound around you (in your room while music is playing, at your workplace, etc.), your sound level meter indicates 70 db or more and you think that the sound is soft, a medical consultation is warranted.

Note: Part of the ear's function, in addition to hearing, is related to balance (equilibrium)—being aware of one's position in space and knowing where the parts of the body (such as the hands and feet) are when the eyes are closed. Tests for such coordination ability (sometimes called labyrinthine tests, because the part of the inner ear that controls these perceptions is called the labyrinth) are discussed under Brain and Nervous System Tests, **Dizziness and Ataxia.**

Reliability

Voice, whisper and ticking watch tests have been shown to be 90 percent accurate in detecting previously unsuspected hearing loss. When tuning fork tests are added, the accuracy increases to better than 95 percent.

BRAIN AND NERVOUS SYSTEM TESTS

DIZZINESS AND ATAXIA
(Possible clues to coordination and/or fainting problems)

Dizziness seems to be an increasingly common complaint, especially among older people. The word *dizziness* can have many different meanings; medically, however, it stands for instability or unsteadiness, along with lightheadedness and a fear of an impending fall. The word is also used frequently for vertigo, which really means either that you feel the room going round and round or that something inside your head seems to be going round and round. Some people also use the word to describe a lack of the sense of balance, when, in fact, the problem is more a loss of coordination—usually referred to as positional imbalance. Ataxia, on the other hand, is a loss of muscle coordination or unexpected, irregular muscle actions; it is often considered as dizziness because it involves difficulty in walking and problems with position sense.

There are many, totally different, diseases that can cause dizziness or ataxia, and these conditions may come on so gradually that they are overlooked until they have reached the point of being extremely difficult to treat. But if dizziness occurs a few times, it is sometimes possible, by applying several basic tests, to help detect the cause of the dizziness while the condition is still in its early stages.

Keep in mind that a great many medicines can, indirectly, be the cause of dizziness; they include: certain antibiotics (see Ear Observations and Hearing Tests, **Hearing Function**), several diuretic drugs, tranquilizers and antidepressants, antihistamines, drugs used to treat high blood pressure and epilepsy, birth control pills, large doses of aspirin, and even excessive amounts of alcohol, caffeine or nicotine. Also, new glasses, allergies and anxiety can all bring on "dizzy spells." In many instances withdrawal of the provocative factor results in relief. The **Orthostatic Blood Pressure** test (see Heart and Circulation Tests) may also offer a clue as to the cause of the problem.

In addition to the possibility of sudden lowered blood pressure upon standing as a cause of dizziness, the blood pressure can also fall markedly after you eat—especially after a large meal, which may prompt blood flow to increase in the intestinal tract as an aid to digestion. Eating may also involve sitting in one position for an hour or more. If you notice dizziness or feel faint after eating, you can check your blood pressure a few minutes before the meal and then from 15 minutes to 30 minutes after eating but while you are still sitting. If you notice a drop in your blood pressure, it warrants a medical consultation. It could be the cause of your dizziness.

And keep in mind that exposure to **carbon monoxide** (CO) (see Environmental Tests) can cause all the signs and symptoms mentioned.

Although you will not be able to make a conclusive diagnosis of the cause of repeated dizziness, vertigo, ataxia or positional imbalance, it is sometimes possible to help discern the origin of the problem by applying six basic dizziness and ataxia tests:

- *The Romberg test:* The individual stands up with feet close together, arms at sides, and then closes both eyes; be sure that someone is ready to catch the person should he or she start to fall.
- *The past-pointing test:* Have the individual sit in front of you with eyes closed, holding out both hands with the index fingers pointing at you; placing your fingertips underneath his or hers so they are resting on yours, tell the person to lift up both arms over his or her head and then return the index fingers to where they were (on your fingertips, which you have kept in place).
- *The finger-to-nose test:* Have the individual stand up and, with eyes closed, extend one arm all the way out to the side, hold it out straight and then quickly bring the index finger back to the tip of his or her nose, keeping the elbow perpendicular to the body; test both arms.
- *The finger coordination test:* Have the individual touch each fingertip with his or her thumb in rapid succession, back and forth; test both hands.
- *The heel-to-knee test:* Have the individual lie down on his or her back and place the heel of one foot on the knee of the opposite leg, first with the eyes open and then with them closed; test both feet.
- *The toe-pointing test:* Have the individual lie down on his or her back and point to various objects with his or her big toe; test both feet.

These are but a few of the various tests that can help locate the area where the problem exists: the inner ear (see Ear Observations and Hearing Tests, **Hearing Function**), the cerebellum (that part of the brain which helps control balance and coordination), or the spinal cord and nerves below the brain level (see Brain and Nervous System Tests, **Reflex Testing** and **Sensory Testing**).

What Is Usual
An individual should not sway or fall when standing up with the eyes closed. All the other tests for coordination and position awareness should be performed without difficulty.

What You Need
The tests require nothing in the way of equipment, although patience and encouragement are helpful.

What to Watch Out For
When performing the Romberg test, be sure that you are physically able to catch the individual should he or she start to fall. Before any testing, be sure to ascertain that drugs are not being used.

What the Test Results Can Mean
A positive Romberg test (falling) and past-pointing test (inability to bring the fingertips back to where they were) usually indicate an inner-ear problem (see the discussion of the Rinne and Weber tests under Ear Observations and Hearing Tests, **Hearing Function**); less often, they point to a loss of positional sense, with the trouble being in the spinal cord. If the foot misses its mark with the heel-to-knee test and keeps slipping down the front of the leg instead of staying on the knee, and there is an inability to perform most of the other tests, this usually signals a cerebellum disorder but can also hint at spinal cord disease. When poor performance on these tests is accompanied by a staggering or lurching type of walk, the symptoms could come from an old spinal cord infection such as syphilis. In general, however, almost all of these tests are positive (the individual is unable to perform them easily and properly) with thyroid disease and other hormone disorders, anemia, deficiencies of some vitamins (especially niacin or B_3), spinal cord involvement (multiple sclerosis), various forms of heart and artery disease, the late consequences of injuries, migraine and as a reflection of a neurosis. Thus, it is easy to see why any abnormal test result warrants a medical consultation. If, of course, the dizziness or ataxia is recurrent and close to disabling, it warrants medical attention. Sometimes, that visit to the doctor results in an immediate cure, such as when the problem is nothing more than a foreign body in the ear (see Ear Observations and Hearing Tests, **Ear Canal and Eardrum Observations**), an allergy, a form of motion sickness, or the consequence of hyperventilation or some other anxiety-type reaction.

Reliability
Abnormal balance and coordination tests are considered 90 percent accurate as an indication of an underlying illness.

REFLEX TESTING
(Screening for brain, nerve and spinal cord problems)

A reflex test is a measure of the body's reaction to stimulation. In effect, it takes into consideration the ability to perceive a stimulus (to the skin, the muscles, the surface of the eye), the efficacy of a nerve to carry recognition of that stimulus to the spinal cord (and sometimes to the brain), the ability of the nervous system to interpret the stimulus, the efficacy of another nerve to carry a response to that stimulus back to the proper organ (usually a muscle) and the organ's ability to respond physically. In other words, a reflex can indicate brain, spinal cord, nerve and muscle well-being, or lack of same.

The most common reflex text is the knee-jerk (shown in Figure 47); tapping the skin over the patellar tendon just below the kneecap (usually with a rubber hammer) stretches the attached upper leg–thigh muscle, and that muscle normally responds by contracting (shortening), lifting the lower leg and foot up suddenly and involuntarily. Virtually every muscle in the body can be tested this way, but only a few such tests are routinely performed. Besides the patellar, or knee-jerk, reflex, they include:

- *The biceps reflex:* Hold the individual's arm partially flexed, with your thumb over the inside bend at the elbow (just about where blood is usually taken for laboratory testing); at this point your thumb is over the tendon from the biceps (the large upper arm muscle), which lifts the lower arm; a tap on your thumb should cause the person's lower arm to lift.
- *The wrist reflex:* Hold the individual's lower arm at the elbow so that the arm is parallel to the floor and the wrist hangs down loosely; tap the upper surface of the lower arm with a rubber hammer about two-thirds of the way down the arm between the elbow and the wrist; when the rubber hammer strikes the main muscle attached to the wrist, it causes that muscle to contract, suddenly raising the wrist and hand.
- *The ankle-jerk (Achilles heel) reflex:* With one hand holding the individual's foot so that the toes point upward, tap the Achilles tendon (in the center of the back of the foot, just above the heel); this contracts the large muscle in the back of the leg and normally causes the foot to point downward.

The above reflexes are called "deep" reflexes, because the force of a light blow is required to stretch a tendon under the skin. In contrast, there are the "superficial" reflexes, for which, to elicit a response, the skin surface need only be gently touched or stroked. A few of these include:

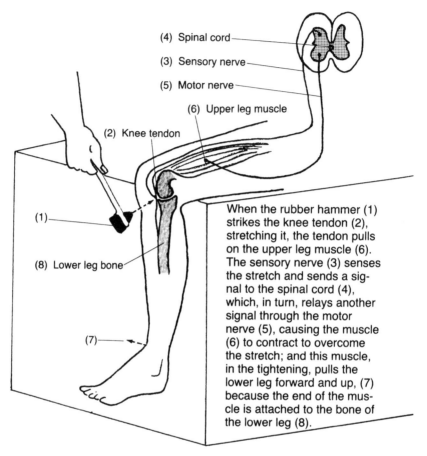

(4) Spinal cord

(3) Sensory nerve

(5) Motor nerve

(6) Upper leg muscle

(2) Knee tendon

(1)

(8) Lower leg bone

(7)

When the rubber hammer (1) strikes the knee tendon (2), stretching it, the tendon pulls on the upper leg muscle (6). The sensory nerve (3) senses the stretch and sends a signal to the spinal cord (4), which, in turn, relays another signal through the motor nerve (5), causing the muscle (6) to contract to overcome the stretch; and this muscle, in the tightening, pulls the lower leg forward and up, (7) because the end of the muscle is attached to the bone of the lower leg (8).

Figure 47. Knee reflex test.

- *The neck-pupil reflex:* If you pinch the skin at the back of the neck, it should cause the pupils to dilate (see Eye and Vision Tests, **Pupil and Pupillary Reflex.**)
- *Corneal reflex:* If you touch the surface of the white part of the eye (the cornea), usually with a tuft of cotton, the eyelids should blink.
- *Abdominal reflexes:* A gentle stroke on the skin above, below or to the side of the umbilicus (navel) should cause the muscles under the skin to pull the umbilicus toward the direction of the stroke.
- *The cremasteric reflex:* A gentle stroke on the skin just inside the upper thigh adjacent to the scrotum (the sac that holds the testicle) should cause the scrotum to rise up, on the side that was stroked, toward the abdomen because of the contraction of the cremasteric muscle.

- *Babinski reflex:* To test this unusual reflex, hold the foot by the ankle and stroke the sole of the foot firmly with a blunt object from heel to toe; usually, the toes curl and point downward.
- *The cold face reflex:* A large ice bag is gently placed over the entire face and held there for one minute; normally, this causes the pulse rate to slow momentarily (see Heart and Circulation Tests, **Pulse Measurements**) through nerve impulses acting on the parasympathetic nervous system (see Heart and Circulation Tests, **Cold Pressor and Finger Wrinkle**).

Muscles to be tested should be relaxed; if they are tense before testing, they may not react normally. One way to induce relaxation in other muscles is to have the individual hold his or her hands together by the fingers and try to pull them apart; this action usually allows the other muscles to relax.

The value of reflex testing is that it not only offers signs of brain, nerve and/or muscle disease but can also give a fairly accurate picture of just where the trouble lies. The more muscles and nerve pathways tested, the more precise the location of the pathology. Reflex testing usually accompanies tests for touch, feel and temperature discrimination (see Brain and Nervous System Tests, **Sensory Testing**) and can also be performed in conjunction with **Smell Function** and **Taste Function** tests (see Brain and Nervous System Tests).

There is now a device quite similar to a doctor's electromyograph test that detects a muscle's specific electrical activity—in reality, its strength. It is called an "Electronic Gym," and by placing over a muscle a pad connected to a measuring gauge, you can determine the muscle's force and follow its progress as a result of exercise. The battery-operated test device is available through most mail-order houses and costs from $70.00 to $80.00. While it performs a more specific muscle measurement than can be done through reflex testing, it is no more revealing of the cause of a disease.

What Is Usual

Reflex reactions should all be present and of a reasonable nature—that is, not too weak nor too strong or forceful. You will have to observe a few reflex reactions to become familiar with "normal," and it might be best to watch your doctor test your own reflexes and those of others to learn what a "normal" response is. The strength of reflex reactions should be the same on both sides of the body.

What You Need

A rubber percussion hammer can make reflex testing easier; it costs from $1.00 to $3.00. One containing a pin and brush (for sensory testing) costs from $4.00 to $5.00. In most instances, however, the edge of the hand and the fingers will serve adequately. You will need an ice bag for the cold face reflex test.

What to Watch Out For

Do not hit too hard; in most instances a gentle tap will suffice. Be sure that the individual being tested is relaxed. If you do not elicit a reflex reaction at first, be sure that you are striking the proper spot. Do not perform the cold face reflex test on someone with known heart disease until you have discussed it with your doctor.

What the Test Results Can Mean

Failure to elicit a reflex reaction with proper technique and relaxed muscles usually indicates a nerve–spinal cord problem; excessive or violent reflex reactions usually indicate brain involvement. At times deep reflexes will be present but superficial ones will be absent; the opposite can also happen. The absence or exaggeration of any reflex warrants medical attention; there are innumerable conditions that can cause these abnormal test results, and the earlier the specific cause is detected, the more efficacious the treatment.

A positive Babinski reflex (where the toes curl upward and spread apart) can be an ominous warning sign of serious brain disease. With the cold face reflex test, failure of the pulse to slow noticeably can be a sign of diabetes or multiple sclerosis or even the consequence of a little stroke that might have gone undetected. Obviously, any doubt about the results of these reflex tests warrants medical attention.

As an incidental observation, many doctors feel that a slow or seemingly momentarily delayed ankle-jerk (Achilles heel) reflex is a reasonable sign of thyroid disease. On the other hand, if repeated testing of the ankle-jerk reflex seems to show an increasing time delay before responding, after an initial normal response, it can be a reasonable sign of diabetes. Either observation warrants medical attention.

Reliability

When testing is properly performed, abnormal reflex reactions are considered 80 percent accurate as an indicator of disease.

SENSORY TESTING
(Sensation screening to detect brain and nervous system disorders)

There are many different tests that help measure your ability to perceive various sensations (pain discrimination and pressure as opposed to light touch, differences in temperature, tuning fork vibrations, position sense and the ability to recognize form and writing when applied to the skin). When these tests are performed along with Reflex Testing (see Brain and Nervous System Tests), they can help diagnose brain, nerve and spinal cord problems. Because a doctor knows just where each nerve functions anatomically, it is usually possible to pinpoint the exact location of the pathology. These tests also help explain some of the many "sensations" that some people complain of: burning, tingling, pins and needles, unexplained pain or the absence of any feeling at all (numbness). And sensory testing can be quite valuable in detecting malingerers.

The following sensory tests are performed with the individual's eyes closed or blindfolded so that the measurements are more objective; they are usually performed on all the body's surfaces, including the trunk and the extremities:

- *Pinprick:* It is usual for an individual to feel the pain of a slight pinprick on the body, and it should feel the same all over; at the same time the individual should be able to discriminate between a pinprick and the push of a pencil eraser.
- *Light-touch discrimination:* An individual should be able to discern the difference between the touch of a piece of cotton, the touch of a small brush and the light stroke of a fingertip, and between coarse cotton and silk.
- *Temperature discrimination:* When two tubes of water, one warm and the other cool, are individually placed against the skin, a person should easily be able to tell the difference.
- *Tuning fork:* When the base of a vibrating tuning fork is placed on a skin covered bony surface (elbow, ankle, spine), an individual should be able to feel the vibrations for as long as the examiner can; some doctors now suggest placing the tip of the vibrating tuning fork over the tip of each finger as a means of detecting the first signs of nerve damage in or near the wrist. A condition called carpal tunnel syndrome (*carpal* is a medical term for wrist), in which there is a numbness and tingling in the hand—especially at night—is being seen much more often. It may reflect thyroid or other hormone disease or simply swelling of the wrist ligaments from excessive use and/or water retention (see Body Observations, **Edema**).
- *Position sense:* An individual should be able to tell when his or her thumb, fingers and big toe have been pointed up or down.
- *Distance discrimination:* When two pins or other objects are placed near each other on the skin, an individual should be able to tell about how far apart they are.
- *Stereognosis:* An individual should be able to recognize and describe the shape of a solid object (coin, button, marble, pencil stub) placed in the hand.

• *Small corks:* This test is best performed on another family member rather than on oneself. Obtain four small corks of different sizes, ranging from ½ inch to 1¼ inches, each varying by ¼ inch; after placing them first in one hand of a blindfolded person and then in the person's other hand, ask that person—using only that one hand and its fingers—to tell how many corks there are and then to hand them back according to size, starting with the largest one (if a cork drops, place it back in the subject's hand and continue with the size discrimination test).

• *Graphesthesia:* An individual should be able to recognize and describe a large letter or numeral traced by the examiner's finger or a pencil on the palm of the hand, the abdomen and the leg.

These sensory tests are but a very few of those that can be performed, but they are sufficient to help identify some early warning signs of disease or hysteria.

What is Usual
"Normal" responses are noted in the description of each test.

What You Need
Other than the tuning fork (the same one used in **Hearing Function** tests; see Ear Observations and Hearing Tests), which costs from $8.00 to $10.00, most other test equipment can be found around the home. Small jars may be used in place of the test tubes. Corks are available at hardware stores.

What to Watch Out For
Be sure that the individual being examined keeps his or her eyes closed at all times; there is a great temptation to "peek," and this, of course, nullifies any test observation. Keep a careful record of your findings; then, when you repeat the same test in the same location, you can tell whether there are changes or whether the individual was trying to mislead you. Some examiners use a washable fabric marker to identify the skin areas tested and thereby facilitate exact repeat testing a short time later.

What the Test Results Can Mean
An abnormal result (failure to perceive what "normal" people can feel and interpret) can be caused by so many different conditions—from disease to dietary deficiencies—that it would be impossible to list them all here; suffice it to say that any lack of sensory function warrants a medical consultation. It takes a physician with years of experience to be able to discern the exact anatomical distribution—the area of activity—of each nerve on the skin's surface (called a dermatome). For example, if the complaint is one of numbness in the knee, the doctor will determine whether that numbness follows

the expected nerve distribution; if it does not, it is just as important to seek the reason for the pretense, which may be hysteria (severe emotional upset) or malingering. An inability to discern the number of corks in one's hand or an inability to pass them back in the proper order according to size can be a sign of a serious nerve disorder and warrants medical attention.

Reliability

Although failure to perceive sensory stimuli, or diminished reactions to sensory stimuli, are considered to be 80 percent accurate as an indication of a nervous system problem, it is not possible to determine the specific cause from these tests alone. If pretense is observed or suspected, and proves to be the case, it is 90 percent indicative of a hysterical-type reaction.

SMELL FUNCTION
(Along with taste function testing, additional tests of your sensory abilities)

If you think it seems superfluous to test for the ability to identify odors normally, then you are not aware of the constant jeopardy in which millions of people live because they cannot detect dangerous chemical fumes, gas escaping from a stove or heater, smoke from a fire or the stench of spoiled or contaminated food. Recent surveys indicate that more than 1 out of every 100 people has a diminished sense of smell or taste, with at least 2 million experiencing smell dysfunction alone.

In some instances the sense of smell is a combination of both smell and taste (see Brain and Nervous System Tests, **Taste Function**). Smell function ability, called olfaction, varies greatly from one person to another: Some people are unable to smell anything at all, called anosmia; some have a decreased ability to smell, called hyposmia; some have perversions of odors, called dysosmia; and others can be extra-sensitive to odors to the point of constant discomfort. Pregnant women are often hypersensitive to the slightest scent.

Because odors are not recognized until they reach the olfactory nerve endings in the uppermost part of the nasal cavity (at or above eye level), as shown in Figure 48, it becomes obvious why someone with sinus problems (see Body Observations, **Sinus Transillumination**), a cold or hay fever can suffer smell impairment at times and then have normal smell function at other times. Smell function should be tested for whenever there is a loss of appetite and diminished enjoyment of food; if there is no obvious allergy or infection affecting the nose, it could be an early warning sign of brain or nerve disease. A sudden aversion to certain food odors usually considered pleasant (chocolate, roast beef, fresh-brewed coffee) can be one of the first

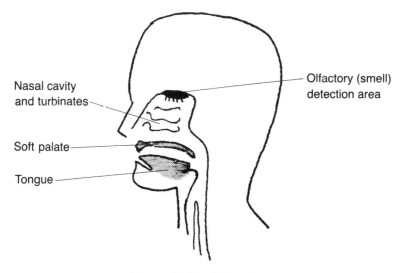

Nasal cavity
and turbinates

Olfactory (smell)
detection area

Soft palate

Tongue

Figure 48. Smell function.

signs of cancer somewhere in the body. Decreased smell function is found with several other diseases, and some people are simply born with smell (and taste) defects.

Many drugs can reduce or temporarily eliminate smell function; cocaine inhaled through the nose can also act as an anesthetic on the olfactory nerves; the excessive use of nose drops and drugs used to treat thyroid disease causes anosmia; and certain antibiotics can, as a side effect, reduce the ability to detect or differentiate odors. Other drugs known to distort or diminish odor perception include appetite suppressants, some of the newer antihypertensive medications and muscle relaxants.

Exposure to X-rays, toxic heavy metals, industrial chemicals and dusts can diminish the sense of smell. And smoking and **air pollution** (smog; see Environmental Tests) can also lessen one's ability to taste as well as smell.

Of unique interest, recent research has revealed that one out of every four people with a sexual performance problem also has a loss of smell function. On the other hand, women's ability to discern odors is most acute in the middle of their menstrual cycles and while they are pregnant. And of even greater interest, the brain and nerve cells that control smell and taste are the only ones that can at times, replace themselves after being damaged.

What Is Usual
With the nasal passages clear, and pressure placed against one of the nostrils to close that side, you should be able to detect and discern different odors—especially familiar ones—through the open side of the nose with the eyes

closed. Both sides of the nose should detect smells equally. The most common aromas used to test smell function include:

- Perfume or fresh flowers; considered the most sensitive indicators of true smell loss.
- Onion or garlic.
- Chocolate.
- Mint (fresh-picked leaves).
- Instant coffee.
- Turpentine.
- Fresh tobacco (usually pipe tobacco, both before and while smoking).
- A burning paper match (or burning paper in an ashtray), usually performed as the last test because of its possible irritating effect.

Do not try to smell ammonia or menthol; they can irritate the nose and give a false-positive reaction that seems to be smell but is not indicative of smell function.

What You Need

At least three of the above-listed items are required. Ideally, with the exception of the burning match, they should be kept in a tightly closed container until the container is opened for two seconds to three seconds. For very precise testing, you can construct a modified Elsberg apparatus (see Figure 49), using a glass jar with a two-holed rubber stopper that allows glass or plastic tubing to be inserted into the jar. Insert the tube gently into one nostril then close off the opposite nostril and breathe in. The jar, tubings and stopper can be obtained at any scientific equipment store for less than $1.00. If one or both sides of the nose seem obstructed due to a cold or allergy and testing is urgent, you might want to drop or spray a nasal decongestant into the nose about a half-hour prior to testing.

What to Watch Out For

If you are testing someone else, occasionally substitute plain water as a test material; it should have no odor and can help eliminate subjective or hallucinatory responses. If nasal decongestants do not open the nasal passageways within 30 minutes, do not repeat their use; put off the testing until another day. It is a good idea to test smell function prior to undergoing any nose operation (rhinoplasty); in that way you will always be aware of any loss of smell as a consequence of surgery.

What the Test Results Can Mean

Any noticeable loss of smell function, not related to temporarily blocked nasal passages, especially if olfaction was previously thought to be "normal," can point to several different diseases. In addition to brain pathology or

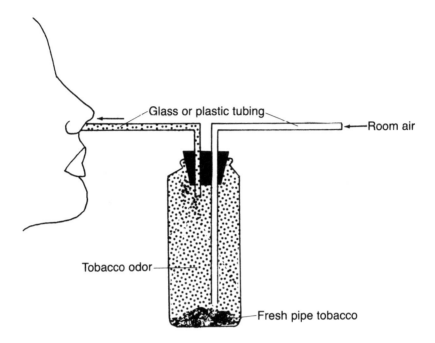

Figure 49. Testing smell function using a modified Elsberg apparatus.

nerve disease, it could be the consequence of a circulatory problem, such as a little stroke; and about 7 percent of all head injuries result in some loss of smell. This is even more likely if smell function is diminished or lost on only one side of the nose; a medical consultation is warranted. Thyroid disease, infections such as encephalitis, pneumonia, many lung conditions, multiple sclerosis, head injuries, nutritional problems and, of course, cancer can also interfere with the ability to detect odors. A sudden noticing of "foul" odors when no one else perceives them can be the first indication of depression or a neurosis (see Breath and Lung Tests, **Breath Odor and Sputum**). A loss of smell and taste can also be attributed to a dietary deficiency of zinc (see Brain and Nervous System Tests, **Zinc Deficiency Taste Test**). And about one out of every five people with a decreased sense of smell ends up with a diagnosis of idiopathic (meaning that the cause cannot be determined) anosmia. Absent or unusual smell function warrants a medical consultation, if for no other reason than to rule out any underlying problem.

If nothing else, testing smell function will let you know whether you are able to perceive odoriferous warnings of possible dangers. If you find that you are unable to notice smoke, it is mandatory that you install smoke detectors throughout your residence. If you have lost the ability to smell spoiled food and have no one around to notice such things, you are better off throwing out questionable leftovers as a form of preventive medicine.

Note: When the 1982 tragedy involving cyanide-adulterated Extra-Strength Tylenol capsules occurred in Chicago, it had always been believed that most people could easily smell the so-called bitter-almond odor of the deadly poison that had been mixed into the capsules. Further investigation revealed that more than half of all laypersons and most doctors in the medical examiner's office were unable to detect cyanide's characteristic odor. Now pathologists are tested for their ability to smell the poison, and if they are unable to do so, they must work with an assistant who is able to recognize a cyanide odor.

Reliability

Home tests for smell (and taste) are merely a rough, qualitative form of sampling but are still considered 80 percent accurate. More precise quantitative testing is available through your doctor to help pinpoint the cause of any abnormalities that may be detected.

The National Geographic smell survey. The September 1986 issue of *National Geographic* magazine carried a unique smell survey using unidentified scratch-and-sniff panels. If you cannot locate a back issue (with the test intact), you can write to the magazine (Washington, D.C. 20036) for a free copy. A fascinating report on the 1.5 million people who sent the magazine their impressions of the smells they detected (or failed to detect) was published in the October 1987 issue of the *National Geographic*—along with a correct identification of the original scratch-and-sniff panels. One unusual finding: Two out of 3 people seem to suffer a temporary loss of smell at times. A second, fascinating, observation was the relationship between smell and memory.

TASTE FUNCTION
(Along with smell function testing, another test of your sensory abilities)

The sense of taste is actually a combination of taste and smell (see Brain and Nervous System Tests, **Smell Function**). Having a stuffy nose can diminish the sense of taste. Although it has always been believed that it was the primary function of the tongue to distinguish saltiness, sweetness, sourness and bitterness, taste buds have since been found not only on the tongue but also on the palate, pharynx, epiglottis, tonsils and even the mucosa of the lips and cheeks. Loss or diminution of taste and smell can be caused by many factors, from ordinary colds to cancer. It is now believed that a loss of taste or changes in the sense of taste can be an early sign of cancer; the taste changes reduce the desire to eat, causing weight loss once thought to be from the cancer itself. It has been estimated that more than 2 million Americans suffer some loss of taste and/or smell. The inability to taste is dangerous in that it can allow the ingestion of tainted foods or poisons, which are usually bitter.

Total loss of taste function is called ageusia; decreased sensitivity to taste or partial loss of taste is called hypogeusia. Hallucinations of taste, called phantogeusia, and distorted taste, called dysgeusia, can occur normally during pregnancy. Many drugs can cause any or all of these problems; some include antifungus preparations, antibiotics and medicines to treat arthritis and muscle pains, Parkinson's disease, thyroid disease and vaginitis, to name but a few. Even toothpaste that contains sodium lauryl sulfate (check the list of ingredients on the label) can cause interference with taste function.

Older people sometimes seem to have a slightly decreased sensitivity to all flavors, especially to salty and sweet flavors, and will often require extra amounts of salt and sugar to make foods taste "right." A number of nutritional deficiencies, especially a lack of zinc in the diet, are also related to taste impairment; saliva must contain a zinc-protein compound to allow normal taste function (see Brain and Nervous System Tests, **Zinc Deficiency Taste Test**).

What Is Usual

Different areas of the tongue are sensitive to different tastes, as shown in Figure 50. The four taste groups and their primary areas are:

- *Bitter*—at the back of the tongue
- *Salty*—on the upper surface, toward the front
- *Sour*—along the edges on either side
- *Sweet*—at the tip

If you place a drop of a corresponding sample solution on the appropriate area of the tongue, you should be able to taste each one distinctly; as a control, there should be no taste perception if a drop of distilled water is used in place of a solution. It is also possible for taste sensations to be noticed when a drop of sample solution is placed somewhere other than in the appropriate area, but initially, the drop should not seem to have as strong a flavor.

What You Need

The test requires an eyedropper and some distilled water to use as a control and to make up applicable solutions:

- *Bitter*—bottled quinine water, undiluted.
- *Salty*—one teaspoon of salt dissolved in four ounces of distilled water.

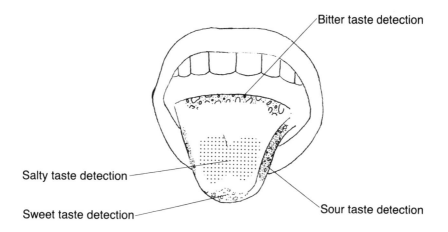

Figure 50. Areas of the tongue involved in tasting selectivity.

- *Sour*—one teaspoon of vinegar dissolved in one ounce of distilled water.
- *Sweet*—one teaspoon of sugar dissolved in four ounces of distilled water.

What to Watch Out For

Do not attempt taste function testing if you have a cold, sinusitis or simply a stuffy nose or if you have recently drunk alcoholic beverages or been smoking. Check with your doctor or pharmacist if you are taking medications; find out whether the drugs are known to alter taste perception. If you are not sure of the results, blindfold yourself and have someone else place the various drops on your tongue to see whether you can correctly perceive the flavors.

What the Test Results Can Mean

The most common cause of ageusia is Bell's palsy (an inflammation of one of the main nerves of the face), but this condition usually makes itself evident because it produces paralysis of the face muscles on one side. Other causes of partial or total taste loss, or taste hallucinations, include: brain, nerve, lung and liver diseases; migraine; diabetes; fungus infections of the mouth; tooth troubles; a deficiency of dietary zinc (excess fiber in the diet can prevent zinc from being absorbed from the intestines); and of course, mental aberrations from a psychotic condition. A decrease in, or the absence of, taste function warrants a medical consultation. A loss of taste function can also mean a loss of the ability to avoid toxic substances such as spoiled food or dangerous chemicals that might otherwise have been detected before damage occurred.

Note: Some conditions can produce a loss or diminution of both smell and taste together. A virus-caused infection, such as influenza, seems to be the most common factor, but kidney, liver and thyroid disorders and even early diabetes can be to blame. If no evident cause is uncovered, consider some environmental condition—especially one that can decrease salivation (for instance, a dry, dusty climate). Other external factors include a wide variety of drugs, such as antibiotics, some pain-relieving products, and many different tranquilizer and sedative medications. Your physician or pharmacist can tell you what drugs will affect both taste and smell simultaneously.

Reliability

Home tests for taste (and smell) are merely rough qualitative sampling measures but are still considered 80 percent accurate in disease detection.

ZINC DEFICIENCY TASTE TEST
(A test to detect the possible reasons for a host of infirmities)

Zinc is an essential dietary mineral needed for good health, just as iodine is required for proper thyroid functioning. Zinc is known to be necessary for fetal and postnatal growth and development, the sense of smell and taste, properly functioning immunity and secondary sexual characteristics. More specifically, a zinc deficiency has been associated with an increased sensitivity to stress, premenstrual tension, presenile dementia (Alzheimer's disease), acne, anorexia nervosa, smaller-than-normal male sex organs, dwarfism, poor healing, greater susceptibility to colds, and a host of other illnesses, including depression, mood changes and the inability to concentrate. The secondary classic sign of a zinc deficiency, after the loss of taste function, is said to be brittle nails that have white horizontal lines across them; another claimed manifestation of insufficient zinc is persistent stretch marks on the skin.

Recent dietary studies indicate that the typical diet contains less than two-thirds of the daily amount of zinc recommended by the National Academy of Sciences. And it is also known that those who drink alcohol, use oral contraceptives, eat vegetarian diets or eat a great deal of fiber tend to need more zinc—and tend to excrete more zinc—than the average person. Some doctors feel that a zinc deficiency causes malabsorption of many food nutrients by damaging the lining of the intestinal tract.

Because zinc is needed to produce testosterone (the male sex hormone), and because the testicles are known to contain the largest amount of zinc of any body organ, and because oysters (and herring) contain more zinc than any other food, the "old wives' tale" about oysters' being a "treatment" for male impotence would seem to have some basis in fact.

Professor Derek Bryce-Smith of Reading University, England, has devised a "taste test"—a simple way to test for zinc deficiency at home using zinc's evident connection with taste ability. One or two teaspoonfuls of a special zinc solution are placed on the tongue and held in the mouth for up to 10 seconds. Depending on the response—no specific taste noted; a definite, not unpleasant taste; or a strong, unpleasant taste—zinc's presence or deficiency is inferred.

What Is Usual

With adequate zinc in the body, an individual should experience a strong, disagreeable taste right away. Some people immediately notice a definite, but not undesirable taste that gets stronger within five seconds.

What You Need

The test is performed using one gram of zinc sulphate heptahydrate dissolved in one liter of distilled water (that is, a 0.1 percent solution). Or a four-ounce bottle of Zinc Challenge can be used; it costs about $10.00 and is available from most health food stores. The same ready-made solution is sold directly to American doctors under the name of Zinc Tally; your doctor may give you a supply for home use. Dr. Bryce-Smith feels that the American solution is a bit stronger than necessary and suggests diluting it with a drop or two of distilled water, but this is not mandatory. A properly diluted solution is available directly from Dietary Products Ltd. (1 Lambert's Rd., Tunbridge Wells, Kent, England) for about $8.00, including airmail shipping.

What to Watch Out For

The test is best performed at least one hour after ingesting one's usual food and beverages. Use only one teaspoonful of the solution at first; if you notice no taste after half a minute, try two teaspoonfuls at once. Do not perform the test after smoking, drinking alcoholic beverages or using anything that might leave its own taste lingering in the mouth. Be sure to check with your doctor or pharmacist if you are taking any medicines; a great many can block taste even in people with adequate zinc in the body (see Brain and Nervous System Tests, **Taste Function**). While not usually considered medicines, nutritional supplements of calcium and iron may lower taste sensitivity. If there is doubt as to whether the solution does or does not cause a particular taste, have someone give you one teaspoonful or two teaspoonfuls of distilled water, alternating the test solution with the water without your knowing which is which; the response, or lack of same, should then be obvious.

What the Test Results Can Mean

If, after two teaspoonfuls of solution have been in the mouth at least 10 seconds, no specific taste or other mouth sensation is noted, a zinc deficiency may be assumed. If only a slight furry-type or dry sensation is noted after 5 seconds, this, too, is suggestive of a deficiency of the mineral. Some doctors recommend that if no taste is noted, zinc supplements be taken for two weeks and the test repeated; it should then result in the test solution's having a more noticeable taste. Failure to detect any improvement after taking zinc warrants a medical consultation to help uncover the reason for the loss of taste function. Many patients note a subjective improvement in mood and a decrease in stress after taking zinc for two weeks. Because the list of symptoms and conditions attributed to zinc deficiency literally runs into the hundreds, it is impossible to stipulate just what problems might be caused by a zinc deficiency. Suffice it to say that many doctors now feel that some zinc deficiency is endemic in contemporary society and that it cannot hurt to be sure one's zinc intake and absorption are adequate. In 1988 the International Atomic Energy Agency began a worldwide study to determine how much zinc really is in the average diet in order to help determine its effects on health.

Reliability

Although the zinc taste test is considered about 80 percent accurate as a means of detecting zinc deficiency, studies have shown that it is at least as accurate as blood, hair, sweat or urine tests. In a recent study relating zinc deficiency to anorexia nervosa and bulimia, the taste test was considered the most valuable. And it must be kept in mind that there can be a great many other causes for conditions that can accompany a zinc deficiency; the zinc problem may simply be coincidental and perhaps even unrelated.

Note: Although a certain amount of zinc is necessary for growth, the performance of many bodily functions and even immunity, recent research seems to indicate that an excessive intake of zinc (estimated to be 300 mg or more of elemental zinc a day) may in fact not be advantageous or safe. There are studies that seem to imply that the copious ingestion of zinc can actually impair one's immune response and may even contribute to heart disease.

MENTAL ABILITY AND PERSONALITY TESTS

ALCOHOLISM
(Helping detect the most common drug abuse problem in the world)

The words *alcoholism* and *alcoholic* relate to compulsive alcohol dependence; they do not necessarily indicate how much alcohol is used, any particular pattern of drinking or the degree of physical damage (brain, heart and liver diseases) resulting from alcohol abuse. A skid-row type of alcoholic may go for many years before alcohol abuse causes physical damage; this sort of drinker occasionally goes for many days without a drink, allowing spasmodic healing. A very heavy drinker who also eats nourishing foods may forestall organ impairment for decades. In contrast, regular "social" drinking of no more than five or six cocktails a day can cause a form of alcoholism that would never be suspected by others.

Medically speaking, alcoholism is said to exist when more than 70 grams of alcohol (seven one-ounce glasses of 86 proof liquor or their equivalent) are regularly consumed daily, either socially or in secrecy; when blood alcohol levels above 0.12 percent (see Breath and Lung Tests, **Breath Alcohol**) do not seem to cause the usual signs of intoxication (lack of coordination, impaired functioning, drowsiness, dizziness, speech difficulties and loss of inhibitions); when there are three or more "yes" answers on the Alcoholism Screening Test questionnaire (shown in Figure 51) developed by the Office of Health Care Programs, Johns Hopkins University Hospital in Baltimore (even two "yes" answers can, at times, indicate alcoholism); or, when a person scores 7 or more on the Mayo Clinic's Self-Administered Alcoholism Screening Test (shown in Figure 52), which denotes possible alcoholism, while a score of 10 or greater is said to denote probable alcoholism.

Lest you dismiss the idea that a simple questionnaire can contribute to the diagnosis of alcoholism, you should know that in a British study of several hundred people designed to detect alcoholics, the use of eight different laboratory tests revealed only 36 percent of those totally dependent on alcohol, while questionnaires uncovered 90 percent. Another, somewhat similar,

Figure 51. The Johns Hopkins University Hospital Alcoholism Screening Test.

	YES	NO
1. Do you lose time from work due to drinking?	☐	☐
2. Is drinking making your home life unhappy?	☐	☐
3. Do you drink because you are shy with other people?	☐	☐
4. Is drinking affecting your reputation?	☐	☐
5. Have you ever felt remorse after drinking?	☐	☐
6. Have you gotten into financial difficulties as a result of drinking?	☐	☐
7. Do you turn to lower companions and an inferior environment when drinking?	☐	☐
8. Does your drinking make you careless of your family's welfare?	☐	☐
9. Has your ambition decreased since drinking?	☐	☐
10. Do you crave a drink at a definite time daily?	☐	☐
11. Do you want a drink the next morning?	☐	☐
12. Does drinking cause you to have difficulty in sleeping?	☐	☐
13. Has your efficiency decreased since drinking?	☐	☐
14. Is drinking jeopardizing your job or business?	☐	☐
15. Do you drink to escape from worries or trouble?	☐	☐
16. Do you drink alone?	☐	☐
17. Have you ever had a complete loss of memory as a result of drinking?	☐	☐
18. Has your physician ever treated you for drinking?	☐	☐
19. Do you drink to build up your self-confidence?	☐	☐
20. Have you ever been to a hospital or institution on account of drinking?	☐	☐

Questions © Johns Hopkins University Hospital. Used with permission

screening program in a Milwaukee, Wisconsin, hospital showed an 80 percent detection rate using questionnaires. This was more than twice as accurate as when the screening was performed using 27 different blood chemical analyses. And the Mayo Clinic's self-administered questionnaire revealed more than twice as many alcoholics as did detailed medical data alone. When the Mayo questionnaire was later compared with drunken-driving arrest records and liver enzyme measurements, it proved to be 95 percent accurate. One thing that all tests for alcoholism seem to have in common, whether the tests

Figure 52. The Mayo Clinic's Self-Administered Alcoholism Screening Test.

	YES	NO
1. Do you enjoy a drink now and then? (If you never drink alcoholic beverages, and have no previous experiences with drinking, do not continue this questionnaire.)	___	___
2. Do you feel you are a normal drinker? (That is, drink no more than average.)	___	___
3. Have you ever awakened the morning after some drinking the night before and found that you could not remember a part of the evening?	___	___
4. Do close relatives ever worry or complain about your drinking?	___	___
5. Can you stop drinking without a struggle after one or two drinks?	___	___
6. Do you ever feel guilty about your drinking?	___	___
7. Do friends or relatives think you are a normal drinker?	___	___
8. Are you always able to stop drinking when you want to?	___	___
9. Have you ever attended a meeting of Alcoholics Anonymous (AA) because of your drinking?	___	___
10. Have you gotten into physical fights when drinking?	___	___
11. Has drinking ever created problems between you and your wife, husband, parent or near relative?	___	___
12. Has your wife, husband or other family member ever gone to anyone for help about your drinking?	___	___
13. Have you ever lost friendships because of your drinking?	___	___
14. Have you ever gotten into trouble at work because of drinking?	___	___
15. Have you ever lost a job because of drinking?	___	___
16. Have you ever neglected your obligations, your family, or your work for two or more days in a row because of drinking?	___	___
17. Do you ever drink in the morning?	___	___
18. Have you ever felt the need to cut down on your drinking?	___	___
19. Have there been times in your adult life when you found it necessary to completely avoid alcohol?	___	___
20. Have you ever been told you have liver trouble? Cirrhosis?	___	___
21. Have you ever had Delirium Tremens (D.T.'s)?	___	___
22. Have you ever had severe shaking, heard voices or seen things that weren't there after heavy drinking?	___	___
23. Have you ever gone to anyone for help about your drinking?	___	___
24. Have you ever been in a hospital because of drinking?	___	___
25. Have you ever been told by a doctor to stop drinking?	___	___
26. A. Have you ever been a patient in a psychiatric hospital or on a psychiatric ward of a general hospital?	___	___
B. Was drinking part of the problem that resulted in your hospitalization?	___	___
27. A. Have you ever been a patient at a psychiatric or mental health clinic or gone to any doctor, social worker, or clergyman for help with any emotional problem?	___	___
B. Was drinking part of the problem?	___	___

28. Have you ever been arrested, even for a few hours, because ____ ____
   of:
   A. Drunken behavior (not driving)?
   B. Driving while intoxicated?   ____ ____
29. Have any of the following relatives ever had problems with ____ ____
   alcohol?
   A. Parents
   B. Brothers or sisters   ____ ____
   C. Husband or wife   ____ ____
   D. Children   ____ ____

Score one point for each YES answer *except* for questions 2, 5, 7 and 8; for these, a
NO answer counts one point.

*A modified version of the Michigan Alcoholism Screening Test (MAST).

consist of blood or sweat analysis in a laboratory or a questionnaire, is that
they indicate that from 5 percent to 10 percent of all people who seek medical care for reasons ostensibly unrelated to alcohol dependency are in actuality suffering from alcoholism. When a patient's complaints refer to the
gastrointestinal system, the chances of alcoholism's being the basis for the
condition rise to 40 percent.

Early detection of alcoholism can prevent a great many subsequent serious
and debilitating—even fatal—diseases, much social suffering and, when the
condition is detected in women prior to pregnancy, congenital malforma-
tions in their future infants. A person who lacks self-awareness regarding
alcoholism may not realize that the resulting high blood alcohol levels can
also dangerously enhance the effect of many other drugs: Excessive consumption of alcohol can cause increased bleeding, especially when aspirin is
used; it will interfere with the proper action of anticonvulsant drugs; it will
markedly increase the sedative effect of antihistamines, tranquilizers, and
other hypnotic or sleeping pills to the point where normal vision and coordination are impaired; and it can so increase the action of anesthetics as to
be fatal.

What Is Usual

Not to be an alcoholic is normal. Alcoholism, however, may be reflected by
inappropriate facial flushing, a dry mouth, spider angiomas over the face
and chest (see Body Observations, **Skin Observations**), a tremor of the hands
and occasional numbness in the arms, hands and feet. As the disease progresses, there can be signs of liver and brain disease, such as the inability to
remember things while still maintaining the ability to lie about not remem-
bering; a limp wrist; a sudden increase in all sorts of injury-causing accidents, with a tendency to bruise and bleed from the slightest trauma; a hos-
tile attitude; and finally, hallucinations (DTs) and epilepsylike convulsions,

especially if the person is deprived of alcohol for more than 24 hours. Again, all these symptoms are usual for an alcoholic, but they are not normal.

What You Need
For self-testing you need to answer the questionnaire and face facts—admittedly not an easy option. A Spanish-language version of the Mayo Clinic's Self-Administered Alcoholism Screening Test is available from Dr. Juan Ramon de la Fuente; write to the Instituto de la Nutricion (Mexico City, Mexico) or telephone (905) 573-1200.

If the test is to be administered to someone else, you may need the support of your doctor, your religious leader, Alcoholics Anonymous (AA) and anyone else who might exert some influence. You will, of course, need the ultimate in patience and a willingness to uncover what brought on the problem in the first place; it might surprise you to learn that it could be an inherited genetic defect or a biochemical imbalance as well as loneliness, competition, peer pressure or senility.

What to Watch Out For
What looks like alcoholism may not be; alcohol is sometimes used to cover up a totally different psychiatric problem or personality disorder or a totally different type of drug abuse (marijuana, heroin, amphetamines, etc.). Some forms of liver, brain and skin diseases that appear to indicate alcoholism can come from environmental toxicity, and autoimmune conditions (in which body cells make antigens and antibodies against themselves rather than against the bacteria or foreign proteins that antibodies usually fight off) can also imitate alcoholism. If the problem is alcoholism, be prepared for rebellion and refusal to admit to the problem.

What the Test Results Can Mean
Unwillingness to take the test can be as obvious an indicator as a positive alcoholism score. Either warrants a medical consultation. If you seek medical help, be sure to inform your doctor as to the reasons; far too many doctors are reluctant to recognize alcoholism as an illness and tend to discount it. Do not argue with such a doctor; find another. Alcoholism can be treated, if not cured, and the result can mean a great reduction in anxiety, greatly improved health and a great savings in money—all of which can contribute to a better life.

Reliability
As already noted, questionnaires to detect alcoholism, when honestly completed, are at least 90 percent accurate.

Note: Also see the discussion of the alcoholism predisposition test in Mental Ability and Personality Tests, **Depression**.

DEPRESSION
(Screening tests that could save your life)

If you feel depressed at times, you are not alone. Research has shown that more than 10 percent of all patients who seek medical help through their family doctor or an internist have some form of depression. In patients with known heart disease, close to 20 percent were found to have depression unrelated to the severity of the heart trouble. If the patient is elderly, at least one out of every three suffers from this affective disorder. Women suffer depression five times as often as men. Unfortunately, the same study that uncovered the extent of the problem also revealed that doctors missed diagnosing depression in three out of every four of their depressed patients. This problem is compounded by the fact that even psychiatrists do not agree on precisely what depression is, how many different kinds of depression there are and just how depression, once diagnosed, should be treated.

In general, depression can take two forms: primary and secondary. Primary, or endogenous, depression is found most often in people over 40 and is usually accompanied by a family history of depression. The external symptoms of primary depression are:

- Insomnia
- Loss of appetite followed by weight loss
- Loss of interest in sex
- Loss of friends
- Loss of energy
- Increased brooding about death
- Guilt
- Hopelessness
- Vague aches and pains
- Increased irritability

Most of all, there is an obvious loss of interest in and avoidance of normal pleasures.

Secondary, or reactive, depression seems to occur in younger people with no family history of depression; rarely do they display the usual symptoms of primary depression, other than sleep disorders. Secondary depression is most likely the consequence of a real or perceived insurmountable obstacle in a person's life. The condition is usually of sudden onset and is most often accompanied by self-pity. It can frequently be successfully treated with nothing more than empathy. In contrast, primary depression seems to be a continuing pattern in the sufferer's life.

Depression can also be manifested in seemingly unrelated ways. The most common disguise is chronic pain in the back or the head. Or it can masquerade as stomach problems such as indigestion, ulcerlike pains, constipation or diarrhea. It can also seem to appear out of nowhere immediately or shortly after pregnancy in spite of the joy of a new baby. When unexplainable symptoms persist and cannot be diagnosed, it is a good idea to consider the possibility of an underlying depression. When other members of a seemingly depressed person's family are observed, they usually show signs of depression as well.

A diagnosis of depression can often be made erroneously in the presence of dementia (see the discussion of the miniobject test in Mental Ability and Personality Tests, **Mental Ability,** Intelligence Tests) and with hormone problems (especially hypothyroidism), certain forms of heart disease, many forms of cancer and kidney disease. A secondary depressive reaction can be caused by many drugs, such as reserpine drugs used to treat high blood pressure, steroid medications, sedatives, tranquilizers, heroin, morphine, marijuana, excessive amounts of alcohol and oral contraceptives. Pills to curb one's appetite can cause depression after they are stopped, as can withdrawal from cocaine use. When in real doubt, your doctor can have you perform the adrenal suppression test (sometimes called the cortisol or dexamethasone suppression test) at home; in this test a tablet of a cortisollike drug is taken at bedtime to see whether it suppresses the body's own cortisol excretion, which it normally should (see the discussion of the saliva depression test later in this entry). Thyroid function testing should be routine when depression is suspected, as should urine catecholamine measurements prior to any form of therapy.

Beck Depression Inventory. It does not seem to matter whether depression is a manifestation of one's mood or a reflection of evident grief, or whether it is an overt symptom of a serious underlying mental illness. Its early diagnosis is necessary to prevent suicide attempts. There are several questionnaires that, when honestly answered, not only can point to the need for immediate medical attention but also can help reveal some latent condition that, when treated, will eliminate the depression as well as the disease. One such test is the Beck Depression Inventory (shown in Figure 53):

Figure 53. Beck Depression Inventory.

On this questionnaire are groups of statements. Please read each group of statements carefully. Then pick out the one statement in each group which best describes the way you have been feeling the PAST WEEK, INCLUDING TODAY! Circle the number beside the statement you picked. If several statements in the group seem to apply equally well, circle each one. **Be sure to read all the statements in each group before making your choice.**

1   0 I do not feel sad.
     1 I feel sad.
     2 I am sad all the time and I can't snap out of it.
     3 I am so sad or unhappy that I can't stand it.

2 0 I am not particularly discouraged about the future.
1 I feel discouraged about the future.
2 I feel I have nothing to look forward to.
3 I feel that the future is hopeless and that things cannot improve.

3 0 I do not feel like a failure.
1 I feel I have failed more than the average person.
2 As I look back on my life, all I can see is a lot of failures.
3 I feel I am a complete failure as a person.

4 0 I get as much satisfaction out of things as I used to.
1 I don't enjoy things the way I used to.
2 I don't get real satisfaction out of anything anymore.
3 I am dissatisfied or bored with everything.

5 0 I don't feel particularly guilty.
1 I feel guilty a good part of the time.
2 I feel quite guilty most of the time.
3 I feel guilty all of the time.

6 0 I don't feel I am being punished.
1 I feel I may be punished.
2 I expect to be punished.
3 I feel I am being punished.

7 0 I don't feel disappointed in myself.
1 I am disappointed in myself.
2 I am disgusted with myself.
3 I hate myself.

8 0 I don't feel I am any worse than anybody else.
1 I am critical of myself for my weaknesses or mistakes.
2 I blame myself all the time for my faults.
3 I blame myself for everything bad that happens.

9 0 I don't have any thoughts of killing myself.
1 I have thoughts of killing myself, but I would not carry them out.
2 I would like to kill myself.
3 I would kill myself if I had the chance.

10 0 I don't cry any more than usual.
1 I cry more now than I used to.
2 I cry all the time now.
3 I used to be able to cry, but now I can't cry even though I want to.

11 0 I am no more irritated now than I ever am.
1 I get annoyed or irritated more easily than I used to.
2 I feel irritated all the time now.
3 I don't get irritated at all by the things that used to irritate me.

12 0 I have not lost interest in other people.
1 I am less interested in other people than I used to be.
2 I have lost most of my interest in other people.
3 I have lost all of my interest in other people.

13 0 I make decisions about as well as I ever could.
    1 I put off making decisions more than I used to.
    2 I have greater difficulty in making decisions than before.
    3 I can't make decisions at all anymore.

14 0 I don't feel I look any worse than I used to.
    1 I am worried that I am looking old or unattractive.
    2 I feel that there are permanent changes in my appearance that make me look unattractive.
    3 I believe that I look ugly.

15 0 I can work about as well as before.
    1 It takes an extra effort to get started at doing something.
    2 I have to push myself very hard to do anything.
    3 I can't do any work at all.

16 0 I can sleep as well as usual.
    1 I don't sleep as well as I used to.
    2 I wake up 1–2 hours earlier than usual and find it hard to get back to sleep.
    3 I wake up several hours earlier than I used to and cannot get back to sleep.

17 0 I don't get more tired than usual.
    1 I get tired more easily than I used to.
    2 I get tired from doing almost anything.
    3 I am too tired to do anything.

18 0 My appetite is no worse than usual.
    1 My appetite is not as good as it used to be.
    2 My appetite is much worse now.
    3 I have no appetite at all anymore.

19 0 I haven't lost much weight, if any, lately.
    1 I have lost more than 5 pounds.   I am purposely trying to lose
    2 I have lost more than 10 pounds.   weight by eating less.
    3 I have lost more than 15 pounds.   Yes _____ No _____

20 0 I am no more worried about my health than usual.
    1 I am worried about physical problems such as aches and pains; or upset stomach; or constipation.
    2 I am very worried about physical problems and it's hard to think of much else.
    3 I am so worried about my physical problems that I cannot think about anything else.

21 0 I have not noticed any recent change in my interest in sex.
    1 I am less interested in sex than I used to be.
    2 I am much less interested in sex now.
    3 I have lost interest in sex completely.

What Is Usual

A depressive mood, while not usually normal, can exist in the face of the loss of a loved one (including separation and divorce), the loss of one's job, the loss of one's social standing, the loss of one's health and money problems. The despondency is usually limited to the situation and its aftereffects. It is not usual to persist in avoiding pleasure and to brood incessantly. Responses to the Beck Depression Inventory (your score is determined by adding all the circled numbers) should total less than 10.

What You Need

You need a willingness to seek a medical consultation should there be any hint of a "blue" mood. A medical consultation is also warranted if you have noticed that you are having trouble sleeping, that you are always tired, that your appetite is gone, that you are always brooding, that you have become indifferent to people and things and that life is just not fun anymore. You owe it to yourself to try to uncover any possible organic or physical cause for your depression.

Insofar as the questionnaire goes, honesty in answering, and appropriate medical consultation or attention if indicated, can be the first step toward relief.

What to Watch Out For

When depression is a problem, be alert to the following pitfalls:

- Self-pity, where you enjoy the attention given to you while you make others miserable.
- Using your depression as an excuse for your failures, misbehavior or inadequacy.
- Drugs that can be to blame; check with your doctor or pharmacist.

What the Test Results Can Mean

A score of 10 or more on the Beck Depression Inventory is suggestive of depression and warrants a medical consultation; a score of 16 or more warrants medical attention; and a score of 20 or more warrants immediate medical attention to the point of seeking out an emergency medical facility if a doctor is not instantly available.

Reliability

When compared with psychiatric evaluations and other scientific determinations of depression, the Beck Depression Inventory is considered 85 per cent accurate.

Saliva depression test. One biochemical way of helping to detect depression, and its possible cause, is by measuring your body's output of the hormone cortisol and how that hormone's production reacts when a similar synthetic hormone is added to the body's own supply. This test has many names, one being the dexamethasone suppression test (DST), since a tablet of dexamethasone (a synthetic cortisol compound) is most commonly used. Normally, when virtually any hormone is taken, the body automatically reduces its own natural output of that hormone; when dexamethasone is ingested, the "normal" person's cortisol level is immediately reduced. In many cases of depression, taking dexamethasone fails to stop the body's cortisol production. While there is some controversy over the test's accuracy, mostly among psychiatrists, many biologically oriented physicians feel that the test is quite valuable; its accuracy rate is considered to be at least 70 percent.

One version of this test, called the Cortitest, is performed at home using saliva. (Saliva testing is considered as accurate as blood serum measurements for many medical tests.) Your doctor gives you six tiny saliva-collection bottles and one tablet of dexamethasone. You collect a sample of saliva at 11:30 one night and then swallow the dexamethasone. A second saliva sample is then collected at 8:00 o'clock the next morning, at noon the same day, at 8:00 o'clock that night and the last at 10:00 o'clock that night. Detailed directions and labeling instructions are included in the kit your doctor gives you. You then return the kit to your doctor or, if so instructed, directly to Psychiatric Diagnostic Laboratories of America (100 Corporate Ct., South Plainfield, N.J. 07080), usually in a prepaid overnight express container also furnished you by your doctor. Your saliva is then analyzed and the results given to your doctor for personal application to your case. The cost is $90.00. This test is sometimes used as a way of measuring hormone changes induced by exercise and as a means of evaluating the body's reaction to stressful situations—physical as well as mental.

Alcoholism predisposition. The saliva depression test may also be used as an indication of a predisposition to alcoholism. Instead of swallowing a tablet of a hormone (dexamethasone), a fairly large amount of alcohol is consumed; the amount is up to your doctor. As with the depression test, a saliva sample is collected prior to drinking the alcohol. Then, saliva samples for cortisone measurements are taken every half-hour for four hours (this test may be performed at any time of day). It does seem that body cortisol levels are much lower—especially after a few hours—in children of known chronic alcoholics than in children of nonalcoholics. Whether this hormone response (or lack of same) is genetic or a natural proclivity has still not been determined. The test can, however, be an early warning sign of an unusual sensitivity to alcoholic beverages and allow appropriate preventive measures.

"BURNOUT" SYNDROME
(A test to help evaluate your response to stress)

One of the many ways to prevent illness is to become aware of the signs and symptoms that could reflect illness while those signs and symptoms are still subtle or latent. The sooner one recognizes warning signals, the sooner one may uncover the cause and reverse the process or begin treatment to overcome the problem. About 10 years ago, the medical profession became aware of a seemingly new syndrome called "burnout." In essence, it is caused by the way the body and mind react to some stresses—primarily related to one's job; most commonly, it is supposed to come from working too hard for too long under too many pressures and, with all that, not feeling successful. While there may be a great many physical and mental reactions to burnout, the condition could be summed up in a word: exhaustion—of the mind, body and spirit. Although it might be assumed that this syndrome is reserved for executives and professionals, even a brand-new employee at the bottom of the ladder can suffer from burnout; all you have to do is be hardworking, have high expectations and strive to do your very best—especially while remaining ethical—and you become a candidate for this condition.

The most common signs and symptoms of burnout are listed in a self-test devised by Alfred A. Messer, M.D., a psychiatrist in Atlanta, Georgia (and reproduced here with his permission; see Figure 54). By completing the test and adding up your score, you can help determine whether you are in danger of coming down with burnout, whether you are in the throes of burnout or even whether medical attention is warranted—not solely for your own benefit but also for the benefit of your family and fellow workers. The test—while primarily designed for physicians, pharmacists and other health care professionals—can apply to anyone highly committed to his or her work.

To determine your burnout potential, note the signs and symptoms in each of the three categories in the left-hand column of Figure 54; yes, almost everyone has one or more of these problems from time to time, but if you feel that they are bothering you at the present time, circle the number of points just to their right. Then, in the adjacent columns, note by the additional point value the answer to the duration, frequency and intensity questions. For example, if you have had insomnia for a week or so, write in 1 point in the appropriate column beneath the time; if you have not been sleeping well for a month or more, write in 2 points; for sleeping problems that have existed for more than a year, write in 3 points. Follow the same point system in each of the next two columns, indicating how often you have the complaint and then how intense the problem is. Add up the circled points and those at the bottom of each of the nine columns to find your grand total.

	How long?			How often?			How intense?		
Points (circle if applicable)	Weeks	Months	Over a year	Sometimes	Frequently	Constantly	Mild	Moderate	Severe
PHYSICAL SYMPTOMS CATEGORY	1	2	3	1	2	3	1	2	3
Fatigue — 2									
Insomnia — 3									
Headache — 2									
Backache — 1									
Stomach or intestinal problems of any kind — 2									
Weight loss or gain — 1									
Shortness of breath — 1									
Lingering cold or flu — 2									
PERSONAL SYMPTOMS CATEGORY									
Bored — 3									
Restless — 2									
Stagnating — 3									
Rationalizing — 4									
Feeling indispensable — 5									
Obsessed — 5									
Depressed — 3									
BEHAVIORAL SYMPTOMS CATEGORY									
Irritable — 4									
Unable to enjoy or compliment colleagues' or associates' successes — 4									
Cynical — 5									
Defensive — 4									
Faultfinding — 4									
Dependent on alcohol — 5									
Dependent on drugs — 5									
SUBTOTALS									

GRAND TOTAL

Figure 54. Burnout Potential Questionnaire.

What Is Usual
It is not unusual to experience unpleasant, illness-imitating symptoms as a consequence of the stress and strain of a job—especially if faced with seemingly inconsistent demands and/or unrealistic expectations. Most people can cope, or learn how to cope, with discouragement and occasional failure—real or imagined. Such people usually end up with a grand total of less than 20 points.

What You Need
In addition to Dr. Messer's questionnaire, you need a willingness to admit to your signs, symptoms and attitudes. Then, depending on your grand total, you will need to accept the possibility that burnout is developing, or already exists, and seek help.

What to Watch Out For
You should be alert for an unwillingness to recognize the possibility that your work or your job can be the cause of your problems. It is all too easy to try to place the blame on home, marriage, children or some other non-occupation-related factor, especially when your work fosters self-importance.

What the Test Results Can Mean
Unfortunately, burnout is usually an insidious illness; rather than occurring suddenly, it more often develops over a period of time so as to disguise the real cause of the sufferer's growing physical and emotional exhaustion. If your grand total is more than 20, this may be an early warning sign that burnout could be a developing problem. If your score is higher in the physical symptoms category, it could also indicate a real physical problem and warrants a medical consultation. If your grand total is more than 56, it is reasonable to assume that you have a problem with your work; if the scores are about equal in each of the three categories, it is an even better bet that your job could be the cause of your difficulties. A score greater than 56 not only warrants a medical consultation, it also warrants a personal inventory of your duties and responsibilities along with your ability or willingness to cope with them (do you need to learn how to relax or take a vacation?). If your score is greater than 103, it warrants medical attention.

Reliability
As a general, nonspecific indicator of an illness, a score greater than 56 is considered to be 80 percent accurate. As to whether the fault lies primarily with your job, the specificity drops to 70 percent.

MENTAL ABILITY
(Clues to proper growth and development)

Mental ability tests encompass a wide variety of evaluations. Although many are interrelated, different forms of these tests are intended to reveal different abilities as well as disabilities. In general, they are categorized as:

- *Intelligence (IQ) tests*—to estimate a person's ability to make use of learning, reasoning, social experience and memory for problem solving; these tests also contribute to understanding learning disabilities and personality problems.
- *Achievement tests*—to evaluate the success or failure of past formal educational experiences; they are designed not simply to compare a child's academic qualifications to those of his or her peers but also to uncover learning disabilities early enough to permit correction.
- *Aptitude tests*—to ferret out latent talents, usually in some specific field such as art, mathematics, mechanics, music, science or stenography.
- *Personality tests*—to evaluate an individual's social actions and adjustment to life; most often administered when a person's attitudes and behavior appear to deviate from what is considered usual or from an expected response.

In the past such appraisals were categorized as "psychological" tests, primarily because they were an outgrowth of clinical psychological studies. Now, however, they have changed to reflect educational and social studies equally as much as psychiatric theories. Tests that employ projective techniques (the examiner's personal decipherment) have not changed over the years and cannot be standardized by objective measurements. In the interpretation of many of these tests, responses to some questions must be filtered through the background, training and prejudices of the examiner; as a consequence of such bias, whether conscious or not, two different examiners can observe identical responses and yet arrive at totally dissimilar conclusions.

It must be kept in mind that the results of any mental ability or personality test reflect only a sample of an individual's performance in response to a question or direction, whether written or spoken, and must never be considered conclusive. Such tests can be compared to X-ray studies. When viewing an X-ray, all that can be seen are expected shadows, possibly unexpected shadows, or a lack of shadows where they should appear. The shadings and shadows do not tell a doctor the diagnosis; rather, after many years of training and experience, the doctor interprets X-ray shadows to infer logical possibilities, which still must be confirmed by concrete evidence before they have any real meaning. According to one study, two or more radiologists looking at X-rays of known cancer disagreed on what the shadows meant almost 50 percent of the time. A mental ability or personality test is but one possible clue (shadow) to an individual's character, individuality, qualifications, peculiarities and other identity traits.

Regardless of just how inconclusive mental ability and personality tests can be, they are an integral part of almost everyone's life. Sooner or later you or your child will be taking one or more of these tests. Depending upon how they are applied, they can be good or bad. One thing is known: The more familiar people become with such tests, the easier they seem to be; testees become more aware of what is expected and are less apprehensive. Therefore, each time a test of this sort is taken, there is an increased possibility of its reflecting true intellectual and academic achievements.

Intelligence tests: intelligence quotient (IQ). Although there is no universal agreement on the definition of intelligence, the present consensus seems to be that it is the ability to make use of learning, reasoning and memory in problem solving. Most intelligence tests measure an individual's ability to learn in comparison with the ability of a similar general population. The intelligence quotient is expressed by dividing the ostensible mental age (as determined by the test) by the chronological age (the individual's actual age in years and months) and multiplying the result by 100. For example, a 10-year-old with test results showing an average mental ability for that age would have an IQ of $10/10 \times 100 = 100$. A 20-year-old with a mental ability score equal to that of a 30-year-old would have an IQ of $30/20 \times 100 = 150$. Many doctors feel that this formula is not applicable after the age of 25, since some mental processes normally seem to diminish after the 20s are reached.

There are numerous forms of intelligence tests; some rely mostly on the individual's verbal ability (Stanford-Binet), while others also take into account physical performance (Wechsler). Performance tests are best for young children, the handicapped and people who have a limited knowledge of the language in which the test is written. Some feel that performance tests are better predictors of social adjustment, while verbal tests are better predictors of educational achievement.

Group tests such as those used by the military and schools are not considered to be as accurate as individual tests, and some states have outlawed group IQ testing. Few group tests take into account the background and environment of the individual, which can seriously distort scoring. For example, a child raised on a farm might identify a picture of a pail as a milk pail, while a child raised in the city might interpret the same picture as a champagne bucket. If the tester does not take into account the child's experiences, the child could be unfairly penalized in the final scoring.

IQ test questions are similar to the following:

• Repeat backward: 9-2-4-6-8 (young children are given three digits, adults up to nine digits).

- Make up a short story about a picture that is shown.
- Describe how certain words are related (for example: *orange, banana;* or *auto, train*).
- Find the missing part in a picture.
- Rearrange the order of several pictures to make them show a story in sequence.

Intelligence tests are no longer used as the sole determination of mental retardation as they once were. Still, they can be helpful in evaluating learning, memory and reasoning powers and in diagnosing learning disorders. They cannot, however, predict how well a person will do in a job, marriage or real life, no matter how high the IQ score.

Intelligence tests: cognitive capacity screening. This variation of IQ testing is used more to help distinguish dementia due to organic disease from functional delirium or an unwillingness to behave properly. Dementia is a physical disease, primarily in older people, that usually results from degeneration of brain substance subsequent to little strokes (caused by tiny blood clots in the brain's circulatory system), which often go unnoticed, or from atherosclerosis of brain arteries, which can accompany diabetes, high blood pressure or heart rhythm disorders; some attribute the condition to a slow-growing virus. A lessening of intellectual functioning, especially in the elderly, frequently comes from the use of prescription drugs. Liver and kidney disease, hypothyroidism and deficiencies of nutrients such as vitamin B_{12} or folic acid may also cause a loss of cognitive abilities. A cognitive capacity test consists of asking several questions that require a certain degree of mental ability:

- Listen to these numbers: 8 - 1 - 4 - 3; now count from 1 to 10 out loud and then repeat the four numbers that you first heard.
- Take 7 away from 100, and what do you have?
- Keep taking 7 away from each answer, and what do you have?
- What is the day of the week, the date, the month and the year?
- Who was president of the United States during World War I? World War II? Today?
- Where were you born? When? What did you have to eat for your last meal?
- Suppose you smelled smoke in your room; what would you do?
- What does the expression "Never one door closes but another opens" mean?

The failure to answer two or more of these questions correctly warrants a medical consultation regarding the possibility of brain disease or an overdose of medicine. There are more than 25 different versions of such mental status tests.

Intelligence tests: the miniobject. This test is a more refined way of screening for dementia, especially senile dementia (one form of which is sometimes called Alzheimer's disease), most often seen in the elderly; an individual with this condition very gradually loses the ability to think, remember, reason and get along socially. All that is required are 15 of the 50 or so 3½-inch-long plastic miniature tools and other objects that come boxed in the game called Jack Straws (a Parker Brothers game that is available in toy shops for about $6.00). Each different object (shovel, saw, wrench, rake, ladder, etc.) is shown to the individual. For each object correctly identified, 1 point is scored. After identification of the object, or even after failure to properly identify the object, the individual is asked to show how the object works or how it is used. Again, 1 additional point is scored for each correct response. A perfect score would be 30 points. Individuals who have problems with abstract thinking, difficulties in sensory perception (see **Brain and Nervous System Tests, Sensory Testing**) or beginning coordination impairment will usually score under 15 points; any score under 24, however, warrants a medical consultation.

Intelligence tests: number connection. This is another form of intelligence testing used to screen individuals whose thought processes appear confused. Although the test is used primarily to see whether a brain problem is the consequence of liver disease, frequently related to alcoholism (see Urine Tests, **Clinical Analysis: Bilirubin;** Mental Ability and Personality Tests, **Alcoholism**), it can also help differentiate a physically caused learning problem from anxiety-provoked learning inabilities. A sequence of numbers, inside small circles, is placed at random on a sheet of paper; the numbers may run from 1 to 10 or even to 20. The individual is asked to connect these numbers with a pencil line in correct sequence; it resembles the children's game in which a picture is formed when dots next to consecutive numbers are properly connected. Failure to connect the numbers in sequence or taking an excessive amount of time to connect them warrants medical attention.

Caution is advised when attempting to draw definitive conclusions about intelligence based on only one test, and some courts have ruled that a person suffering embarrassment or unfairness as a result of an IQ rating can be compensated by a monetary award.

Intelligence tests: growth and development observations. Growth and development observations during the first year of a child's life are another indication of intelligence coupled with physical skills. The age at which a baby rolls over, sits up without help, walks, smiles, says words and understands what a parent says can be the earliest signs of learning ability. Within the first 2 months of life, a baby should:

• Be quiet when hearing a parent's voice
• Watch an object moving back and forth in front of his or her eyes

• Look you in the eye
• Smile
• Make sounds

At 3 months to 4 months, a baby should:

• Hold up his or her head when in a sitting position
• Roll to one side
• Turn the head in response to a distinct sound, music or a voice
• Coo and even laugh

By 6 months a baby should:

• Reach for a toy with eyes fixed on the toy
• Respond to people

From 9 months to 11 months of age, a baby should:

• Sit, crawl or creep
• Wave bye-bye
• Say "mama" and "dada"
• Understand what is said
• Play peekaboo

By 1 year a baby should:

• Stand alone
• Say meaningful words

While your doctor can give you a much more detailed list of what infants usually do in their first 12 months, and also what behavior is typical up to the age of 3, constant observations of such skills or the lack of same can help detect a developmental problem. Not all babies develop at the same rate, and failure to perform some expected task at a certain age may still be quite normal. At the same time failure to observe an expected action warrants a medical consultation, if only for reassurance. If an infant seems irritable all the time, or even too quiet all the time, or moves parts of his or her body without evident purpose, a medical consultation is warranted. This is also the time to start eye observations for **strabismus** (see Eye and Vision Tests). One general observation that has been made repeatedly: An infant who does not seem to perform properly at, say, 3 months of age may suddenly, at 6 months, start doing all the things a 9-month-old child should do. And performances during the first year of life do not seem to reflect what IQ scores will be after the age of 6.

Achievement tests. While intelligence tests are supposed to measure one's ability to learn, achievement tests are constructed to measure how well past educational experiences were understood and remembered. For example, reading readiness tests, usually given to children in kindergarten or just prior to entering the first grade, will reveal whether the child can distinguish capital from lowercase letters, can recognize printed words with similar sounds and can remember words a short while after they have been taught. As a child grows older, there are specific achievement tests covering various academic subjects, such as reading comprehension, mathematics understanding and application, spelling ability and how much was learned in relation to grade standing in science, social studies and vocabulary. Most of these tests derive their questions and answers from the typical curriculum taught throughout the United States at each grade level and are based primarily on what a child should have learned by his or her age and grade. Many schools require children to take achievement tests every few years.

Until recently, a child's ability to learn, especially as observed in the school environment, was considered a nonmedical condition. It is now known that a child's inability to understand and remember equally as well as his or her peers can result from inherited developmental defects that cause mental retardation (see Urine Tests, **Phenylketonuria Screening**); eye and ear difficulties (see Ear Observations and Hearing Tests, **Hearing Function,** and Eye and Vision Tests, **Visual Acuity**); muscle incoordination (see Brain and Nervous System Tests, **Dizziness and Ataxia** and **Reflex Testing**); hormone disorders; plumbism, or **lead** poisoning (see Environmental Tests); and even allergies (see Allergy Tests, **Patch Testing** and **Elimination Diet**), especially those that cause hyperactivity. And many medicines that children take for seemingly unrelated conditions in turn cause impaired learning as a side effect. Dyslexia, or difficulty in understanding the written word because of a brain problem in which the child sees printed letters reversed (a *b* is seen as a *d*, or *dog* is read as *god*), is probably the most common learning disability. At the same time, a child can have a condition that distorts the meaning of words in a sentence, preventing comprehension, and still can excel in mathematical ability. Achievement test results, especially the reading readiness tests, can be the very first indication of a learning disability in a child whose close preschool relationship with his or her parents obscured some slight mental or physical defect.

Some standard achievement tests used by schools are the *Metropolitan* and *Stanford;* these usually comprise several different subjects and measure learning for each year from kindergarten through the 12th grade. There are many other commercial tests to measure a child's reading ability and skills in specific subjects, and there are related tests that evaluate an adult's past academic achievements; the latter are used mostly by personnel departments considering the employment of workers who did not complete formal education.

The *Bender-Gestalt test* is one specific test that measures the ability of the eyes to see, the brain to understand, and the muscles and nerves to be able to coordinate and carry out the brain's directions. Here the child is shown geometric designs, from simple squares to complex patterns, and is then asked to copy them. Some examiners leave the drawing in front of the child; others ask the child to reproduce the figures from memory. Noting how well the drawings are reproduced, taking into consideration how much time is required, can help detect a learning disability.

A simple home screening test along the same lines is to show a child age 5 or older the symbols on the aces in a pack of *playing cards* and ask him or her to copy them onto another piece of paper. By comparing the child's copies to the originals—and if possible, to the artistic efforts of another child of similar age—it is sometimes possible to detect a learning disorder at its earliest stages and start corrective measures.

Aptitude tests. Intelligence tests are general in nature; that is, they measure a combination of all one's abilities working together. Aptitude tests, on the other hand, are essentially intelligence tests that evaluate the integral fragments that comprise overall intellectual abilities. One child may have an uncanny ability to discern musical notes; another, while unable to distinguish a high tone from a low one, can glance at a picture of a complicated piece of machinery and immediately delineate its workings as well as notice any possible flaw concealed in the illustration. Thus, an individual could have a low IQ score and yet be a musical virtuoso or possess exceptional mechanical reasoning, both of which could be overlooked by routine IQ testing. There are individuals who fail the IQ test, figuratively speaking, and yet have extraordinary powers of abstract reasoning; their creativity would go unnoticed unless deliberately sought out.

Related aptitude tests are available that attempt first to assess one's capacity to grasp unusual, ostensibly difficult training and then to foretell success in one of the professions, such as medicine, nursing, law and accounting. Most of these tests try to measure the ability to interpret offered facts, memorize them and then follow a logical sequence to a conclusion not actually stipulated in the facts. Tests of vocational interests and career-planning tests also fall into this category.

Personality tests. Unlike intelligence, achievement or aptitude tests, which attempt to measure something of a more positive nature, personality tests (now more commonly called personality inventories) are intended to uncover negative behavioral traits and the reasons behind them. Although it has been claimed that personality inventories can differentiate between neurosis and psychosis, specify a psychosis, detect hypochondriasis and even discern sociopathic disturbances, such as sexual identity conflicts and other forms of dyssocial reactions, the usefulness of these tests has never been scientifically documented in controlled studies. Almost all personality evaluations depend not only on the examiner's interpretation but also on the honesty of the responses of the individual taking the test. For example, a test may ask whether the individual wishes that he or she could be as happy as others seem to be. The score for that question depends not only on what the test creators felt a "normal" response should be but also on what the person taking the test feels would be regarded as the most appropriate answer for him or her to give. The test may require nothing more than a "yes" or "no" reply, or there may be a graded choice of responses, but the variables of pleasing oneself and the examiner, along with indeterminate prejudices, make an objective evaluation of personality virtually impossible.

Still, personality inventories abound, and many people are forced to come face-to-face with them in connection with employment opportunities, educational situations, medical or psychiatric diagnosis and prognosis, or as a means of avoiding the consequences of the law. Someday you may be induced to take a Minnesota Multiphasic Personality Inventory (MMPI), in which you will be given a box of 550 statements, each printed on a separate card, and asked to sort them into piles on the basis of whether you agree with each statement, disagree or "cannot say." An approximate example: "Sometimes I think my friends are talking about me behind my back." Based on your answers, the examiner will categorize you as being normal, hypochondriacal, hysterical, paranoid, schizophrenic, homosexual, psychopathic or simply weak in the mind.

Other personality inventories range from describing what you see in smudges of inkblots to placing characters on a miniature stage (designating that stage as a house or a particular room in the house or simply as a theater) and describing the characters' actions. Some other personality inventories include: the Rorschach technique (which uses 10 inkblots), the Holtzman inkblot technique (which uses 90 inkblots), the make-a-picture story (in which the stage setting is used to construct a scene), the draw-a-person test (in which you are asked to draw one person and then a person of the opposite sex, emphasizing the "best" and "worst" parts of the body), the thematic apperception test (in which you look at pictures and make up stories about what you think the people in the pictures are thinking, doing and intending to do; there are children's versions that use animals in place of people) and the Rotter incomplete sentence blank test (in which you are told the first word or two of 40 sentences and asked to complete each one). These are only a few examples; all these tests are alleged to reveal your attitudes, desires, fears and wishes, thus unmasking your personality.

The threat of privacy invasion is only one problem associated with personality testing; many people find such tests threatening to their self-image as well. Before you voluntarily take any type of personality test, be sure that you understand the reason you are being given the test and that the results will be kept confidential.

What Is Usual

IQ scores have been standardized by compiling the results from testing people of all ages the world over. In general, an IQ score of from 90 to 110 is considered average. Below 83 is suggestive of a slight degree of mental retardation, and below 70 is suggestive of mild retardation; a score in either range warrants a medical consultation. Between 83 and 90 is considered borderline and warrants repeat testing. A score greater than 140 is considered "genius" level, and when a person's score is over 130, he or she becomes eligible to join Mensa, the international high-IQ society. A Wechsler score 7 points lower than a Stanford-Binet score is considered equivalent.

Achievement tests are generally scored as to grade level; when tested, a child in the 6th grade should reflect knowledge equal to that attained by most children who have completed the 5th grade. Some schools only require children to show that they have acquired knowledge equivalent to a 7th-grade level before they are allowed to graduate from high school (12th grade). The Bender-Gestalt test is usually not given until a child reaches the age of 5. By the age of 7 he or she should be able to copy at least two designs; and by age 10, all of them.

There are no normal or abnormal results for aptitude testing; the individual either does or does not show some particular talent or ability.

Since virtually all personality tests require projection or interpretation, "normal" is in the mind of the beholder—in this case, the person giving the test. Among psychometrists (those who specialize in testing), individuals who end up with "good" scores (showing few or no abnormalities) are all too often considered overly eager to please the examiner.

What You Need

Just about every kind of test is available in books from a library or bookstore. Ask your librarian or bookseller to show you the current edition of *Medical Books and Serials in Print;* in the "Subject Index" section of that book, check for appropriate titles under the following headings: "Ability—Testing," "Intelligence Tests," "Learning Ability," "Learning Disabilities," "Personality Assessment," "Personality Tests," "Psychological Tests" and "Self-Evaluation." In most instances copies of actual tests along with expected answers, scoring and interpretation are given; otherwise, reasonable facsimiles of the real tests are shown. A few titles and sources include:

- *Know Your Own I.Q.* and *Check Your Own I.Q.*, by H. J. Eysenck (these are also paperback books published by Penguin).
- The Standard I.Q. Test, obtainable by mail from Mensa Headquarters (1701 West Third St., Brooklyn, N.Y. 11223).
- Test workbooks similar to reading readiness and achievement tests can usually be found in school supply stores.
- The Guided Career Exploration test material, which reveals aptitudes in

relation to career possibilities, is available from The Psychological Corporation (757 Third Ave., New York, N.Y. 10017).

- Sample aptitude tests for almost every job and profession have been published by Arco Publishing Company, which also puts out many different achievement tests.
- *Check Yourself Out,* by Craig Norback—a personality test published by Times Books.
- *Adult Assessment: A Source Book of Tests and Measures of Human Behavior,* by Richard S. Andrulis—a paperback published by C. C. Thomas.
- *How to Beat Personality Tests,* by Charles Alex—published by Arco Publishing Company as a paperback (it may be out of print but can still be obtained in libraries or through book-finding services and is well worth the effort to locate).
- *Big Secrets,* by William Poundstone—published by William Morrow & Co.; it presents the uncensored truth about the Rorschach test.

While a great many tests are available directly to individuals to perform and interpret at home, some must be acquired through schools, employment personnel offices, psychologists or physicians. Many are still completed at home, but some must be interpreted by the professional tester. The largest single source of testing material is The Psychological Corporation (noted above). Other test sources can be found in the telephone company's yellow pages under the headings of "Aptitude and Employment Testing" and "Psychologists."

What to Watch Out For
Your own personal bias can be a problem, as can the temptation to cheat by not following instructions to the letter or by not answering the questions honestly. Do not accept the test results at face value without considering your background, education and environment. Be sure that any unusual test results are not caused by drugs; even many nonprescription products such as antihistamines and other cold preparations can dull the senses; other medicines can help bring on hypoglycemia (see Blood Tests, **Glucose**), and even large doses of aspirin and some weight-reducing aids can cause temporary mental incapacity. Anticholinergic drugs—many of which are used to treat allergies, gastrointestinal problems and Parkinson's disease—can cause memory defects.

What the Test Results Can Mean
Although tests of mental ability and personality are not considered hard evidence of a medical condition, they can suggest the need for further diagnostic investigations, especially in children with apparent learning problems. They have been used to assess the effect of an illness or injury on

intellectual functioning. Test results that vary significantly from what is expected warrant a medical consultation. When appropriate tests were performed on patients thought to have incurable senile dementia, more than 50 percent of them showed that they really had easily treatable behavioral problems. More than anything else, familiarity with such tests can prevent subsequent misinterpretation of test results and avoid erroneous or unnecessary therapies.

Reliability

Unfortunately, most of these tests are nothing more than possible clues to learning difficulties or aberrant behavior. Their accuracy can only be rated at 50 percent. Tests to help detect dementia, however, are felt to be 75 percent accurate. While growth and development observations are not definite and can vary by several months to a year, failure to show at least half of the expected reactions is considered about 80 percent accurate as a problem warning sign. When used by an individual to gain familiarity prior to more formal testing, the tests can be considered 100 percent worthwhile.

Type-A behavior (related to heart disease). While the psychological makeup of an individual has long been suspected as a possible cause of illness, a particular pattern of behavior called type A—characterized by aggressiveness, competitiveness, hostility and being extremely time-conscious—has been reported to increase the risk of having a heart attack. And it seems such behavior is unrelated to one's diet. Although many studies have since refuted this general concept, and especially certain aspects of the theory such as the "sense of urgency," the association between being angry all the time and being predisposed to heart disease remains plausible. In contrast, a person with a type-B personality is, at least outwardly, relaxed; is seldom impatient or belligerent; and takes time for recreational activities.

The primary way of labeling a patient's personality as to being type A or B is through a physician's interview, in which the physician notes the manner and speed of the person's speech, the response to feigned hostility on the doctor's part and the general attitude that the individual has toward life and work, and also assesses the person's written responses to the Jenkins Activity Survey (a questionnaire available from most doctors).

A relatively simple home test that can point toward a type-A personality is the Bortner test, in which you sit down and write a short phrase, such as a familiar proverb, the way you usually would with respect to speed and style. Then you tell yourself to rewrite that same phrase more slowly. Finally, you tell yourself to rewrite it a third time even more slowly. It does seem that type-A personalities cannot write slowly no matter how hard they try, while type Bs perform this task with ease.

The initial studies of the relationship between personality and heart disease did report that type As had five to seven times as many heart attacks as type Bs. More recently, however, there have been studies that indicate that type-A personalities, if they do suffer a heart attack, live longer than type Bs recovering from the same illness, indicating that type-A behavior does not necessarily harm one's chances of surviving a heart attack. Some attribute this evident contradiction with respect to how one's personality affects one's health to the fact that type As are more compulsive about following their doctor's orders, something that type Bs seem reluctant to do blindly.

In general, then, no real accuracy rate can be applied to type A–type B testing. The A-B classification also fails to take into account people who do not fall into either category absolutely. And there are, in fact, people who fall unquestionably into the type-A category but who are quite content to work under pressure on their jobs, get great satisfaction out of their achievements and show no signs of heart disease during their lifetime. In contrast, there are evident type Bs who are bored with their jobs and disappointed with their lives and their lack of achievement and who show an unusually high rate of heart disease. Perhaps the results of the Bortner test, along with your score on the **"Burnout" Syndrome** test (see Mental Ability and Personality Tests), may help you better understand yourself—and your attitude toward your job. Although there is no absolute proof at present, recognizing yourself as a type-A personality and attempting to become more like a type B could lessen your risk of heart disease.

DENTAL TESTS

DENTAL PLAQUE DISCLOSURE
(Screening to prevent tooth loss)

Tooth plaques are really colonies of bacteria. They secrete two substances: a gluelike material that allows them to adhere to the surface of the teeth and an enzyme that breaks down complex sugars and white flour, causing acid to be produced. It is the acid that can erode the tooth's surface (enamel) and also dissolve the calcium that comprises the hard tooth substance. The end result may be a cavity or loss of the tooth. Once plaques are established, and ignored, they can last for years and continually damage the teeth. They also contribute to periodontal disease: gingivitis, or an infection of the gums (the first stage of periodontal disease), and pyorrhea, or an infection of all the tissues around the teeth, which can destroy the bones that hold the teeth in place, causing the teeth to rot and fall out—not to mention bad breath. After a while plaque can turn into tartar, the whitish, hard bits of plasterlike material whose rough surface can cause bleeding gums and loose teeth. In fact, a "pink toothbrush" (reflecting gums that bleed easily even with mild brushing), is considered a diagnostic sign of tooth and gum disease.

Preventing the initial plaque formation can be one of the most effective means of preventing tooth decay and avoiding both periodontal disease (loss of bone that supports the teeth) and the eventual need for dentures. Periodontal disease is the prime cause of tooth loss in people over the age of 35. Plaque prevention really involves proper cleaning of the teeth and gums—not simply brushing, but using the right toothbrush (with small enough bristles), cleaning between the teeth with dental floss and adequate irrigation (rinsing) of the teeth and gums to remove the plaque and food particles after they have been loosened. The success of regular preventive tooth care can then be tested by applying disclosing substances, which will reveal any remaining plaque.

What Is Usual

Plaques in their natural state are virtually invisible to the naked eye—even on close inspection. Home plaque-disclosing preparations may consist of tablets

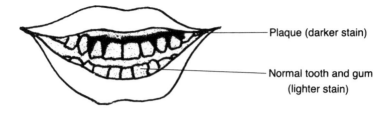

Plaque (darker stain)

Normal tooth and gum
(lighter stain)

Figure 55. Dental plaque detection.

or solutions of erythrosine—the federal government's FD&C (Food, Drug and Cosmetic) red No. 3 dye—or other colorings—and when a tablet is chewed, or a solution rinsed throughout the mouth, the plaque will usually show up as a vivid color (see Figure 55). Obviously, no evidence of any stain is normal, albeit absence of such staining is not always usual.

What You Need

The test requires disclosing tablets, which average $4.00 for a package of 125 tablets; most dentists will give their patients, without charge, sample packages of 4 tablets for home use. Packages of 1,000 cost less than $10.00 (you only use 1 tablet at a time). Several companies make disclosing tablets; disclosing solutions cost about $1.50 for a two-ounce bottle, but you only use 10 drops at a time diluted in an ounce of water. Some companies combine the discloser in gels.

A new, and slightly different, plaque-disclosing solution is now available through dentists or pharmacies. It is called 2-TONE and is painted on the teeth with a cotton-tipped applicator. After the teeth are painted and the mouth rinsed with water, areas with old, thicker plaque will stain dark blue, while new, thin plaque formations will stain red. The dark blue areas show where the teeth have been neglected for a long time, while the red stain will reveal any recent poor oral hygiene. The 2-TONE solution also contains much less red No. 3 dye than other solutions and costs $4.50 for a two-ounce bottle. TRACE-28, which costs $2.95 for one ounce and contains no red No. 3 dye, is a flavored concentrate that can be used to make a solution to swish in the mouth prior to brushing the teeth; it stains plaque red. Household bleach or detergent will remove its stains from clothes.

A solution that will not stain the teeth or clothing, and is not obvious when in the mouth, comes in the Lactona Plaque Detector Kit (1330 Industry Rd., Hatfield, Pa. 19440). The kit, costing about $10.00, also includes a small flashlight with a special blue optical filter that reveals the plaque and an attachable mouth mirror to enable you to view all tooth surfaces more easily.

What to Watch Out For

Do not be surprised if your whole mouth seems to turn color, especially the first time you use some plaque disclosers; the color will disappear in a short while with rinsing. Many people test for plaque at bedtime, so the color will be gone by morning. If you are not sure what you see (what is stained plaque and what is not), have your dentist demonstrate the procedure for you; he or she can also show you the best way to remove your plaque. If you have a thyroid problem or know that you are unusually sensitive to iodine, check with your doctor before using dental plaque disclosers that may contain iodine. Erythrosine contains iodine as part of its chemical makeup; it could affect any thyroid function tests, so be sure to tell your doctor if you are using plaque disclosers before any medical testing.

What the Test Results Can Mean

The appearance of distinct dark red, blue or yellow stains on the teeth and along the gum line usually means plaque. It also means that your tooth cleaning and mouth care are probably inadequate. If you can reclean your teeth, removing the red stains—especially those that go in between the teeth—using floss, you are markedly diminishing your chances for cavities and other dental disease. If you find that home cleaning does not seem effective, you may already have formed hard tartar, which is best removed by your dentist. You will also learn just what areas of your teeth you have usually ignored, and this alone will improve your dental hygiene.

Reliability

Studies have indicated that plaque detection and removal can be at least 80 percent effective in reducing tooth decay and preventing periodontal disease.

Periodontal disease detection. Some dentists advise their patients to insert the tip of a thin, wedge-shaped stick (Dental Pic, Stim-u-dent—available at most pharmacies for from $1.40 to $1.90 per 100) between all the teeth at the gum line on a weekly basis. If gums bleed right after pushing the sticks against them for a second or two, it could indicate the beginning of periodontal disease (involving gum inflammation and destruction of the underlying bone). Normally, such poking will not provoke bleeding. If bleeding does occur easily and does not stop after you practice more careful dental hygiene for a few weeks, it warrants a dental consultation.

Tooth sensitivity. Many people have pain in their teeth after contact with hot and/or cold foods or beverages. You can detect which teeth are so sensitive by placing your toothbrush in hot and cold water and then touching each tooth. Should a tooth become painful after a temperature change, apply a desensitizing toothpaste (some contain formaldehyde, some strontium, some nitrates and others a form of fluoride) at least twice a day using a cotton swab. If the tooth pain disappears within two weeks, you may have solved your problem; if not, a dental consultation is warranted. *Note:* Not all desensitizing dentifrices are equally effective; you may have to try different brands.

Cavity susceptibility. Because tooth *cavities (caries,* to your dentist) primarily need an acid environment for plaques to grow, and because saliva is usually alkaline (neutralizes acid), measuring the pH of saliva has been used as a means of identifying those who might be more predisposed to cavity formation.

Placing a drop of saliva on a strip of litmus paper (see Urine Tests, **Clinical Analysis: pH**) will show whether the saliva is acid or alkaline; the more alkaline the better. The multiple-test dipsticks used to test urine can also be used for saliva and will give a more precise reading. While saliva should be alkaline two hours after eating, for some as yet unexplained reason, it may be slightly acid in the morning hours. If the saliva is always acid, it could mean a greater susceptibility to both plaque and cavities. Incidentally, the amount of saliva produced also seems to have an effect on cavity prevention; the more saliva, the less bacteria can grow on teeth. People who have little or no saliva, such as those with Sjogren's syndrome (dry eyes, dry mouth) or those whose salivary glands have been removed by surgery or destroyed by radiation (X-rays), suffer a prodigious amount of cavities regardless of diet (even with a marked reduction in sugar-containing foods).

MOUTH, THROAT AND GASTROINTESTINAL TESTS

FECES OBSERVATIONS
(A worthwhile, if unpleasant, guide to health)

Although some people find it disturbing simply to look at a bowel move-ment, the observation of feces (or stool, as they are sometimes called) can be one of the simplest, yet best, sources of health information, second only to urine testing. Feces, like urine, are a waste product and primarily reflect digestion as opposed to metabolism; normally, they consist of food material that could not be digested, some remnants of bile from the liver, intestinal secretions and bacteria. Abnormal constituents such as blood, foul odor or the absence of certain pigments can be the first clue to pathology and, when detected early enough in the course of disease, can lead to simple, efficient treatment.

Most people on a typical diet produce approximately 100 grams to 300 grams (from 3 ounces to 10 ounces) of feces a day, close to 70 percent of which is water. The rest is about two-thirds fiber such as cellulose, the skin and seeds of fruits and vegetables and one-third normal intestinal bacteria, which are supposed to be present. Home tests on feces include: observing color and consistency, odor and whether the feces float in the water or sink to the bottom of the bowl; determining whether or not blood (both visible, called hematochezia, or invisible, called occult), white blood cells (leukocytes) or glucose is present; determining the degree of acidity; and indirectly, searching for pinworms and other parasites.

What Is Usual
Although more than 70 percent of people studied by the federal govern-ment say that they have a bowel movement daily, having more than one a day or only one every two days or three days may still not be abnormal. Most doctors define constipation as having only one bowel movement in

four or more days; many patients, however, especially the elderly, consider constipation as straining, regardless of the frequency. Women complain of constipation twice as much as men do, and inactive men complain 15 times as much as men who exercise (inactive women complain only twice as much).

If the amount of feces remains reasonably related to the diet (large quantities of fruits, vegetables and whole grains tend to increase the amount of feces, while proteins and liquids tend to decrease it), little attention need be paid to feces volume. The color should be from medium to dark brown and homogenous (of uniform color) throughout; but again, diet and drugs must be considered: Eating large amounts of green vegetables can give feces a greenish hue, and some antibiotics can cause feces to have a yellowish tinge. Food coloring or dyes in drugs can also alter stool color. The consistency should be firm, but not hard or watery; each segment should be from one-half inch to one inch in diameter. A diet high in fiber will usually cause the feces to float. The odor, while never described as pleasant, should not be too obtrusive. The pH should be close to neutral (7); large amounts of meat in the diet can make it more alkaline (7–8.5), while large quantities of carbohydrates make it more acid (6–7). There should be little or no glucose and no evidence of blood, white blood cells or parasites. Eating rare meats, certain vegetables and fruits, and vigorous brushing of the teeth are a few of the things that can cause a false-positive blood test.

What You Need

A willingness to observe a feces sample is all that is really required. More specific tests are performed with dipsticks used for urine testing, such as: Chemstrip 3 or Combistix (which also includes glucose and pH testing), costing from $17.00 to $20.00 for 100 dipsticks; Chemstrip 5L (which includes all the tests in Chemstrip 3 and Combistix plus the test for white blood cells), costing about $23.00 for 100 dipsticks; or Chemstrip L (which includes only the white blood cell test), costing $8.00 for 100 dipsticks.

A pocket-size microscope, such as the Panasonic 30-power light scope, which costs from $7.95 to $30.00, can be used to identify pinworms and some other worm eggs (ova) or segments of parasites such as tapeworms. A few drops of normal or physiological saline (salt solution) are best to dilute a bit of feces for microscopic examination; it costs about $0.60 to $0.75 for a one-ounce bottle.

A bedpan or a very widemouthed, dry, clean jar is needed to collect a feces specimen for testing for pH, glucose, white blood cells and parasites. As with some tests to detect occult blood, for these tests to give accurate results, the feces should not come in contact with toilet paper, urine or water. The **Occult Blood** test is described separately (see Mouth, Throat and Gastrointestinal Tests).

What to Watch Out For

Do not test feces from a toilet bowl that contains any chemical bowl cleaner. Should the feces specimen be very dry, place a drop or two of normal saline on the area of the specimen to be tested and wait 30 seconds before testing.

What the Test Results Can Mean

If feces seem very light brown or gray or even appear to be without color, and you have not been limiting your diet to unusually large amounts of milk, medical attention is warranted; this can mean liver or gallbladder trouble. If there is any red color of the feces not related to eating beets, it could mean rectal bleeding and certainly warrants medical attention. Black or tarry-colored stools not related to large doses of iron must be considered as suspicious evidence of bleeding in the upper portions of the gastrointestinal tract (esophagus, stomach and small intestines); while it could be the consequence of taking large amounts of aspirin, it could also mean some serious gastrointestinal condition, and it warrants medical attention. Greenish-colored feces can accompany diarrhea but are not a specific indication of any one condition. Silver or aluminum-colored feces, especially if accompanied by jaundice, could come from a growth blocking the pancreas gland duct and warrant medical attention.

If the consistency of the feces suddenly seems to change, particularly if the diameter seems to be much smaller than usual, medical attention is warranted, since this can be one of the first signs of an obstructed bowel. Repeated watery feces, especially if mucus is seen, can mean a chronic irritable bowel or an infection by bacteria or parasites such as amebiasis, giardiasis (see Figure 56) or typhoid—especially if you have recently been camping out or traveling away from home (see Mouth, Throat and Gastrointestinal Tests, **String Test**). Infections or parasitic infestations are usually accompanied by feces with a very foul odor, and feces with such an odor should make one think of giardiasis. In addition, Peace Corps workers have noticed that people with giardiasis give off a very offensive belch that they call the "purple burps" (see Breath and Lung Tests, **Breath Odor and Sputum**). Repeated episodes of very hard, dry feces mean constipation, most often from a faulty diet, but they could also result from disease, especially in young children, and warrant a medical consultation.

If there is a suspicion that drinking milk is causing problems (see Mouth, Throat and Gastrointestinal System Tests, **Milk Products (Lactose) Intolerance**), insert a dipstick into the feces sample to test for pH and glucose, wait 10 seconds, rinse the dipstick and then compare the colors on the container to see whether the feces are very acid (5–6) and glucose is present (it should not be); this helps confirm intolerance to the milk sugar lactose.

The white blood cell test is usually performed when there are chronic

Figure 56. Parasites, or their eggs, that can cause intestinal diseases. The six illustrations are as they might be observed through a 30-power pocket light microscope. All but the *Giardia* can sometimes be seen with the naked eye.

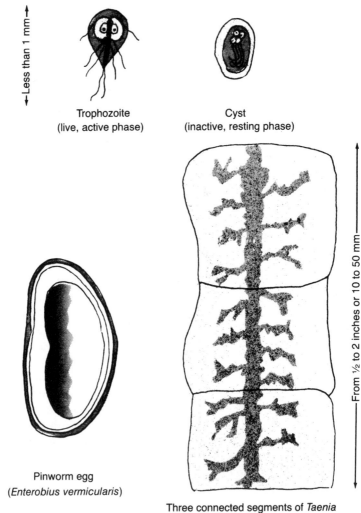

Giardia lamblia, the cause of giardiasis.

Trophozoite
(live, active phase)

Cyst
(inactive, resting phase)

Less than 1 mm

Approximately 2 mm

From ½ to 2 inches or 10 to 50 mm

Pinworm egg
(*Enterobius vermicularis*)

Three connected segments of *Taenia solium*, the pork tapeworm. Beef and fish tapeworms are similar in appearance. The entire pork tapeworm is from 6 to 12 feet long; a beef tapeworm is from 12 to 35 feet; and a fish tapeworm from 10 to 40 feet. All can be composed of hundreds of segments.

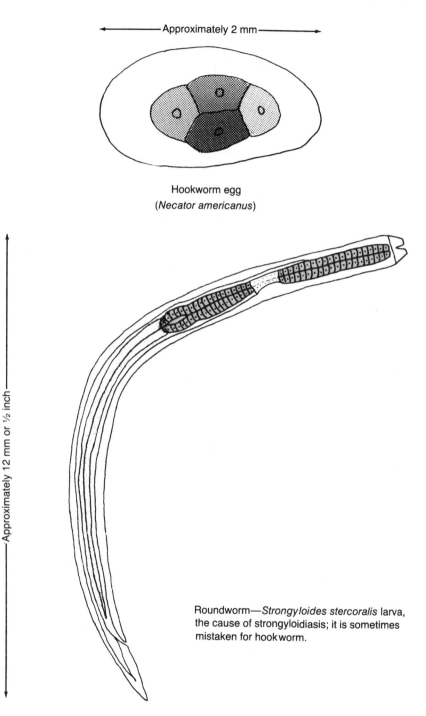

Approximately 2 mm

Hookworm egg
(*Necator americanus*)

Approximately 12 mm or ½ inch

Roundworm—*Strongyloides stercoralis* larva,
the cause of strongyloidiasis; it is sometimes
mistaken for hookworm.

intestinal problems, most often involving repeated bouts of diarrhea, frequently showing mucus along with lower bowel cramping. When a dipstick that tests for white blood cells is inserted into a feces specimen for 10 seconds and then rinsed off, a positive test (indicating that white blood cells are present) can mean a parasitic infestation, typhoid fever or some other salmonella-type infection, or it can indicate ulcerative colitis. A negative white blood cell test suggests giardiasis, a virus infection or cholera. But then, this much chronic bowel trouble should already have prompted a medical consultation.

When children are persistently scratching their buttocks, and usually the nose as well, think of pinworms as a possible cause; they are the most common worm infestation. In a study of California elementary school children between 5 years and 10 years of age, 1 out of 5 was found to be infected with pinworms; projecting this figure, at least 4.5 million young children in the United States may be carrying these worms. Pinworm infestation often imitates appendicitis in children.

To detect this infestation, wind a piece of Scotch Tape, sticky side out, around the eraser end of a pencil and during the night touch the sticky surface to and around the child's anal area (the worms come out at night to lay their eggs after the child has been under a blanket and warmed the buttocks). Spread the Scotch Tape out on a glass slide and search for the eggs (shown in Figure 56) through a pocket microscope; they are quite distinctive. You may have to repeat this test for several nights before the pinworm eggs are detected. If what looks like eggs are seen, a medical consultation is warranted. Egglike objects from other parasites and even some worm segments may sometimes be seen on the Scotch Tape or when a piece of feces about the size of a match head is placed on a glass slide and mixed with two or three drops of normal saline; a feces sample is more apt to show evidence of worms if it is taken from the surface of either end of the segment or adjacent to a speck of mucus.

Tapeworms (see Figure 56) can come from eating raw or inadequately cooked meat (steak tartare) or raw fish (sashimi or some sushi preparations), or by unconsciously tasting raw food during preparation (such as when making gefilte fish). Hookworm infestation and strongyloidiasis (a form of roundworm), both shown in Figure 56, can come from going barefoot on ground (or pavement) where dogs have deposited excrement containing worms or where bird droppings are found; the worms burrow through the skin of the feet to enter the body. Both of these worms can cause skin lesions, but hookworms also cause anemia (see Blood Tests, **Hemoglobin**), while strongyloidiasis can cause a cough and other symptoms similar to asthma. Any suggestion or even suspicion of parasites in the feces warrants a medical consultation.

Reliability
Direct feces observations are about 75 percent accurate as clues to internal disease; professional testing for parasites has about the same rate of accuracy.

OCCULT BLOOD (FECES)
(Though *not* a specific test for cancer, this test can help detect a gastrointestinal tumor, among other bowel problems.)

The word *occult* in medicine, when referring to blood, means that blood is present but not visible to the naked eye. Feces occult blood testing is a rough screening measure to see whether a bowel movement contains blood—which it should not. As noted in **Feces Observations** (see Mouth, Throat and Gastrointestinal Tests), a black-colored stool usually indicates bleeding in the esophagus, stomach or upper intestines; the black color comes from the action of the stomach's acid on the normally red blood. Bright red blood in the stool, or accompanying a bowel movement, usually indicates bleeding from the lower or large intestines, the rectum or the anus. Hidden blood in the stool, when tested for regularly—at least twice a year, especially after the age of 50—can provide the earliest warning signs of intestinal disease, albeit the possibility of such a test, when positive, indicating cancer is only from 5 percent to 10 percent. There are a great many other factors, ranging from one's diet and medicines to simple hemorrhoids, that will cause a positive result. Still, a past president of the American Cancer Society has said that of the 130,000 cases of colon and rectum cancers that are diagnosed every year, more than 75 percent could be cured if everyone over the age of 50 regularly tested himself or herself for feces occult blood.

What Is Usual
Despite the fact that some doctors believe that feces can, at times, contain a minuscule amount of blood and still be normal, the amount of blood, if present at all, in a typical bowel movement should never cause a positive result when the feces are tested for occult blood by any one of the home tests.

What You Need
At present there are more than a dozen different home tests for occult blood. They vary primarily in the technique for obtaining a sample; some, however, are much less sensitive to dietary factors. The most commonly used tests require you to use a thin wooden stick to obtain a tiny portion of the feces and place it on a special collecting paper or plastic. Some tests require

you to take the sample to your doctor; others allow you to apply a chemical "developer" to the sample and look for a color change (if positive). The simplest of all the tests allows you to drop a specially treated piece of paper into the toilet bowl and watch for a distinctive reaction (that is, the appearance of a color change). These tests usually have "controls" built in—that is, they will show you whether something went wrong or whether the test ingredients are not working properly. One such test paper, called the Colo-Screen or CS-T, claims it is not affected by many foods or iron compounds; it costs a doctor about $1.50 for a three-test kit (Helena Laboratories, P.O. Box 752, Beaumont, TX 77204).

Most tests are available at pharmacies at a cost of from $3.00 to $7.00 for a three test kit. Whatever type you choose, you should obtain sufficient test material to perform three different tests on three consecutive days; this is to catch bleeding that is only occasional. You might ask your doctor for the test material; many offer this material to their patients without charge. And at times various hospitals, drugstore chains and even health agencies supply the test material free of charge. Virtually all of the tests (there are one or two exceptions), whether performed at home or in a professional setting, employ the same analytical process. When using a test that requires a tiny sample of feces, it is best to take two samples for testing—one from the surface of the stool (to aid in detecting lower bowel bleeding) and one from the inside center of the specimen (to help detect possible upper intestinal bleeding).

What to Watch Out For

Follow the directions carefully; many test kits seem to be alike, but they can differ with respect to the procedure that must be followed.

The most common problem with fecal occult blood testing comes from foods, vitamins, drugs and brushing one's teeth (even the slightest amount of blood from the gums, when swallowed, can cause a positive test result). For four days prior to performing the test, and certainly on the day before, avoid consuming red or rare-cooked meat, artichokes, broccoli, cantaloupe (or other melons), citrus juices, horseradish, radishes, raw mushrooms or turnips; there are substances in these foods that can chemically affect the test, causing a false-positive reaction. Some test manufacturers also request that you take no iron supplements, such as may be contained in vitamin compounds or tonics. Other manufacturers proscribe alcohol as well as nutritional supplements containing calcium, copper, and even iodine.

In contrast, some doctors insist that you eat a lot of fruits and vegetables (apples, corn, lettuce, peanuts, prunes) and even bran in order to increase the stool's bulk and roughage.

Avoid a great many drugs such as aspirin (which can cause stomach irritation and non-disease-related bleeding). Nonsteroidal anti-inflammatory drugs that may be substituted for aspirin as pain relievers (ibuprofen, naproxen, etc.), while known to irritate the stomach, have not always been shown to interfere with the fecal occult blood test; if you are taking one of these drugs, check with your doctor prior to performing the test.

Most of all, avoid taking vitamin C for several days prior to testing; it can cause a false-negative result—hiding the fact that there really is blood in the stool. Some antacids and antiulcer medicines, Pepto-Bismol, simethicone (used to help relieve gas pains) and even red wine have also been reported to cause a false-negative test result.

Obviously, any bleeding in or near the intestinal tract (nosebleed, menstruation) will cause a false-positive results. And even exercise can, at times, cause a false-positive reaction; the more vigorous the physical exertion, the greater the chance that there may be gastrointestinal bleeding. Recently, there have been reports that even chlorophyll (in some breath deodorizers) can cause a false-positive result.

If you use drop-in-the-bowl test paper, do not perform the test in a toilet bowl that contains chemical cleaners.

What the Test Results Can Mean

A positive occult blood test, especially after you have been on a proper diet and avoided all other interfering substances, warrants medical attention. It does not, however, automatically mean cancer. There are a great many other conditions—outside of those that can interfere with the test, such as diet, drugs and exercise—that can cause blood in the feces. Diverticulitis, hemorrhoids, hookworms or simple polyps may be at fault. Repeated negative tests, in the presence of any bowel discomfort or symptoms, still warrant a medical consultation.

Reliability

When all extraneous factors are taken into consideration, the test is 90 percent accurate as an indication of blood coming from somewhere in the bowel. The test does not reveal the precise location or the specific cause. In one study, of all those under the age of 50 who had a confirmed positive test result, only 3 percent had cancer. Over the age of 50, cancer was found in only 10 percent; over 70 years of age, it was found in 23 percent.

Occult blood (Stomach Contents) There are times when it can be valuable to test for occult (hidden) blood from stomach bleeding, especially if you are taking stomach-irritating drugs such as aspirin or if a stomach ulcer is suspected. Usually, vomitus is tested, but even slight regurgitation may be revealing.

The test is similar to that for occult blood in the feces; only the name of the test is different. It is called Gastroccult and is available from your doctor for home use whenever vomiting occurs. It costs the doctor about $0.60 a test. Only one drop of vomitus or regurgitation is applied to the test card, followed by the addition of two drops of a developing chemical. The test also shows the pH, or acidity, of the test material to help pinpoint from what portion of the upper bowel the sample came.

MILK PRODUCTS (LACTOSE) INTOLERANCE
(Helping to distinguish between an enzyme deficiency and an allergy)

Most milk products contain lactose, a form of sugar, which requires an enzyme, lactase, to metabolize it. Many people, primarily after the age of 20—although the condition can occur in very young children—do not naturally produce sufficient lactase to break down the ingested milk sugar adequately, and as a result, they may suffer uncomfortable symptoms after drinking milk or eating foods containing milk products, such as ice cream, commercially prepared bakery products, desserts, soups, frozen fruits and vegetables, baby foods, candies, liqueurs, artificial sweeteners, chocolate drink mix powders and foods that have "milk solids," "caseinates" or "whey" listed as ingredients on the label. Some other commercial products—such as instant coffee; powdered beverages; breaded foods; hot dogs; bologna (kosher meat products are lactose-free); canned fruits and vegetables; cookie, cake and pancake mix; and prepared sauces (although some lactase-deficient people can tolerate certain yogurts)—can also contain lactose as an ingredient, but it may not appear on the label. Soft cheeses contain lactose, too, however the sugar is usually broken down and disappears in the making of hard cheese. And lactose is commonly used as a binder in the manufacture of medicine tablets and vitamin pills. A list of all medications containing lactose can be obtained from your regional Food and Drug Administration office.

The most common symptoms of lactose intolerance include:

• Bloating and flatulence—excessive and uncomfortable amounts of gas in the abdomen, which can cause the abdomen to swell.
• Borborygmi—rumbling abdominal noises.
• Diarrhea.
• Intestinal cramps.

For people with a lactase deficiency, some or all of these symptoms usually appear within 30 minutes to 90 minutes after the ingestion of a full glass of whole milk or the equivalent in milk products; some people can tolerate a very small amount of lactose (a teaspoon of cream in their coffee), so the quantity of milk products must also be taken into account. If you happen to be of Mediterranean origin, Arab, black, Oriental, of Ashkenazi Jewish (Central and Eastern European) ancestry or American Indian, your chances of suffering from lactose intolerance are much greater (from 10 to 20 times greater) than if your forebears came from Northern Europe; the problem is primarily an inherited one.

The essence of the illness seems to be that individuals with insufficient lactase cannot break down the milk sugar lactose into more simple sugar molecules (glucose and galactose), and therefore, it cannot be properly digested. Undigested lactose then causes excess body fluids to be drawn into the upper portion of the intestines, and when the heavily watered food moves through the bowel, it causes increased acidity and an increased amount of gas along with a watery bowel movement. Milk product intolerance is not the same as milk allergy (see Allergy Tests, **Patch Testing** and **Elimination Diet**); it rarely causes a rash or other skin manifestations of hypersensitivity.

The simplest way to test for lactose intolerance is to eliminate as many lactose-containing products from the diet as possible. If formerly frequent gastrointestinal symptoms disappear or even lessen considerably within two days to three days, this is the first step; the second step is to drink a glass or two of whole or skim milk (use only one-quarter glass of milk for children) and wait to see whether bloating or cramps recur, usually followed by a bout of diarrhea within the next 12 hours to 24 hours.

A more definitive test, if drinking milk does cause symptoms, is to add LactAid, a commercial preparation of lactase, to the milk and again wait to see whether symptoms develop. When discomfort occurs after drinking milk without LactAid but not after drinking milk with LactAid, this should confirm the condition, and the treatment is to eliminate lactose-containing products where possible and to make LactAid part of your diet where lactose cannot be avoided.

Other confirmatory measures include dipstick-type testing for pH and glucose (see Mouth, Throat and Gastrointestinal Tests, **Feces Observations**).

What Is Usual

While most people have no trouble digesting milk and milk products, it is believed that more than 30 million Americans are unable to digest lactose completely; in the rest of the world, the problem is found in 2 out of 3 people. Again, the intolerance to lactose in milk can also be one of degree; some people have no uncomfortable symptoms until they exceed a certain quantity of the milk sugar.

What You Need

A willingness to try to identify foods containing lactose and a desire to avoid those foods are required. Or you can obtain a small quantity of LactAid; a supply sufficient to "treat" 12 quarts of milk costs from $2.75 to $3.00 and is available without a prescription. In some parts of the country, dairies offer milk and soft cheeses already treated with LactAid. LactAid is also available in the form of tiny tablets for direct swallowing, at a cost of about $0.02 a tablet, or as LACTRASE capsules, which can be opened and sprinkled on food. These can be quite useful when you are eating out.

What to Watch Out For

Do not attempt the test if you have any sort of intestinal infection or upset, if you have undergone surgery or X-rays of your abdomen within the past two months or if you are taking antibiotics, especially penicillin or neomycin; these interfering factors tend to give temporary false-positive reactions.

If you do avoid lactose-containing foods, be sure to supplement your diet with other foods containing calcium (hard cheese, green leafy vegetables, sardines, etc.) and vitamin D.

If you have diabetes, do not use LactAid until you talk with your physician; it can add a bit more glucose to your system.

What the Test Results Can Mean

Avoidance of milk and milk products containing lactose followed by the relief of gastrointestinal discomfort is a result sufficient unto itself. The use of LactAid can prevent your having to eliminate many favorite foods from your diet. If avoidance of lactose or the use of LactAid does not give obvious relief, there is always the rare possibility that the gastrointestinal symptoms are caused by allergy (see Allergy Tests, **Patch Testing** and **Elimination Diet**). Should nothing seem to help, a medical consultation is warranted; other conditions that can imitate milk product intolerance include: thyroid disease, Crohn's disease (an inflammation of the lower part of the small intestines), sprue (a malabsorption problem) and kwashiorkor (primarily a protein deficiency that can cause mental irritation and apathy in addition to symptoms resembling those of lactose intolerance).

Reliability

When eliminating milk and milk products relieves related signs and symptoms, the test is close to 100 percent accurate. The use of LactAid usually offers relief 90 percent of the time where true lactose deficiency exists. Always keep in mind that even after discomfort disappears, it is still possible to have other intestinal problems unrelated to milk product intolerance.

MOUTH, TONGUE AND THROAT OBSERVATIONS
(Detecting early signs of several serious diseases)

It cannot be emphasized enough that it is as much of a medical test to look for abnormalities in and on the body as it is to detect the presence of some abnormal substance in the blood or urine. To examine the inside of the mouth and notice the sudden presence of a new white spot that will not wipe away could be a most valuable test result, especially if it turns out to be a sign of cancer detected early enough to allow simple, effective treatment. Nearly 20 percent of mouth cancers start out as a white patch, or leukoplakia. On the other hand, similar-looking white patches could also be lichen planus, a disease with no known cause that does not require specific treatment, other than symptomatic relief of any irritation. White patches in the mouth could also mean thrush (candidiasis or moniliasis), a fungus infection that commonly comes about while a person is taking antibiotics or cortisone drugs, or they might also signal diabetes or leukemia.

It is not that you can be expected to diagnose unusual mouth lesions, but if you regularly examine the mouth, tongue and throat so that you become aware of what these areas normally look like, you can then notice an unusual lesion almost as soon as it appears. And when it comes to spotting tumors and other illnesses that can reveal themselves through mouth, tongue and throat manifestations, observation alone is far superior to the most sophisticated chemical analysis or X-ray.

Start by inspecting the lips; blisterlike lesions are most often the result of herpes (see Body Observations, **Skin Observations**), but also look for any irregularities, cracking, drying or dark blue patches on the lip surfaces. Next, using a bright flashlight and, if necessary, a wooden tongue depressor (see Figure 57), look at the gums and then at and under the tongue. Then inspect the inside of the cheeks. Continue your visual observation over the palate (roof of the mouth) and then back toward the throat, comparing both sides where the tonsils are (or were); also note the color and size of the uvula (the small flap of tissue that hangs down from the middle of the top of the back of the mouth; it looks somewhat like a tonsil). Finally, survey the back of the throat (the pharynx), looking particularly for redness, any mucus drippings, sores or a membrane (a thin film that seems to be covering the throat). After observation comes palpation. Slowly but firmly slide your fingers over the top and under the tongue and then sweep them over the inner cheek surfaces; see whether you can feel any small bump or irregularity, even when nothing is evident to the eye. The simple secret of effective mouth and throat observation is to learn by practicing on an individual who has no fever, no mouth complaints or symptoms, and no sore throat.

What Is Usual

The lips should be moist and without any lesions or discoloration. The gums should be uniformly pink and show no signs of bleeding. The tongue and the inside of the mouth should be smooth, with no bumps or plaques (small flat patches) either seen or felt. There should be no swelling, dryness or tremor of the tongue. No heavy white coating or other discoloration should be evident. When the tongue is protruded (stuck out), it should come out

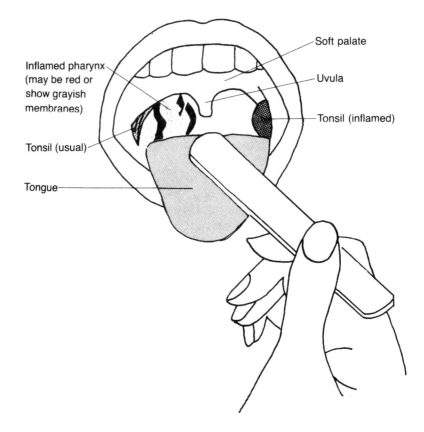

Soft palate

Inflamed pharynx
(may be red or
show grayish
membranes)

Uvula

Tonsil (inflamed)

Tonsil (usual)

Tongue

Figure 57. Mouth and throat observations.

Note: The adenoids (tonsillar tissue) are usually not seen, as they lie behind and above the soft palate.

straight and not lean toward one side or the other. On some people the tongue will show furrows (little valleys) crossways (from side to side), or it may show patches of red, brighter than the rest of the tongue (called geographic tongue, because it almost looks like a relief map); these manifestations are usually inherited and are probably normal. Because the surface of the tongue is open to injury from the teeth (biting one's tongue), from hot (high-temperature) or spicy foods, or from fish bones, red or sore spots may occur occasionally.

The tonsils, if still present, should be pink and of equal size, and they should have thin grooves running up and down; sometimes tonsils, even though present, are difficult to see in their natural pockets. After a tonsillectomy the pockets where the tonsils once were should be hollowed out, pink and smooth. The uvula should be small and pink, and it should hang straight down. The back of the throat should look evenly pink over the entire surface, and there should be no evidence of any mucus dripping down from the nasal cavity.

What You Need
These observations require a bright flashlight and some tongue depressors (also called tongue blades), which come in two sizes: adult and children's; they cost $3.00 for a box of 100. If you have an otoscope (see Ear Observations and Hearing Tests, **Ear Canal and Eardrum Observations**), it may have come with an attachment that holds a tongue depressor in place just under the light bulb. If not, special tongue blade light sets (one is called Oralume) are available at a cost of $15.00. The Sears, Roebuck Orotoscope, which includes an otoscope, also has a fiber-optic-lighted tongue depressor (you do not need the wooden tongue depressors); it costs $17.00.

What to Watch Out For
Do not use a spoon or something similar in place of a tongue depressor; sudden biting down could chip a tooth. If it is difficult to see the back of the throat, grasp the tip of the tongue with a dry gauze pad; it will keep the tongue from slipping. If the individual being examined tends to gag when saying "aaaah" or while you are trying to see the back of the mouth and throat, tell the person to stick out his or her tongue and pant like a dog; this can help eliminate the gag reflex.

What the Test Results Can Mean
Any obvious lesion on the lips or in the mouth or throat—especially the sudden appearance of a new, pigmented one that does not go away after a few days—warrants a medical consultation. Even herpeslike lesions (unless they have been recurring almost all your life) warrant a medical consultation to be sure that the disease is limited to the mouth. Dark blue dots over the lips could be a sign of an intestinal disorder and warrant a medical consultation. Bleeding gums most often come from overzealous brushing of the teeth, but they may also come from poor tooth care (see Dental Tests). Unfortunately, bleeding gums can also be the first sign of several blood disorders, especially bleeding tendencies (see Heart and Circulation Tests, **Capillary Fragility**); leukemia, infections (especially trench mouth); toxic metal poisoning (see Body Observations, **Hair Observations**); and insufficient vitamin C in the diet. Certain drugs such as Dilantin can cause swollen, bleeding gums, and at times toxic metal poisoning will show itself by a thin, dark line adjacent to the gum line.

If you should feel a bump while rubbing under the tongue and inside the cheeks with your finger, it could be a calcified stone in one of the salivary glands, but these usually pass out with time; if, however, there is any discomfort or any hard round bump, no matter how small, it warrants a medical consultation. If the tongue has a smooth, glossy surface or appears unusually dry (without thirst), these could be signs of various anemias or vitamin deficiencies; furrows that run only from front to back could mean an infection such as syphilis; a hairy tongue (one that looks dark and furry at the back surface) usually comes from a fungus infection that can occur while taking antibiotic drugs. If the tongue seems larger than usual, it could come from a hormone disorder, an infection, toxic metal poisoning or blocked veins (varicose veins under the tongue are not unusual after 60 years of age). A swollen, red tongue that is painful can indicate inflammation, anemia or the glossitis of severe vitamin B deficiency. Occasional swelling of the tongue can be seen with edema, glossitis and cellulitis. The tongue grows larger as amyloidosis and acromegaly develop. An enlarged tongue is generally seen with Down's syndrome and hypothyroidism (cretinism and myxedema). A burning sensation in the tongue may come from smoking, and it seems to be quite common in women during the menopause; it can also come from toxic metal poisoning. The tongue should not have a thick white coating, which may indicate precancerous lesions. Dryness of the tongue without swelling or longitudinal lines is one symptom of Sjogrens syndrome (an autoimmune disease found primarily in women past the menopause). Tremor of the tongue occurs with nervousness, thyroid problems (thyrotoxicosis), alcoholism and syphilis. Observation of any deviations from what is usual warrants a medical consultation.

If one or both tonsils look enlarged (the grooves disappear, look fiery red or have yellow or white dots over them), they are probably infected. Because tonsillitis could easily turn into an abscess, it warrants immediate medical attention. Any other swelling, especially if seen in only one tonsil, warrants a medical consultation. If the uvula is red and swollen, it is more apt to be from an allergic reaction; it should return to normal color and size as the allergy is controlled. If, however, it swells to the point where it could interfere with breathing or swallowing, immediate medical attention is warranted.

A red throat (redder than usual) means some sort of throat infection (pharyngitis); very bright, shiny red usually accompanies a streptococcus infection (see Mouth, Throat and Gastrointestinal Tests, **"Strep" Throat**), while a dull red usually accompanies a virus infection or could be from infectious **mononucleosis** (see Blood Tests). If there seems to be a pale membrane or film over the reddened throat, it could mean diphtheria—even in today's world, where all children should have been immunized against this disease. A membrane or film could also be a sign of trench mouth, or Vincent's angina (a severe mouth infection), especially if other areas of the mouth seem to have spots of membrane. Any suspicion of a membrane warrants immediate medical attention. Since a red-looking throat without fever or other symptoms can come from gonorrhea, any red throat that lasts more than one day warrants a medical consultation; if fever occurs and goes above 102 F (38.9 C), immediate medical attention is warranted.

Reliability

As with other observational tests, the early detection of disease, especially precancerous lesions, makes these examinations close to 100 percent effective. When unusual lesions do appear, there is a 90 percent chance that they are abnormal.

"STREP" THROAT
(Detecting streptococcus to prevent rheumatic fever)

While just about everyone has heard of "strep" throat (pharyngitis caused by a particular form of the streptococcus bacteria called group A), not too many people associate the consequences of that throat infection with rheumatic fever—a severe form of heart disease that can also be accompanied by arthritis, kidney infections, skin rashes and lumps under the skin. Once a common, often fatal illness, primarily in children, it seemed to disappear in the late 1950s; since 1985, however, there has been a marked resurgence of rheumatic fever in adults as well as children all over the country. In some areas the number of cases in one year has increased up to eight times greater than the number normally diagnosed. The American Heart Association claims that more than 10,000 people will die of rheumatic fever each year because of the failure to diagnose group A streptococcal infections. This is the same bacteria that also causes scarlet fever.

Not all sore throats are caused by group A streptococcus; in general, except for epidemics, a dangerous strep throat is at fault only about 10 percent of the time. The likelihood of pharyngitis's being from group A streptococcus increases when swallowing is excruciatingly painful, the throat is red and beefy-looking, the tonsils (if they are still present) give off dots of yellow pus and the patient has a high fever, little or no cough and tender, swollen glands alongside the neck. If the condition is diagnosed early enough, and adequate and proper treatment begun, the chances of suffering from rheumatic fever are reduced to almost zero.

At present there are more than three dozen different, relatively simple tests to detect group A streptococcus ("strep A") in the throat. A throat swab (a cotton/dacron swab at the end of a long stick used to touch the back of the throat) is treated with two or more chemicals, and if strep A is present, a color change is seen. The time required to perform the test ranges from five minutes to several hours, depending on the manufacturer's technique; it can take less than two minutes to swab the throat and apply the chemicals and less than 10 minutes for the color change to take place.

What Is Usual
Although few sore throats are caused by strep A, one out of three children may still carry strep A in their throats with no symptoms whatsoever. And recently it has been discovered that house pets can also be carriers and reservoirs of strep A; they may not show symptoms, but they can transmit the bacteria to family members.

What You Need
The test can be performed with any one of the many available throat swab strep A tests. With such a variety offered, it might be best to ask your physician for his or her preference. As a matter of fact, although no prescription is required for the tests, and several companies admit that they are quite simple to perform at home, it may be difficult to obtain them except through your doctor. At present the simplest test of all is called Chroma Chex (Henry Schein Inc., 5 Harbor Park Dr., Port Washington, N.Y. 11050), in which two chemicals are dropped onto the throat swab; it takes only a few minutes and costs the doctor less than $2.00 per test. Other tests cost the doctor from $1.40 to $3.00

What to Watch Out For
If a strep A sore throat is just starting, there may not be enough bacteria to give a positive result; repeat the test again each day if the signs and symptoms indicate a strep throat. Be sure that you know how to take a throat swab; have your doctor show you the proper place and technique. If someone with any sore throat has difficulty breathing, immediate medical attention is warranted.

What the Test Results Can Mean
Strep throat testing at home is primarily for children, and occasionally adults, who are known to have repeated strep throats or are known to be very susceptible to streptococcus infections. Many doctors give such patients several strep A test kits along with the appropriate medicine to take whenever a sore throat occurs and the strep A test is positive. Such a plan is the best known preventive medicine against rheumatic fever. Other doctors recommend home strep testing for families with small children as a routine measure whenever a child complains of a sore throat. But unless you work with

your doctor in such a program, any sore throat, especially with a high fever, deserves medical attention.

Reliability
It does seem that the easiest-to-perform tests and the ones that take the least time are not as accurate as those that are more complicated. However, in general, all of these tests are from 80 percent to 90 percent accurate.

STRING TEST
(A way to help distinguish heartburn from heart trouble)

It has been reported in the medical literature that at least 10 percent of the population suffer from heartburn (sometimes called pyrosis), a burning sensation in the chest just behind the sternum, or breastbone. This painful, aching discomfort is often caused by gastroesophageal reflux, in which stomach acid refluxes, or regurgitates, back into the lower section of the esophagus. The lining of the esophagus is not the same as the lining of the stomach and cannot stand the acid's irritation.

It is now believed that the lower esophageal sphincter (LES)—a sphincter is a band of muscle tissue that opens and closes entrances to body cavities— loses its ability to stay closed against the pressure of the stomach's contents, especially when a person is lying down. Thus, the pain—sometimes described as pressure or cramping—occurs most often about an hour after a meal or during sleep. The condition may be related to hiatal hernia, in which, because of an ostensible defect in the diaphragm muscles, a portion of the stomach is sometimes pushed up into the chest area, causing similar discomfort.

At times the pain can be so acute that a heart attack is erroneously suspected. When 100 consecutive patients with severe chest pains were studied, 77 complained of pain that was identical to that of angina (reduced oxygen to the heart); 16 of the 77 were ultimately diagnosed as having an esophageal problem.

Most doctors feel that 90 percent of the time the diagnosis of gastroesophageal reflux can be made by listening to the patient's history of the pain and noting whether the pain can be relieved with antacids, smaller meals, standing and drinking water, or sleeping with the head of the bed elevated at least eight inches. At times stopping a certain medication, a particular food (chocolate, coffee, tea, tomatoes) or smoking will relieve the discomfort. There are doctors who feel that all alcoholic beverages relax the lower esophageal sphincter sufficiently to cause reflux. There are also doctors who have patients with this problem swallow a lot of saliva (sometimes chewing gum or sucking on candy can help increase salivation); the alkaline pH of the saliva neutralizes the stomach's acid, and this can help confirm the diagnosis.

Another way to help determine whether gastroesophageal reflux could be the cause of chest pain is to perform the string test. A gelatin capsule filled with a 55-inch nylon string that has a loop on its free end is swallowed with a small amount of water—much as a capsule of medicine is taken—after the looped end of the string is fastened to the cheek by adhesive tape. Usually, two string tests are performed—one upon awakening or after fasting for at least four hours and the second about an hour following a filling meal. After 10 minutes to 15 minutes, the string is pulled back up (the capsule at the end is made to detach at the slightest tug and then dissolves), and the string is tested for its pH, or acidity. It can also reveal bleeding in the upper portion of the gastrointestinal tract—esophagus, stomach or duodenum (the beginning of the small intestine)—by showing flecks of red blood on the string as it is withdrawn (see Figure 58).

A point of interest: The string, when left in place for three hours to four hours, can also be used to help detect certain parasites that are difficult to find in feces (see Mouth, Throat and Gastrointestinal Tests, **Feces Observations**), giardiasis in particular—probably the most common cause of episodic diarrhea. Many doctors also send the recovered string to a commercial laboratory to be examined for cancer cells and other intestinal infections.

You can estimate where portions of the string were located by measuring the distance from the teeth to the xiphoid process (the lowest point of the sternum), which lies over the esophagus. That part of the string which went through the stomach into the small intestine is usually a greenish brown color after having been stained by bile. The portion of the string in between the two designated areas will have been in the stomach. For an average-size adult, the first 15 inches of string from the teeth usually correspond to the esophagus; from 15 inches to 21 inches, the stomach; and the stained remainder, the duodenum (the first part of the small intestine).

What Is Usual

After the string has remained in the upper gastrointestinal tract for 15 minutes and has been retrieved, it is immediately stroked with a special pH (acidity-detecting) indicator stick, which comes with the string, and compared to an accompanying color chart. That portion of the string that rested in the esophagus should show a pH close to neutral, or a numerical value of 7. The length of string that was in the stomach should be acid—a value of 5 or less. The end of the string that passed through the stomach into the duodenum, where it should have been exposed to bile, is usually alkaline—a value of 7 or greater. If no food had been eaten for several hours prior to the test, the string should remain white (except for possible bile staining);

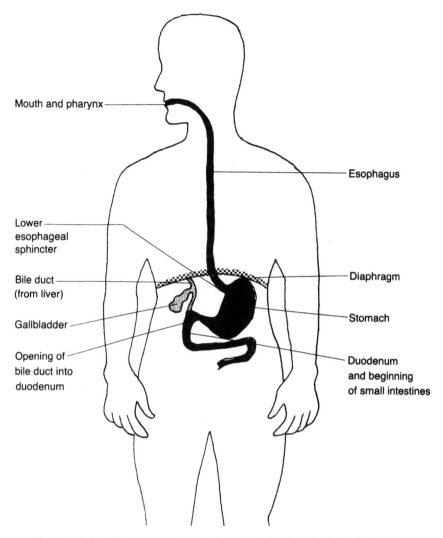

Figure 58. Bodily areas and locations involved with the string test.

eating within an hour before the test can cause flecks of partially digested food to stick to the string, but this does not interfere with acid testing.

What You Need

You use an Entero-Test, containing the capsule, string, pH indicator stick and pH color chart; it costs your doctor or a hospital about $3.50. A pediatric Entero-Test is also available at the same cost, using a smaller-size capsule and a shorter string (36 inches); this version can be used by adults for gastroesophageal reflux or blood testing, but the longer string should be used when searching for parasites in adults. If testing is to be limited to the detection of blood and/or acidity, the Gastro-Test is available at the same price; this test takes only 15 minutes. At the present time the string test may require a prescription or be obtained from your physician to be performed at home before and after a meal. You will need a pocket light microscope should you wish to search for parasites; they cost from $7.95 to $30.00.

What to Watch Out For

If you have had, or are having, severe chest pain, do not attempt the string test until you have obtained medical attention and a doctor has ruled out heart, liver, gallbladder or lung disease. Be sure to tape the loose, looped end of the string to your cheek before swallowing the capsule. If you are going to leave the string in place for more than three hours to search for parasites, be sure to fast for at least four hours prior to testing and sip only water, if necessary, during the test period. Should the string seem impossible to retrieve, simply cut it off at the mouth and swallow it. No ill effects should occur, and you can repeat the test later.

What the Test Results Can Mean

If that portion of the string which was limited to the esophagus shows acidity (a pH of 6 or less), it usually means that stomach acid is escaping into the esophagus. Such a finding, especially if accompanied by heartburnlike symptoms, warrants a medical consultation. If the portion of the string that was in the stomach shows little or no evidence of any acid (a pH of 6 or greater), it could be a sign of pernicious anemia and also warrants a medical consultation. Thyroid disease, adrenal gland dysfunction and growths in the stomach can also cause a lack of acid in the stomach. Failure to see bile staining on that part of the string which should have gone through the stomach into the small intestines could indicate a gallbladder or liver problems (see Urine Tests, **Clinical Analysis: Bilirubin**). Any sign of bleeding on the string, no matter where, warrants medical attention. If there is any doubt about whether a pink or red stain on the string is blood, a Hemastix dipstick (see Urine Tests, **Clinical Analysis: Blood**) can be touched to the suspicious area. If parasites are suspected, a medical consultation should already have been sought. If the parasites have not been identified, rubbing that portion of the string which was in the small intestines on a glass slide and viewing the slide through a pocket light microscope could reveal a live parasite or its cyst (egg form); see Figure 56. Identification of a parasite warrants medical attention.

Reliability

The string test is considered to be 90 percent accurate in determining pH measurements. Many doctors feel that it is the best test for giardiasis.

GENITOURINARY SYSTEM TESTS

MURPHY'S KIDNEY PUNCH
(An aid in locating the cause of a backache)

Many people simply endure what seems to be a chronic backache—uncomfortable, but not painful enough for them to seek a medical consultation. In many instances the cause is a muscle strain from overexertion or exercise. But a backache can also signal the beginning of kidney disease, most likely an infection in or around the outside of the kidney. The sooner a kidney problem is detected and treated, the less chance there is for permanent kidney damage and uremia—an extremely toxic condition that can require dialysis and even be fatal. Repeated testing by performing Murphy's kidney punch whenever a backache occurs can be lifesaving.

The kidneys are located within the abdominal portion of the body toward the back and just under the ribs. To be more specific, they lie just beneath the skin of the back where the lowest (12th) rib joins the spinal column; the area is called the costovertebral angle (*costo* pertains to the ribs; *vertebral* refers to the spinal column). Some doctors call this area the costophrenic angle, because it is also where the 12th rib lies adjacent to the diaphragm (*phrenic* refers to the diaphragm). Usually, the left kidney is a bit higher than the right, because of the liver's location just above the right kidney.

If the kidney is infected, it usually swells, and a mild blow over the costovertebral angle with the side of a closed fist will likely elicit a sensation of pain or severe discomfort (see Figure 59). Some doctors now use short jabs with the thumb or the heel of the palm instead of the fist; the end result is the same.

What Is Usual
A moderate thump or jab over the costovertebral angle (whether self-administered or performed by another) should elicit no discomfort at all.

What You Need
A few minutes are required to feel your back and locate the costovertebral angle; follow the bottom edge of the lowest rib until it joins the spine.

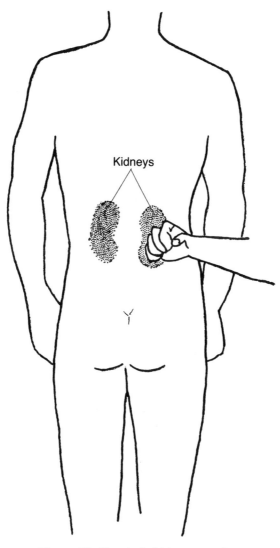

Figure 59. Murphy's kidney punch.

What to Watch Out For

Do not hit too hard; a forceful blow is not necessary when the kidney is infected. Of course, if you are very obese, it may be hard to pinpoint the costovertebral angle, but a blow to the general area should still elicit acute discomfort different from the dull ache of muscle strain.

What the Test Results Can Mean

A positive Murphy's kidney punch sign (a sharp pain when the costovertebral angle is thumped) warrants medical attention. Most often this means a kidney infection; but it could also reflect other kidney pathology. (See Urine Tests, **Clinical Analysis: Blood, Clinical Analysis: Leukocytes** and **Clinical Analysis: Nitrite.**) A colicky pain in the same area (intermittent and not necessarily related to movement) that occurs without thumping is one sign of kidney stones.

Reliability

Pain elicited by Murphy's kidney punch is considered 80 percent accurate as an indication of kidney disease.

Note: Originally, this test was called Murphy's sign. Now most physicians use the term *Murphy's sign* for yet another physical examination test: They push their fingers under the right front ribs and have the patient take a deep breath; if this causes pain, it can mean gallbladder disease. A third similar-named test devised by a Dr. John Benjamin Murphy, a Chicago surgeon who practiced in the late 1800s to 1916, is drumming the fingers—as if playing a piano—over the appendix area; if the usual resonant sound is not heard, it can indicate appendicitis.

NOCTURNAL PENILE TUMESCENCE MONITORING
(An inexpensive way to help ascertain the cause of impotence)

Impotence means the inability to achieve an erection of the penis; it has nothing to do with fertility, or the ability to cause pregnancy. Some doctors refine the definition and limit it to the inability to achieve an erection for a long enough period of time to permit successful sexual intercourse. Although the condition was once thought to be almost always psychological, it has now been shown that a substantial number of men suffer impotence due to an organic or physical problem; the most recent study revealed that one out of every eight men over the age of 40 suffers from some degree of medically treatable impotence.

- Impotence may be secondary to a seemingly unrelated disease, such as diabetes, in which subsequent atherosclerosis can interfere with the blood supply to the penis or diabetes-caused impairment of nerve impulse transmission occurs; leukemia, Peyronie's disease and even sickle-cell anemia can also be to blame.
- In one study heart disease was the specific cause in 1.5 million men.
- The problem can be caused by testosterone deficiency, which can be the result of normal aging but can also come from pituitary disease; thyroid imbalance; adrenal conditions that interfere with cortisone production; or simply testicle dysfunction.

- An old, seemingly unrelated injury or previous surgery on the pelvis or spinal cord can be the underlying cause.
- Prostate problems—especially growths, but also as a consequence of some sexually transmitted disease—can also be responsible.
- Smoking and other lung problems have been shown to be associated with impotence (see Breath and Lung Tests, **Pulmonary Function Measurements;** Environmental Tests, **Carbon Monoxide**).
- The repeated use of certain hair preparations, especially those that claim to promote hair growth, may be an overlooked factor; some contain estrogens (female hormones).
- Drugs are probably the most common cause; anything from large amounts of alcohol (colloquially referred to as "distiller's droop"), to normal doses of sedatives, tranquilizers, antianxiety and antidepressant medicines, small amounts of narcotics and most—but not all—drugs used to treat high blood pressure have been shown to prevent erection as a side effect. Some other medications also known to be at fault, although not as frequently, include: anticholinergics and other atropinelike drugs; decongestant nose drops; antihistamines; estrogens (which may be found in certain meats if the animals were fattened by hormones); toxin-producing fungi (mycotoxins such as zearalenone), which can grow on improperly stored grains such as corn or wheat and, if eaten, act as if they were estrogens (some doctors feel that the oil in certain vitamin E capsules could contain the toxin); some preparations used to treat cancer, glaucoma and parasites; a few antibiotics; Cimetedine (a form of antihistamine used to treat ulcers); and drugs used to treat parkinsonism (incidentally, many of these drugs can also cause frigidity in women).

The basic test to help distinguish physical from psychological causes for impotence is nocturnal penile tumescence monitoring, usually performed in hospital sleep-disorder centers, where measuring devices record whether penile erections occur during sleep and, if so, their number and degree. It is considered normal for a man to have from one to four penile erections intermittently throughout the night during the deepest stage of sleep—called REM sleep because it is accompanied by *rapid eye movements*. Such professional testing is quite expensive, and many doctors suggest that patients worried about impotence first perform the stamp test version of nocturnal penile tumescence monitoring at home.

Just prior to retiring, a strip of several stamps connected only by perforations at each side is placed around the base of the flaccid penis so that the first stamp is glued over the last to make a closed ring. The stamps are then examined the next morning, upon awakening, to see whether any of the perforations along the sides were torn open—an indication that at least one erection probably took place during sleep (see Figure 60). The test should be repeated for three nights.

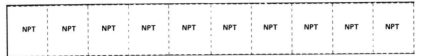

Strip of Nocturnal penile tumescence stamps as manufactured at the Oregon Health Sciences University

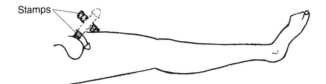

Figure 60. Nocturnal penile tumescence screening.

What Is Usual

It is considered normal for the stamps to tear during the night (indicating an erection during sleep). Nocturnal erections usually tend to lessen after the age of 50 but should still occur occasionally.

What You Need

A strip of stamps or segments of glue-backed paper connected only by perforations at the side is required; while the post office sells a ready-made roll of five hundred 1-cent stamps for $5.00, you can make a similar, far-less-expensive device by asking a postal clerk to tear off one or more horizontal strips of 1-cent stamps from their standard sheets of 100. An article in a medical journal (*Urology*, February 1980) reports that postal officials require you to obtain permission from the Secret Service in the Treasury Department in order to use postage stamps for such testing; the office of the Chief Postal Inspector, however, says that there are no legal restrictions on using postage stamps to test for impotence. That same medical article also notes that use of Christmas Seals for this purpose requires permission from the American Lung Association. Some stationery stores carry glue-backed or gummed sheets of address labels that are separated by perforations. And as of now there seem to be no restrictions on the use of trading stamps.

The Oregon Health Sciences University Printing Service (Portland, Ore. 97201) sells nocturnal penile tumescence (NPT) screening stamps; a minimum order of 10 sheets of 90 stamps at a cost of $1.00 per sheet is required. Checks should be made out to the Urology Gift Account, No. 70-262-2846; the cost is tax-deductible.

For those who simply cannot bring themselves to consider strips of stamps as professional scientific equipment, there is the Dacomed Snap-Gauge, a specially designed, padded, cloth and plastic band that is fastened around the penis with Velcro straps. The device not only reacts to an enlargement of the penis, it also contains three separately colored built-in snap elements that are set to break at different levels of rigidity, thus providing a much more precise measure of intercourse capability, which is considered perfectly normal if all three snap elements break during the night. Although this device does not require a prescription, and can be used in the privacy of one's home, it is advisable to obtain the Snap-Gauge through a physician or sex counselor. The cost to the doctor is $20.00 each. The Snap-Gauge is made by the Dacomed Corporation (1701 East 79th St., Minneapolis, Minn. 55420). When compared to the usual $1,000.00-a-night charge by professional impotence-testing (sleep) laboratories, the cost is relatively minor; some health insurance companies will reimburse you for the cost of the Snap-Gauge when used under a doctor's direction.

A unique, much more technical device for home use is the Life-Tech Bedside Monitor; a doctor usually leases this book-size box to the patient for a few nights. This monitor records the presence and degree of erections on graphs and shows the difference between the strength of the erection at the base of the penis, between the base and the tip and at the tip, along with the times of occurrence. A particular feature of this monitor is an alarm that wakes the patient when an erection occurs so that its presence can be confirmed. The rental fee is up to the doctor but seems to average $300.00 for three nights' use; health insurance companies and Medicare reimburse from 80 percent to 100 percent of the rental fee.

What to Watch Out For

Check that the stamp perforations tear easily; some postage stamps today are difficult to tear apart. Do not use alcohol or take any sedatives or sleeping medicines for at least two days before testing; these drugs tend to prevent REM sleep, during which nocturnal erections are most apt to occur.

What the Test Results Can Mean

Tearing apart of the strip of stamps during the night usually means that an erection took place. If erections are impossible at other times, there is the possibility that the problem is psychological, and a medical consultation is warranted. Failure of the stamps to tear over a three-night period can mean that some physical condition or drug interference is causing the impotence, and a medical consultation is warranted to help detect the underlying condition or uncover the dastardly drug. If the Dacomed Snap-Gauge is used, the results are best interpreted by your physician.

One possible reason for a false-positive result (indicating impotence when none may exist) may be the fact that as one ages, the amount of REM sleep during the night normally decreases. In other words, it may also become necessary to evaluate one's sleep patterns independently of ostensible impotence. And recent research hints that nocturnal erections may not always be related to a strictly sexual erection.

Reliability

Most doctors consider the stamp test 80 percent accurate in detecting nocturnal erections. The Dacomed Snap-Gauge is better than 90 percent accurate. The ability to have any nocturnal erection is considered to be 90 percent reliable as an indication that an impotence problem is treatable.

PROSTATE OBSERVATIONS
(One way to help detect a common cancer in men)

The prostate, a small gland found only in men, is considered an integral part of the reproductive system because of its chemical and enzyme secretions, which increase during sexual activity. It is located just under the bladder at the point adjacent to where the urethra begins (the urethra is the tube that carries urine from the bladder through the penis to the outside). The prostate is also adjacent to the wall of the rectum, about three inches from the anus (see Figure 61).

Normally, the prostate stays the same size until around the age of 50, after which it almost always grows larger, so that by the age of 70 virtually every man has some degree of enlargement. Unfortunately, such enlargement sometimes makes urination difficult in various ways. It may be a strain to start urinating; the normal force of urination may be lessened (most men become consciously aware when the force of urination seems less than usual); or it may seem that the amount of urine is diminished, causing a need to urinate more often. Such conditions can cause urine to remain in the bladder for longer periods than normal and can lead to bladder or kidney infection. (See Urine Tests, **Clinical Analysis: Leukocytes** and **Clinical Analysis: Nitrite.**) An enlarged or infected prostate may also be the cause of blood in the urine (see Urine Tests, **Clinical Analysis: Blood**). Then there is the possibility of cancer's developing in the gland; it is estimated that 90,000 American men will have such a cancer diagnosed each year (it is the second most common cancer in men), and no one knows how many go undiagnosed. The earlier any enlarged or nodular prostate gland is detected, the easier the treatment and the less serious the consequences; when cancer is found to be limited to within the prostate gland, it is curable.

While there are many sophisticated chemical blood and urine tests to help diagnose prostate disease, the digital rectal examination is still considered the most sensitive and efficient of all prostate tests. Many partners have learned to perform this simple examination semiannually to the satisfaction and inner security of all parties. Some doctors even teach their male patients to perform the test on themselves; sometimes this self-examination is more easily performed lying on one's back.

What Is Usual

After the person whose prostate is to be examined bends over a table or bed with the stomach and chest down on the surface (the knees may be bent to suit the height of the table or bed), the examiner lubricates a gloved finger and gently presses it against the anus at first, without trying to insert it (see Figure 61). Repeated light pressure will allow the finger to enter the rectum more easily than a sudden, forceful insertion attempt. The process is similar to the insertion of an enema tip or a suppository. Once the finger is inside the rectum to its full length, it is moved lightly back and forth over the anterior rectal surface (toward the abdominal side). The prostate gland should be obvious and feel about 1 inch to 1¼ inches in size (some doctors describe it as walnut-size), and it usually protrudes against the wall of the rectum. With a normal-size prostate, a shallow vertical groove is commonly felt in the midline between the two lobes on either side that make up the smooth posterior surface of the gland. If you make a very tight fist and feel the soft but firm area between the base of the thumb and the base of the index finger, it approximates normal prostate consistency (see Figure 62).

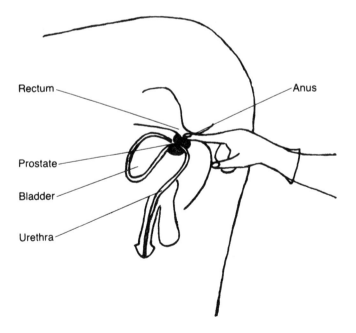

Figure 61. Prostate examination.

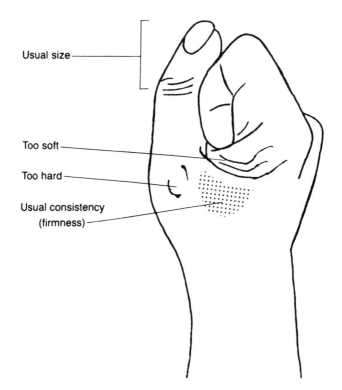

Usual size

Too soft

Too hard

Usual consistency
(firmness)

Figure 62. Making a fist to approximate the prostate gland's size and consistency.

When the finger is lightly pressed from the outer margins of the prostate toward the center or midline portion repeatedly, it simulates a prostate massage, often employed when performing the urine **Two/Three-Glass Test** (see Urine Tests, **Urine Observations**).

What You Need

The test requires a thin latex, rubber or plastic glove (disposable plastic gloves that fit any size hand are best; latex gloves cost $10.00 per 100, and disposables cost $5.00 per 100); some lubricant such as glycerine, plain (not carbolated) petroleum jelly or petrolatum (Vaseline is one brand name; greaseless K-Y Jelly, which doctors prefer, costs $1.00 a tube and is another similar product); and patience and understanding between examiner and examinee.

What to Watch Out For

The following cautions apply when performing the test:

- The bladder and the bowels should be emptied prior to examination.
- The examining finger should not have a long, sharp fingernail.
- Do not use any medicated ointment for a lubricant.
- Do not force the entrance of the examining finger; if strong resistance is felt, do not attempt the examination.

What the Test Results Can Mean

If the size of the prostate does not seem larger than the distance between the tip of the thumb and the first joint, if the consistency is not soft or mushy, if the midline groove can be felt and if there are no nodules that feel like a hard, bony thumb joint, the chances are reasonable that the prostate is as it should be. If, however, there is any suspicion of something abnormal in terms of size, shape, texture or smoothness, that is the time to seek medical attention. Many doctors will use this examination to verify a partner's observations and confirm the findings for future testing. Some doctors will use a routine medical checkup to teach the prostate examination—but usually only on request.

Note: Many doctors will touch the gloved finger used for prostate examination to occult blood testing material (see Mouth, Throat and Gastrointestinal Tests, **Occult Blood [Feces]**) to perform a feces occult blood test at the same time. You can do so, too.

Reliability

The finding of any enlargement or hard area in or on the prostate gland is almost always (90 percent) abnormal. The chance of cancer, however, is less than 5 percent. Most often such an abnormality will be benign hypertrophy (a very slow-growing, noncancerous enlargement).

OVULATION TIME
(Primarily for the woman having difficulty becoming pregnant)

One out of every six couples who want to have children find it almost impossible to do so. While the causes for an inability to become pregnant can be diverse and multiple, there is a common belief that failure to have intercourse at the "right" time is a major factor—the "right" time being within 24 hours after ovulation, or when, in the normal menstrual cycle, the ovary gives off an egg to be fertilized (ovulates); this is called ovulation time. Medical observations show that a potentially fertilizable egg will live a day or two, while sperm will live inside the vagina and uterus for about three days. Thus, since the time for conception is relatively limited, the more precise one can be about ovulation time, the better the opportunity for a pregnancy—assuming, of course, that timing is the only problem affecting the couple's inability to conceive.

Basal body temperature. Prior to 1985 ovulation time was primarily determined through regular body temperature measurements. Known commonly as basal body temperature (BBT) testing, the technique is still quite commonly used. (It is also employed as a family-planning device, and here intercourse is purposely *avoided* for several days after ovulation.) To determine ovulation time using basal body temperature, you simply take your temperature every morning, immediately upon awakening and before getting out of bed, and keep a regular chart record of the results (see Figure 63). If ovulation occurs—and it does not always happen every single month—a small, but definite rise in temperature can be detected, usually involving about a one-degree rise that takes place midway between menstrual periods.

Lutenizing hormone detection. Since 1985 a host of new, simpler and relatively more accurate tests have become available to detect ovulation time. Virtually all are based on the same principle: an expected surge in a particular body hormone called lutenizing hormone (LH), which, within 24 hours, will prompt the ovary to give off an egg and send it on its course to the uterus. The sudden excess of LH is almost immediately excreted in the urine, where it can be detected through special testing.

There are several different types of kits using dipsticks or test tube solutions to detect LH; all are supposed to show ovulation by a color change. Some of the kits allow for 5 days of testing, some for six days and some for up to 10 days; the more days the test is performed, the more apt one is to spot the exact day of ovulation. Some require that only the first morning urine be tested, while others allow testing at any time of the day. At present there are many different brand-name kits, and they are all about equally sensitive; the primary differences are in the number of days that the test can be performed and the complexity of the technique. If you cannot decide on a particular kit, you might ask your doctor for the benefit of his or her experience.

Cervical mucus. Another far less high-tech but nonetheless long-standing test for ovulation time involves the change in the viscosity (thickness or thinness) of the mucus normally secreted by the cervix during a menstrual cycle; it is sometimes called the *spinnbarkeit* test (the word means "threadiness"). To perform the test, a woman removes some mucus from the vagina with a finger and then places it between the thumb and forefinger. She then slowly spreads the thumb and finger apart; most of the time during the menstrual cycle, the mucus is thick and sticky and will not stretch for more than an inch across the spreading fingers without breaking. A day before ovulation, and for a day or two afterward, the mucus suddenly becomes thin and watery and will stretch easily, without breaking, as a long string between widely separated fingers. There are doctors who consider this test more accurate

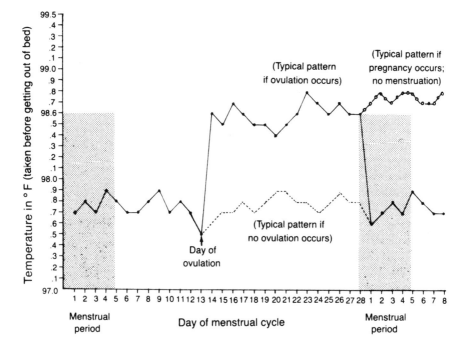

Note: During childbearing years the usual body temperature of a nonpregnant woman ranges between 97.5 F and 98 F.

Figure 63. Typical ovulation time (basal body temperature) test pattern.

than basal body temperature, and in fact, mucus viscosity has become incorporated into new high-technology ovulation-time-detection devices.

Salivary/vaginal secretions. Present state-of-the-art at-home ovulation-time-detection devices now measure electrolyte (sodium, calcium, potassium) changes in saliva that are known to occur during the menstrual cycle while at the same time evaluating changes in cervical mucus in the vagina. Usually, detectable saliva changes occur five days to six days before ovulation, and this allows a more precise evaluation of mucus changes in the vagina; this not only permits a more accurate ovulation-time determination but also markedly reduces the emotional anxiety and physical strain affecting the couple, who now have several days to plan their intercourse as opposed to the less-than-24-hour notice offered by most other tests. Such computer devices look like small, hand-held calculators with separate sensors (probes) for the mouth and vagina. The battery-powered computers evaluate all the data detected by the two probes and then visually display the expected day of ovulation.

What Is Usual

While it is usual for a woman to have a menstrual cycle every 28 days, it is not abnormal for that cycle to run from 24 days to 35 days. And just as it is usual for a woman to ovulate once each cycle, it is not abnormal for a cycle to go by where ovulation does not occur. The usual temperature and vaginal mucus findings have already been described.

What You Need

For basal body temperature testing, an ordinary fever-detecting thermometer is quite adequate. Today's easier-to-read digital thermometers now cost about $6.00. Special glass ovulation thermometers (easier to read than fever thermometers) are available for about $4.00; these usually come with special graph paper for daily charting of temperature readings. There are relatively expensive automated and computerized thermometers that remind you to take your temperature and then translate the findings into your expected ovulation time; they can cost up to $160.00.

Ovulation-time dipstick or test tube kits cost from $20.00 to $70.00, with the price depending mostly on the number of daily test that can be performed. Computerized ovulation-time predictors may be rented or purchased, usually through a physician. The rent is about $50.00 per month, and the purchase price runs from $400.00 to $500.00.

What to Watch Out For

In most instances the tests are predicated on a reasonably normal menstrual cycle; if your time between menstrual periods varies considerably, it warrants a medical consultation prior to ovulation-time testing. The test devices usually require following directions exactly; timing, time of day and measurements must be precise. Obviously, basal body temperature readings are useless if you have a fever. And certain drugs can interfere with some test kit results; check with your doctor or pharmacist.

What the Test Results Can Mean

When ovulation is pinpointed, it permits the best possible timing for sperm and egg to meet to produce pregnancy. But that is all; the test does not indicate any of the other myriad causes of infertility. Most doctors, however, consider this test the first and least expensive approach to overcoming conception problems. There are some doctors, though, who decry ovulation-time test kits; they feel that the marital and sexual disharmony that can come from attempting to adhere to a specific time schedule for intercourse far outweighs their possible benefits.

Reliability

There seems to be some disagreement between doctors and the manufacturers of the LH-detection test kits. The companies that make the kits claim a 98 percent accuracy rate, but there have been studies indicating that at least 15 percent of the test results are false-negative; that is, they fail to show when ovulation will occur. Other studies indicate that the test kit may show the hormone surge, but ovulation does not follow. In general, the kits are accurate enough for a home-use trial prior to seeking professional help.

Basal body temperature tests, especially if performed along with cervical mucus observations, are considered to be from 22 percent to 75 percent accurate, depending on which medical study you accept. Computerized ovulation-time predictors are considered at least 90 percent accurate in determining ovulation time but not necessarily in helping couples achieve pregnancy.

An important fact to consider, when it comes to suspected infertility, is that most gynecologists who specialize in this field feel that testing for infertility should not be started until a couple has gone at least one year deliberately but unsuccessfully attempting pregnancy (without any sort of contraceptive).

Seminal fluid (sperm) screening. Infertility may come from the failure of the man to produce sperm. One simple test, performed in the privacy of one's home under a doctor's directions, is the detection of semen—the whitish fluid from the penis that carries sperm—in the vagina following intercourse. Specifically, this is a test to determine whether the enzyme acid phosphatase (a normal constituent of semen) is present. It is a simple, three-minute procedure, and while not absolutely diagnostic, it can help your doctor help you. A kit called Seminal-Screen that allows you to perform the test twice is available through your doctor from David Diagnostics (4601 Broadway, Astoria, N.Y. 11103) for $4.50. In general, the test is close to 100 percent accurate when used within 24 hours after intercourse and where, of course, semen was present.

Home seminal fluid collection. When sperm are produced, such as may be indicated by the semen Seminal-Screen test, but fertility is still primarily a male problem, microscopic study of that sperm may be indicated. Since collection of a semen sample can be embarrassing, your doctor can now supply you with an Apex Medical Technologies home collection kit that allows proper deposition, storage and transportation of the semen sample; the kits cost $4.00.

ALLERGY TESTS

PATCH TESTING
(Screening for allergic reactions of the skin and other body organs)

Patch testing to detect allergic or hypersensitivity reactions was first tried nearly 100 years ago; it is still considered a valuable, if not precise, evaluation of an individual's immune system response to provocation. When an antigen (bacteria, virus, parasite, poison, pollen, animal dander, chemical or unfamiliar protein such as may be found in food) enters or touches the body, it can provoke the production of specific antibodies by certain body organs. These antibodies, now known to be immunoglobulins, circulate through the blood to where the antigens have settled; in the case of allergy, it may be in the lungs, causing asthma; in the skin, causing a rash; in the bowels, causing diarrhea; or in the nose, causing sneezing and mucus production—to name but a very few manifestations. If one's immunity is in good working order, the antibodies help prevent disease and/or allergic symptoms.

The patch test is a means of applying a suspected allergy-causing antigen to the skin's surface to see whether it provokes an antibody response. Although this test really only measures the response of the skin, some doctors feel that it can offer valuable clues to other allergic-type bodily responses—asthma, bloodshot eyes, eczema, hay fever, headaches, hyperactivity, runny nose, sinusitis, stomach cramps, diarrhea, urticaria (hives), rheumatoid arthritis and even personality changes such as learning difficulties and bizarre behavior.

The patch test is almost identical to the doctor's intradermal skin test, the exception being that no needle injection is made just under the surface of the skin. Instead, place a very small amount of the potentially allergenic substance (about the size of the head of a paper match) on a half-inch circle or square of gauze; if it is not already in liquid form, mix it well into one or two drops of water or mineral oil—the oil will not evaporate, as water sometimes does. Then place the wet patch of gauze against the skin and cover it with adhesive tape; unmedicated Band-Aid-type adhesive bandages have the gauze patch built in and work well. Use skin surfaces where there is no hair, such as the inside of the arm or the back. Leave the patch in place for two days (48 hours), and try not to let it become wet. If, however, the skin under the patch starts to itch, burn, ache or feel irritated in any way, no matter how slight, remove the patch immediately and wash the area well with water. Should the irritation continue, apply a nonprescription cortisone ointment and consult your physician.

After the patch is removed, your susceptibility to the substance applied is supposedly indicated by the extent to which redness, swelling, papules (pimples), vesicles (blisters) and itching are observed (see Figure 64) on the skin

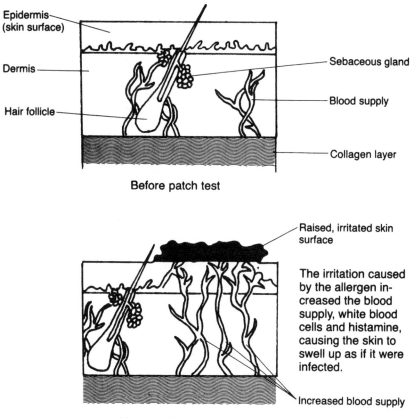

Epidermis
(skin surface)

Dermis

Hair follicle

Sebaceous gland

Blood supply

Collagen layer

Before patch test

Raised, irritated skin surface

The irritation caused by the allergen increased the blood supply, white blood cells and histamine, causing the skin to swell up as if it were infected.

Increased blood supply

After positive patch test

Figure 64. Allergy patch testing—diagrammatic cross-section view of the skin before patch test is applied and after positive patch test. The skin consists of two distinct layers, with the epidermis being the surface layer. Under the dermis layer is subcutaneous tissue, which includes collagen (the protein fibers that act as a matrix to hold tissues and organs together).

where it was in contact with the antigen (see Body Observations, **Skin Observations**). A skin response (positive reaction, in which the surface of the skin is raised and usually red where it came into contact with the allergy-provoking substance) may not appear for anywhere from one hour to two additional days after the patch is removed, so the skin test site should be examined for up to two days afterward. If no signs of irritation are seen, it is then considered a negative reaction (see Figure 64). It has been observed that positive reactions that appear immediately (irritation before the patch was supposed to be removed) are more apt to come from allergies to drugs or foods, while allergies to plants, pollens and pets seem to take longer to show themselves. Positive delayed reactions are also thought to be indicative of a poorly functioning immune system and may suggest an increased susceptibility to disease in general.

Should you attempt patch testing for the first time, always place two additional identical patches, one patch completely dry and another soaked with the water or oil used to mix with the test substance—but both without the test substance—on different areas of the skin to be sure that you are not allergic to the gauze, adhesive tape or diluting liquid. If either of the "control" patches shows a positive reaction, the allergy test cannot be considered accurate, and different material should be tried.

It is quite possible to test for several different allergy-provoking substances at the same time, but each patch should be kept well separated from the others. If a negative response appears in the face of a very suspicious substance, it may be that the amount of test material was insufficient to provoke a reaction; try the test again a week later with twice as much material.

When selecting test material for allergy patch testing, start out with the most common allergy-causing substances. Foods frequently to blame are milk, eggs (most often only the white part) and wheat flour. Should a piece of bread provoke a positive reaction, you may have to retest using the specific grains from which the flour was made; then again, an allergy can come from the bread's other added ingredients. In some cases it turns out not to be the food that causes the allergy but rather the chemicals that restaurants and food processors use on and in foods to keep them looking fresh, enhance flavor, provide color and prevent spoilage; for example, **sulfites** (see Environmental Tests); tartrazine, or FD&C yellow No. 5—a food coloring; and monosodium glutamate (MSG).

Testing for an allergy to pets requires a bit of animal hair or feathers; sometimes a drop or two of the animal's saliva will provoke a more specific reaction. Birds seem to cause far more allergies than is generally suspected; they spread their symptom-producing substances throughout a room every time they preen themselves and flap their wings—even while in their cages.

Pollen testing may be difficult when grasses, trees and weeds are involved, so it is best to try to isolate the specific pollen; if this is not possible, you can use a bit of grass or leaves, but be sure that they have not been sprayed with pesticides, fertilizers or other chemicals. Obtaining pollen from house plants and flowers should be less of a problem.

While drugs are the most common cause of allergic reactions, drug allergies are also the easiest to test for. You must use extreme caution, however, when evaluating sensitivity to medicines, for sometimes the tiniest trace of a drug—especially a penicillin product—can cause a severe reaction. In addition, animal feed can contain several drugs, especially antibiotics, and at times animals (especially chickens and fish) are dipped in antibiotic solutions before being marketed; eating meat from such animals can also provoke an allergic reaction. Never test yourself for a drug allergy if you already know that you are allergic to any other drug.

Other common allergy-provoking substances include: house dust, cotton linters and other upholstery—and mattress-stuffing materials—even the stuffing in toys, various fabrics, tobacco smoke, insecticides, paints, cosmetics, deodorants, toothpaste, detergents, molds, cockroach body parts (more common than previously believed) and smog (see Environmental Tests, **Air Pollution**); the list is virtually endless.

The purpose of patch testing is not only to detect allergy-provoking substances but, more important, to enable you to eliminate them from your life if at all possible. This, of course, is not always easy; if the family pet turns out to be the guilty party, simply putting that pet in another home might not result in any improvements until all traces of the animal's hair and saliva and everything that the hair or saliva came in contact with are also removed. It is usually easier to change the environment of the allergic person on a trial basis to one in which no pets are kept and see what happens in a week or so. If a specific household product turns out to be the cause of an allergy, removal of the substance might be rewarded by symptom relief within days. With pollen-type allergies, desensitization by your doctor may be attempted, but it is not always successful; avoiding the pollen by filtering the air (see Environmental Tests, **Indoor Air Pollution**) may help, but usually total removal of the pollen source is the only truly effective treatment.

What Is Usual
Any allergy is not really normal; unfortunately, many people seem to inherit their allergic tendency, and while not normal, it is still "usual" for such an individual.

What You Need
The patch test requires small, square or round gauze pads and adhesive tape (if you already know that you are allergic to adhesive tape, you might try hypoallergenic tapes). Band-Aids and similar brands of spot or square

bandages are preferable because they have adhesive tape all around the gauze, but strip Band-aid types work very well. A tube of a cortisone skin cream or ointment may also be needed should skin irritation occur.

What to Watch Out For

You should be alert for any intense allergic response; do not leave a patch test on if any irritation, no matter how slight, occurs. Use a patch that will not allow easy evaporation of the liquid—that is, one that is not too porous. If at all possible, try to keep the test substance free of any contamination. Never leave a patch test on for more than 48 hours, but be sure to continue watching the test area for at least two days after removing the patch. If you already know that you are allergic, or seem to have allergy-type reactions, to any substances, check with your doctor before attempting any patch test. Do not attempt patch testing if you have any skin irritation, such as a sunburn or skin infection. Do not rub or put any pressure either on the patch while it is in place or on the test area after the patch has been removed; it can cause a false-positive reaction. If you are taking any antiallergy medicine, such as an antihistamine or a cortisone product, check with your doctor before testing; such drugs can cause false-negative reactions.

Keep in mind that certain areas of your body may be more sensitive than others; many people find the back twice as sensitive as the inner part of the upper arm. Some people find that when they apply patch tests early in the morning, they seem to have a greater, more immediate, response than when they are applied in the afternoon. Many allergies are known to be active to a greater or lesser extent at different times of the day; asthma, for example, is frequently worse at night. If the patches are placed too near each other, a positive test with one patch can cause an adjacent patch to test false-positive.

What the Test Results Can Mean

A positive patch test usually, but not always, indicates an allergy to the test material. When subsequent avoidance or elimination of that substance brings relief from allergy symptoms, the test has been successful. Again, a positive patch test may reflect only the skin's allergic response; it may not always be of value in pinpointing the cause of other allergic symptoms. And a negative patch test does not always rule out an allergy. Evidence of allergy that cannot be controlled by avoidance or elimination warrants a medical consultation. Patch tests that show a positive (allergic) response within minutes, or even within an hour, warrant medical attention; you could be so unusually sensitive that you require an antiallergy protection kit on hand at all times, together with knowledge of how to use it. Other indications of allergy such as dermatographism or a seemingly allergic response to water warrant a medical consultation to search for some possible underlying disease; itching after a bath is a common symptom of polycythemia (too many red blood cells). (For further information, see the discussion of supplementary tests at the end of this entry.)

Many people who are allergic to tartrazine are also allergic to aspirin and aspirin-containing medicines. Conversely, those with a known allergy to aspirin are frequently allergic to tartrazine.

Should you ultimately prove to suffer from an allergy, be sure to carry with you, or wear, some sort of identification to notify others of that fact. This is particularly important if you are allergic to a drug such as penicillin, and it can also help you avoid other problems related to hypersensitivity.

Reliability
A positive skin test reaction indicating an allergy to egg whites is 90 percent accurate; positive (allergy-indicating) reactions to other foods range from 30 percent to 80 percent accurate. For other (nonfood) allergies many allergists feel that patch testing is the best method available, although it is considered only about 70 percent accurate. In general, a positive patch test result should be considered suggestive rather than definitive, with the elimination diet (below) or avoidance of nonfood allergens being the deciding factor.

Supplementary tests. Some other simple tests that can hint at an underlying allergy include:

- *Tang:* After drinking a six-ounce glass of Tang (or any other product whose label lists the coloring "FD&C yellow No. 5," which is really tartrazine), hypersensitive individuals will usually show an allergic reaction such as wheezing. Tartrazine is contained in hundreds of food products: commercial desserts, cake mixes, candies, seasonings, packaged dinners, ice creams and sherbets, salad dressings, the coatings around medicines and vitamin pills, etc.
- *Dermatographism:* Stroking the skin, usually on the back, with a dull instrument may produce weltlike urticarial lesions (raised white plaques or flat patches surrounded by red areas) where the instrument stroked.
- *Cold response:* Ice placed against the skin for a few seconds may produce an urticarial rash similar to dermatographism.
- *Sunlight response:* Sunlight may cause a dermatographism-type rash. When people are suspected of having an allergic reaction to sunlight, they are usually asked to expose themselves to bright sunlight through a window pane to see whether the glass blocks out the sun's allergy-causing rays.
- *Stress response:* People who develop a dermatographism-type rash when they are upset or subject to anxiety usually develop a similar allergic rash after strenuous physical activity; a stress-type allergy can sometimes be confirmed by having the patient exercise vigorously and then noting the appearance of a rash immediately afterward.

- *Pressure response:* A dermatographism-type rash may develop on the arms after heavy bundles have been carried; a similar rash may develop on the buttocks after a person has been sitting for several hours.
- *Water response:* A dermatographism-type rash may appear over the upper part of the body within 15 minutes after a warm bath.

Allergic reactions must sometimes be differentiated from other types of skin reactions such as herpes (see Body Observations, **Skin Observations**), parasite infestations (see Body Observations, **Skin Infestations: Flea Bites, Pediculosis** and **Skin Infestations: Scabies**), eczema, generalized itching from sweat or high humidity (prickly heat), and manifestations of some type of systemic disease (liver disease, certain cancers, kidney disease, thyroid disease and polycythemia, a disease involving the production of too many red blood cells).

Elimination diet. When it comes to food allergies, the logical next step after a positive patch test for a specific food is to eliminate the suspect food, foods or food additives (such as MSG) from the diet and see whether annoying or irritating symptoms disappear. Elimination diet testing can also be performed without previous patch testing, especially if there are strong suspicions about one or more foods. A successful elimination diet test not only requires eliminating the suspect food for a few weeks but seems to work best if, during the first few days, the person eats only foods that are commonly known to rarely provoke allergy, such as rice and tea (only beet sugar should be used; cane sugar is a known allergen). A careful written record should be kept of all foods eaten along with allergy symptoms. A food and symptom diary has allowed many a diagnosis to be made after all high-tech testing turned out to be useless.

After four days to seven days, one suspect food is introduced back into the diet every two days, and symptomatic allergic reactions, if they occur, are noted. The most common symptoms provoked by this test particularly include: indigestion, stomach cramps, heartburn, headache, hyperactivity, runny nose, skin rash, unusual behavior and even **edema** (water retention, causing puffiness of the face, hands or feet; see Body Observations). In the face of an allergic reaction that appears within 1 hour to 10 hours after eating a suspect food, omit that food again for four days and then try it once more; another allergic response justifies permanently eliminating that food from the diet. Of course, the degree of symptom aggravation must be weighed against the degree of pleasure derived from the food, and only the allergic individual can make such a decision. When milk products are reintroduced into the diet, a distinction must be made between milk allergy and milk intolerance (see Mouth, Throat and Gastrointestinal Tests, **Milk Products (Lactose) Intolerance**).

TESTS TO COME

It would not be at all surprising if, between the time the manuscript for this book is given to the publisher and the time it is actually published—about one year—at least a dozen new home medical tests will become available to the public. Just two weeks before the manuscript was completed, two different home cholesterol tests were announced. And it is just as likely that some do-it-yourself medical tests already being marketed will be withdrawn—some simply because they did not perform as promised, some because there turned out to be no public demand for them and some because the Food and Drug Administration (FDA) objected to a self-test device's being sold without prior government permission. To be sure, the FDA does approve all medical tests prior to sale—both to the profession as well as to the public; but keep in mind that the FDA does not review any medical test—whether to be performed by a physician, a laboratory technician or a layperson—for accuracy. The FDA simply reviews the manufacturer's claims and then decides whether the public may purchase that test or whether its sale will be restricted to doctors.

A good example of a home test that did not work out is one to detect salmonella bacteria in food; salmonellosis is a severe, even fatal, intestinal infection that comes primarily from improperly stored and/or inadequately cooked poultry, eggs and egg-containing products. This test came to the marketplace with a great deal of publicity and promise: Many of the tens of thousands of foodborne diseases could now be prevented. The trouble was, it did not always work properly. Foods with known salmonella contamination failed to test positive for this deadly typhoid-type bacteria; other foods free of any of this bacteria showed a positive test reaction. The end result: After a great many salmonella-detection test kits were sold, they suddenly disappeared.

But for every home test that does not live up to expectations, there will probably be two or three that will survive—and even perform a valuable service.

Some of the tests on the horizon include:

- A simple allergy test, using a drop of fingertip blood, that will reveal not only whether an allergy is present but even the specific substance causing the allergic symptoms. For information contact the Quidel Company (11077 North Torrey Pines Rd., La Jolla, Calif. 92037).

- A do-it-yourself Pap test in which a woman obtains a sample of vaginal fluid—and hopefully cells from the cervix—at home and sends it directly to a laboratory for evaluation, with the reported result being a strictly private matter. For information contact MedTech Diagnostics Inc. (355A Central Ave., Bohemia, N.Y. 11716).
- A simple urine test to detect the presence of the AIDS virus antibody. For information contact Dr. Alvin Friedman-Kien, Professor of Dermatology (New York University Medical Center, New York, N.Y.).

APPENDIX

HEALTH MAINTENANCE INDEX

Many medical tests can be performed to keep a check on the state of one's health as well as to uncover dormant diseases. Preventive medicine means more than avoiding illness; it also includes the detection of early warning signs of impending ailments, thereby permitting one to prevent or lessen subsequent disability. The following tests, when performed routinely, should help reduce the number and severity of many medical maladies. The value of many of these tests lies as much in an individual test result as in providing a record over a period of time, so that any change can be noted. See the Index to locate the tests listed below.

DAILY

Carbon Monoxide

WEEKLY

Visual Acuity—Amsler Grid (especially if over the age of 40)

MONTHLY

Blood Pressure
Breast Self-Examination
Dental Plaque Disclosure
Pulmonary Function Measurements—Forced Vital Capacity (FVC) Test
Skin Observations
Skin Saltiness
Testicle Self-Examination
Urine Tests—using a multiple-test dipstick. These screening tests will provide a check on whether urine contains bilirubin, blood, glucose, ketones, nitrite, protein and urobilinogen as well as its pH. Although it is not necessary to regularly perform some of the tests included on these dipsticks

on a monthly basis, the cost-effectiveness factor makes it worthwhile to use them all.

Weight Measurements (weight alone)

QUARTERLY (Every Three Months)

Hearing Function—Voice, Whisper or Ticking Watch
Hemoglobin
Mouth, Tongue and Throat Observations
Visual Acuity
Visual Field

SEMIANNUALLY (Every Six Months)

Dizziness and Ataxia—Finger-to-Nose, Romberg
Feces Observations—Occult Blood
Prostate Observations (especially if over the age of 40)
Pupil and Pupillary Reflex
Reflex Testing—Knee-Jerk, Wrist
Smell Function

ANNUALLY (Once a Year)

Calcium (urine)
Glucose (blood)
Hair Observations—Anagen-Telogen
Hearing Function—Rinne, Weber
Sensory Testing—Graphesthesia

SPECIAL CIRCUMSTANCES

Before taking any prescription drug and monthly for six months after taking it; monthly if taking drugs regularly:

Dizziness and Ataxia—Romberg
Hemoglobin
Occult Blood (feces)
Pupil and Pupillary Reflex
Urine Tests—using a multiple-test dipstick

Before and monthly for six months after taking drugs known to affect hearing or suspected of affecting it:

Hearing Function—Audiometer (if possible), Stethoscope, Ticking Watch, Voice and Whisper

Before (and once a month for two months after) a woman of childbearing
   age takes any medicine known to affect a fetus or suspected of affecting
   it or before undergoing any X-ray examination:

Breast Self-Examination

Pregnancy

Protein

On a newborn once a week for the first six weeks of life:

Phenylketonuria Screening

ABOUT THE AUTHORS

Cathey (Catherine Larkum) Pinckney was a regular book reviewer for "Parade of Books," a weekly column distributed by King Features Syndicate. Trained in psychology and microbiology (New York University, Syracuse University, The New School for Social Research), she is health and medical editor for "Vector TV Consumer News," a program prepared for cable TV stations throughout the United States that reports on health, food and other related consumer matters.

Dr. Edward R. Pinckney's academic positions have included: chairman of the Department of Preventive Medicine and director of the Comprehensive Medical Clinic at Northwestern University College of Medicine, Chicago; lecturer, School of Public Health, University of California, Berkeley; and associate clinical professor of medicine at Loma Linda College of Medicine, Los Angeles. He is a regular book and film reviewer for the American Association for the Advancement of Science. Dr. Pinckney also has additional graduate degrees in law (LL.B.) and public health (M.P.H.) and is certified as a specialist (Diplomate) in Preventive Medicine and Public Health by the American Board of Preventive Medicine. In 1970 he was requested to prepare comprehensive information, and to testify directly, for two U.S. Senate committees on the cost and quality of medical care and on problems in the drug industry. He was a consultant to the California Assembly Committee on Malpractice.

Among the many professional organizations with which he is affiliated, Dr. Pinckney is a Fellow of the American College of Physicians, a Fellow of the American Association for the Advancement of Science and a Fellow of the American College of Preventive Medicine, on whose Committee on Policy and Legislation he once served.

Dr. Pinckney has also authored: *You Can Prevent Illness* and *How to Make the Most of Your Doctor and Medicine.* Other writing included a regular health column in *Blue Print for Health,* the magazine of the Blue Cross Association; multiple contributions for *Encyclopedia International;* 134 screenplays for postgraduate medical teaching films distributed by Encyclopaedia Britannica

Films; and more than 100 scientific articles in professional medical journals. Editorial positions have included: associate editor of *The Journal of the American Medical Association;* editor of *The New Physician* (received the 1960 American Medical Writers' Association Honor Award in Journalism for this editorship); executive editor of *Trauma* (a medical journal for the legal profession); and associate editor of *Physician's Management.*

Dr. and Mrs. Pinckney together have authored: *Medical Encyclopedia of Common Illnesses, The Fallacy of Freud and Psychoanalysis, The Cholesterol Controversy* and *The Patient's Guide to Medical Tests* (also from Facts On File).

For many years they wrote the syndicated daily newspaper medical column "Mirror of Your Mind," distributed to 110 U.S. and foreign newspapers by King Features Syndicate. They have also coauthored articles in *The Saturday Review, Media & Consumer* (where they were contributing editors), *Consumer Newsletter* and various newspapers.

The Pinckneys live in Beverly Hills, California.

INDEX